Innovations in Drug Manufacturing

Kuldeep Vinchurkar • Sheetal Mane
Editors

Innovations in Drug Manufacturing

FDM 3D Printing for Pharmaceuticals

Springer

Editors
Kuldeep Vinchurkar
Department of Pharmaceutics
Sandip Institute of Pharmaceutical Sciences
(SIPS), Affiliated To Savitribai Phule Pune
University (SPPU, Pune)
Nashik, Maharashtra, India

Sheetal Mane
NMT Gujrati College of Pharmacy
Indore, Madhya Pradesh, India

ISBN 978-981-96-9074-9 ISBN 978-981-96-9075-6 (eBook)
https://doi.org/10.1007/978-981-96-9075-6

This Springer imprint is published by the registered company Springer Nature Singapore Pte Ltd.
The registered company address is: 152 Beach Road, #21-01/04 Gateway East, Singapore 189721, Singapore

Contents

3D Printing in Pharmaceuticals: An Introduction

1

Palanirajan Vijayaraj Kumar,
Sharon Anthea Simeon Anthony, Ng Ru Yun,
Choo Choy Foong, Koh Xin Yu, Jyoti Kumari,
Krishna Kant Jangde, and Dinesh Kumar Mishra

Abstract

Three-dimensional (3D) printing is a rapidly developing manufacturing technique that emerged in the 1980s. This technology is now being integrated into healthcare settings to ease processes in the pharmaceutical industry and clinical practice. It enables the exact layer-by-layer deposition of materials to produce customizable dosage forms and drug delivery systems, such as transdermal patches, microneedles, implants, capsules, and tablets. 3D printing can also be used to produce customized prescriptions, solve supply chain problems, and minimize product waste and waiting times. This chapter focuses on the fabrication of customized 3D-printed dosage forms tailored to patient needs, materials, procedures, advantages, and challenges in the dispensing and pharmaceutical industries.

Keywords

3D printing · Pharmaceutical compounding · Materials · Personalized medicine · 3D-printed drug delivery systems

P. V. Kumar (✉) · S. A. S. Anthony · N. R. Yun · C. C. Foong · K. X. Yu
Faculty of Pharmaceutical Sciences, Department of Pharmaceutical Technology, UCSI University, Kuala Lumpur, Malaysia
e-mail: palanirajan@ucsiuniversity.edu.my

J. Kumari · K. K. Jangde · D. K. Mishra
Department of Pharmacy, Guru Ghasidas Vishwavidyalaya (A Central University), Bilaspur, Chhattisgarh, India

K. Vinchurkar, S. Mane (eds.), *Innovations in Drug Manufacturing*,
https://doi.org/10.1007/978-981-96-9075-6_1

1.1 Introduction

Three-dimensional (3D) printing technology, a rapidly developing manufacturing technique, emerged in the 1980s. In general, there are four basic components to 3D printing technology: G code file translation, digital slicing, digital model design and development, and 3D printer manufacturing. This method provides a significant advantage over traditional manufacturing techniques for designing complicated structures and fabricating customized drug delivery devices [1].

Three-dimensional printing is a technology for creating 3D objects by layering through a computer-created design. It is known as additive manufacturing (AM) and is now being integrated into healthcare settings to ease many processes in the pharmaceutical industry and clinical practice. This technology has become robust since the concept of personalized medicine became known from a study in the UK showing that the traditional mass manufacturing method is ineffective for approximately 70% of patients, with 90% of drugs working for only 30–50% of the population and 7% of patients having adverse drug reactions leading to hospital admissions. Due to differences in genetic make-up, lifestyle, environmental factors, and disease states among patients, the "one-size-fits-all" approach cannot be implemented, and more personalized treatment is required to achieve the best efficacy [2].

The 3D printing method enables the exact layer-by-layer deposition of materials to produce various customisable dosage forms and drug delivery systems, such as transdermal patches, implants, immediate-release, and controlled-release tablets [3]. In addition, this technology can be used to produce tablets of various forms and shapes to allow precise dosing by controlling the release of an active ingredient. Moreover, pharmaceutical firms may employ 3D printers to produce customized prescriptions as needed. Therefore, supply chain problems can be solved, especially for drugs with short life spans, and product waste and waiting times can be minimized and reduced [2, 4].

The principles of 3D printing technology can be divided into four main categories: sheet lamination-based systems, liquid-based systems, powder-based systems (Fig. 1.1a), and extrusion-based systems (Fig. 1.1b). In the pharmaceutical field, the most commonly used 3D printing technologies are fused deposition modelling (FDM), semisolid extrusion (SSE), and melt extrusion deposition (MED). In 2013, the first FDA-approved 3D-printed drug was Spritam® (levetiracetam tablets). It possesses an antiepileptic effect and is used as an adjunct to the treatment of seizures. It is a porous formulation created through 3D printing to achieve rapid disintegration of tablets [5].

The process of developing 3D-printed medications is highly challenging because it requires the expertise of not only mechanical engineers and pharmacy researchers but also specialists in materials science, software, and information engineering, in addition to having to navigate the stringent legal requirements of the pharmaceutical industry. For instance, extrusion-based solutions are limited

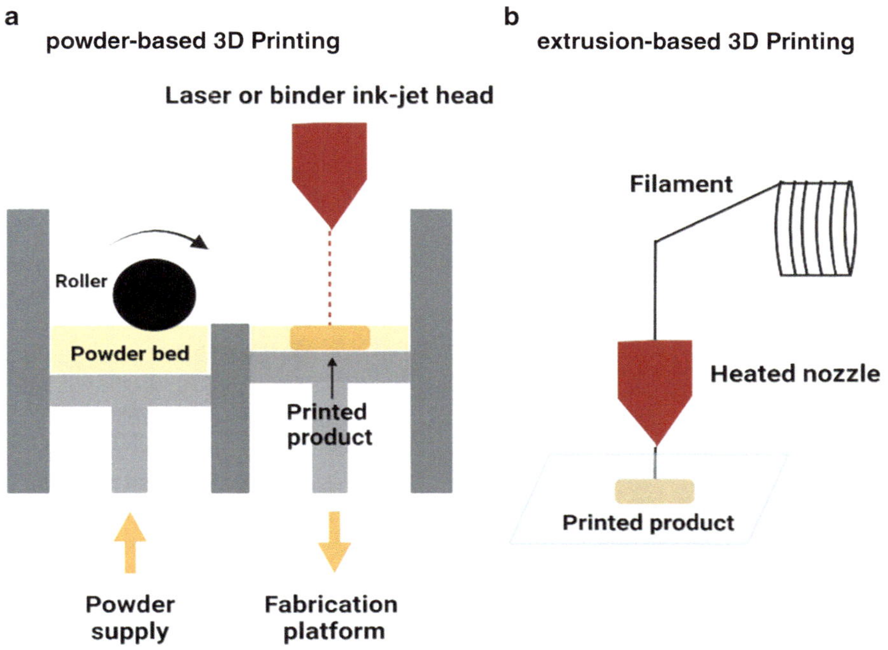

Fig. 1.1 Types of 3D printing (**a**) Powder-based 3D printing (**b**) Extrusion-based 3D printing

to thermostable active ingredients because heat is required in the process. Thus, the market for 3D-printed drugs is currently limited despite an increase in business and cutting-edge research. The leading medical technology companies in the 3D medicine printing field are Doser, Aprecia Pharmaceuticals, Exentis, FabRx, MB Therapeutics, Merck, and Triastek [6].

1.2 The Benefits of 3D Printing Technology in Pharmaceuticals

3D printing technology can create personalized drug formulations and dosages for patients, addressing variations such as genetics, age, sex, and disease state, as shown in Fig. 1.2. It can deliver precise dosages with minimal toxic effects and maximize therapeutic benefits. This is especially important for paediatricians and geriatricians, as children have specific sensitivity and reactivity, while elderly people have lower absorption and metabolism. 3D printing also allows for personalized medicines with unique shapes and colours, lower doses, and porous formulations for elderly patients. It also addresses complex dosage forms and drug delivery systems, enabling the creation of advanced drug delivery systems [7].

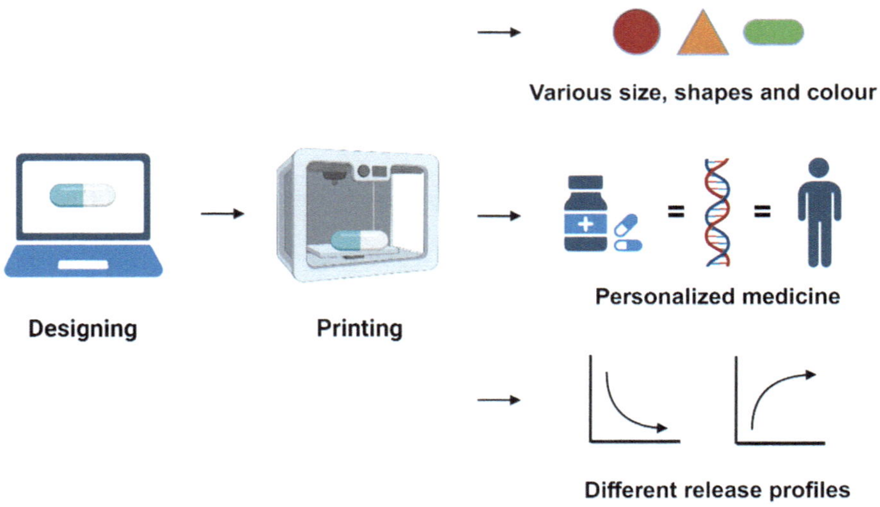

Fig. 1.2 Benefits of 3D printing in customizable formulations

3D printing technology offers rapid and automatic production of products, allowing for faster prototyping and development. This process reduces labour and costs, as it only uses what is needed to print, reducing material waste. This technology is particularly useful in fields such as aircraft and sports cars, where lightweight metal items are crucial. Additionally, 3D printing can be used to produce personalized medicines at a lower cost, as minimal effort and cost are required for altering digital files. Furthermore, 3D printing enables on-demand manufacturing, reducing inventory costs and allowing for more efficient production [8]. Table 1.1 summarizes the advantages and disadvantages of 3D printing technologies in the pharmaceutical industry.

3D printing has significantly improved patient care and medical treatments by creating diagnostic, educational, and clinical tools based on a patient's anatomy. This reduces discomfort, improves health outcomes, and minimizes complication risks. Customizable medical devices such as dental and orthopaedic implants and surgical instruments are available. 3D printing is also crucial in the surgical field for training, simulation, and preoperative planning. It helps surgeons become familiar with anatomical structures and procedures before surgery. 3D printing also educates patients about their body conditions and helps them make informed decisions about treatment options [10, 11].

Table 1.1 Advantages and disadvantages of 3D printing methods in the pharmaceutical industry [9]

Method		Advantages	Disadvantages
Powder based	BJ-3D printing	Wide range of excipients available for use	Postprocessing procedure is relatively complex (curing and densification)
		High drug loading capacity	Lacking in product design specificity
Extrusion deposition	FDM	Widely available and affordable	Layer lines may be visible on the finished object
		Wide choice of suitable thermoplastic materials	Limited resolution compared to SLA
		Suitable for rapid prototyping and functional parts	High printing temperature deems it unsuitable for thermolabile products
3D printing photopolymerization	SLA	Higher product resolution	Depends on the viscosity and general resin chemistry
		Suitable for thermolabile ingredients as it can be printed at room temperature	Limited use of conventional polymers with prospective solutions
	DLP and CLIP	High product resolution	Low material availability
		Wavelength multiplexing	Complex postprocessing

BJ-3D printing binder jet 3D printing, *SLA* stereolithography, *DLP* digital light processing, *CLIP* continuous liquid interface production

1.3 Materials for 3D Printing

1.3.1 Polymers

Due to the different release patterns of the medication needed, the polymer used will also vary during the formulation development process. Each release pattern, such as instant, immediate, or extended release, has a different therapeutic effect. To select the proper polymer, several aspects need to be considered, including the compatibility between the drug and the polymer, the polymer's melting point, and its extrudability. Table 1.2 provides a brief idea about the different types of polymers used in 3D printing. First, polyvinyl alcohol (PVA) is a type of synthetic polymer that is soluble in water and has no odour but is thermally unstable. It will undergo degradation when the temperature reaches 350–450 °C. PVA can undergo more polymerization and less hydrolysis, resulting in a water-soluble and crystallizable polymer. PVA can be employed in inkjet-based or extrusion-based techniques. In inkjet printing, PVA is used for smooth printing by minimizing the chance of nozzle clogging and mixing the ink with glycerine during layering. PVA is suitable and stable for printing because it is economical and has good physicochemical properties [1, 16]. Sustained-release formulations and suppositories can be printed with PVA. Spritam® is a drug produced using 3D printing with PVA as a material [17].

Table 1.2 Various kinds of polymer used in 3D printing technology [12–15]

Category	Polymer	Printing technology	Significance
Synthetic polymer	ABS	FDM	Dimensional stability, resilience to chemicals, great hardness even at low temperatures, and high resistance to impact
	PLA	FDM, SLA, MDM, LDM, PEM	Highly biocompatible, biodegradable, good tensile strength and modulus, melting temperature 150–160 °C
	PEG	SLA, DLP, FDM, DIW, inkjet bioprinting	Highly biocompatible, biodegradable, low tensile strength
	PVA	FDM, inkjet printing	Moderate mechanical strength, melting temperature ~180–230°C
	PLGA	FDM, SLA	Tunable degradation rate, good, adjustable by altering lactic/glycolic acid ratio, melting temperature ~130–170°C
	PEGDA	FDM, SLA, DLP, SLS, inkjet printing	Biocompatible, biodegradable, hydrophilic, non-toxic
	PP	FDM, SLS, SLA, MJF	Resistant to chemicals, non-toxic, hydrophobic, requires high extruder temperature
	PETG	FDM, SLS, SLA, MJF	High strength and durability, tougher than PLA and can withstand stress without cracking or breaking
	PCL	SLS, SLA, FDM	Slow degradation rate, good flexibility, low melting temperature ~60 °C
	PHEMA	FDM, SLS, SLA, MJF	Optically transparent, inert, less toxicity, cytocompatibility, and hydrophilicity
	PEEK	SLS, SLA, FDM	High tensile strength and stiffness with excellent dimensional stability, melting point around 343 °C
Natural polymer	Hydrogels	FDM, SLS, SLA, DLP, inkjet printing	Transparent, soft, flexible, and retain large amounts of water
	Hyaluronic acid	FDM, SLS, SLA	Extracellular matrix, biocompatible, highly acidic polysaccharide, viscoelastic
	Sodium alginate	FDM, SLS, SLA, inkjet printing	Derived from seaweed, non-toxic, biocompatible, hydrophilic, gel-like texture when hydrated
	Gelatin	FDM, SLS, SLA, DLP, inkjet printing	Dissolvable, biocompatible, non-toxic, hydrophilic, thermoreversible (can be melted and reformed multiple times), can be crosslinked with other polymers or chemicals
	Chitosan	FDM, SLS, SLA	Cationic polyelectrolyte, biodegradable and biocompatible, non-immunogenic

ABS acrylonitrile butadiene styrene, *PLGA* poly(lactic-co-glycolic acid), *PP* polypropylene, *PETG* polyethylene terephthalate glycol, *PCL* polycaprolactone, *PEEK* polyether ether ketone, *MDM* materialise dental module, *LDM* liquid deposition modeling, *PEM* paste extrusion modelling, *DIW* direct ink writing, *MJF* multi-jet fusion

Another polymer known as polylactic acid (PLA) is the most commonly used biodegradable polymer for implants and drug delivery systems. Once PLA enters the human body, it is converted into alpha-hydroxylic acid by hydrolysis and is subsequently excreted via metabolism. Thus, its noncarcinogenic and nontoxic features make it suitable for FDA approval. In addition, it degrades in the body slowly, so it can be formulated for extended release for prolonged in vivo use. However, the solubility of PLA in water and alcohol is low, but it has good solubility in organic solvents such as chloroform. By increasing the temperature of the water or alcohol to the boiling point, its solubility in those solvents can be improved. At approximately 150–175 °C, the sample melts [16, 18]. For instance, a combination of paracetamol and caffeine can be produced by hot melt extrusion techniques that use PLA as the material [19]. In addition, polymers such as polyvinyl pyrrolidone (PVP), polyethylene glycol [20], polyethylene glycol diacrylate (PEGDA), poly (2-hydroxyethyl methacrylate) (PHEMA), and polyurethane are often used in pharmaceutical 3D printing. PVP is ideal for immediate-release formulations due to its low printing temperature, which is approximately 100–110 °C. For printing of tablets, PEG can improve the solubility, stability, and compatibility of tablets. FDM employs polyurethane to produce personalized medicine because it is thermoplastic, and a wide variety of dosage forms can be developed [20, 21].

1.3.2 Hydrogels

In addition, hydrogels are hydrophilic polymers that allow for water or biological fluid absorption without bursting, because they are composed of a 3D network structure. They are classified into various categories, such as natural, synthetic, and hybrid. For instance, natural hydrogels are obtained from chitosan, alginate, and collagen, while synthetic hydrogels are derived from PEG, PVA, and polyacrylamide. Since natural hydrogels are obtained from natural polymers, they are mostly biocompatible and bioactive. It can mimic human soft tissues and thus be used for bone tissue regeneration. In addition, they also serve as matrices for controlled drug delivery systems, infection control, wound care, and cultural heritage preservation. Hydrogels can encapsulate active pharmaceutical ingredients, provide a controlled drug release profile, and allow precise spatial and temporal control over drug delivery to target sites [22].

1.3.3 Ceramics

Ceramics can also be used to produce implants and drug delivery systems. Upon the completion of the printing process, the model was settled within a dense layer of finely powdered alumina silica ceramic, providing substantial support. The properties of ceramics are what cause them to be applied in pharmaceutical 3D printing; they have a particular mechanical strength, are biocompatible, and exhibit controlled release properties. In addition, ceramics enable personalized dosage forms by accurately printing the product into complex geometric shapes. With a controlled release profile, 3D-printed ceramic tablets or implants are formed to release drugs gradually over time. Adverse drug reactions can be minimized because ceramics are biocompatible with the body. There are various ceramics used in the 3D printing of medical implants, such as alumina-toughened zirconia (ATZ), hydroxyapatite (HA), and tricalcium phosphate (TCP). Due to its high mechanical strength, abrasion resistance, and hardness, ATZ is suitable for manufacturing permanent implants by 3D printing, such as femoral head implants and dental implants. TCP and HA are often used in alloplastic bone substitution because they have a degree of similarity to the chemical composition of human bone. Its strong biocompatibility allows for potential resorption and remodelling into bone tissue post implantation [23].

1.3.4 Metal Alloys

Moreover, some metals are suitable for 3D-printed medical implants, such as stainless-steel alloys, pure titanium, and Ti6Al4V alloys. These materials can be used to produce orthopaedic implants with 3D printing technology, where complex bone implants are fabricated and act like real human bone. To be suitable candidates, metals must have high resistance to corrosion and good biocompatibility. Therefore, it will not easily oxidize when exposed to those oxidizing media. The Ti6Al4V alloy, also known as the titanium-aluminium-vanadium alloy, has good properties from titanium, vanadium, and aluminium, in which the vanadium and aluminium are light in weight while titanium has good strength. Thus, this material is suitable for printing prosthetic joints to aid in patient mobility [24].

1.3.5 Sugar-Based Materials

In addition, due to their biocompatibility and versatility, sugar-based materials such as isomalt can be used as materials in 3D printing technology to create various drug delivery systems and personalized medicine. With this material, a porous formulation can be formed to enhance the dissolution of tablets. Moreover, it can act as a binder to increase the binding and mechanical strength between drug particles within a dosage range, which will then enhance the stability of the formulation [25]. In addition to sugar-based materials, lipid-based materials such as microalgae-derived lipids and functionalized lipid-based inks can be used in 3D printing. By incorporating these lipids into drug delivery systems, the pattern of drug release can be improved. These lipids can also be applied in the process of printing tissue scaffolds and regenerative medicine, as they provide a certain degree of support and protection to the tissue structure [26, 27].

1.4 3D Printing Techniques

Conventional pharmaceutical manufacturing methods are mostly confined to subtractive manufacturing, considering that changes in the already solidified production line may cause cost and demand concerns for the product manufactured. Nonetheless, the desire for a controlled drug release profile and personalized medicine fuels the change from subtractive manufacturing to AM processes through the incorporation of 3D printing into medicine [28]. Several 3D printing techniques, such as the drop-on solid powder-based method, extrusion-based method, and photopolymerization method, have been heavily studied for their suitability for different dosage forms. Among these methods are the drop-on solid powder-based method, which has successfully introduced the drug Spritam® into the market, as well as the FDM method, which is currently the most popularized and researched 3D printing technology in the industry [28]. Table 1.3 displays many 3D printing applications in pharmaceutical company operations.

1.4.1 Fundamental Steps for 3D Printing Techniques

3D printing is the process of building an object "layer-by-layer" while following instructions from computer-aided design (CAD) software. This ability to present an automated printed build of any possible designed structure in a wide range of material options is what makes 3D printing flexible for manufacturer [39].

Depending on the materials used and the particular requirements of the newly designed product, different techniques may be used [6]. All of these techniques for different dosage forms in the pharmaceutical industries have different principles but employ a common fundamental steps of 3D printing as shown in Fig. 1.3:

- *Designing*—The use of computer-aided design software to design a file for 3D objects.
- *Stereolithography (SLA)*—The designed file will be converted into an STL file having an extension ".stl".
- *Slicing*—The STL file is transformed by the slicer into a sequence of thin layers with instructions on how to print the 3D object.
- *G-code*—The layered file is then converted into G-code which is in printer readable form and transferred to the printer.
- *Material processing*—Depending on the technique being utilized, pharmaceutical ink is created in the form of a paste, granule, or filament binder solution.
- *Printing*—On a substrate, the formulation ink that is delivered to the printer head solidifies layer by layer.
- *Post printing*—The final product requires redusting, polishing, sintering, etc., after printing a product.

Table 1.3 Applications of 3D printing in the pharmaceutical industry

Method		Dosage forms	Drugs	Materials	Reference
Powder-based	BJ-3D printing	Powder mould	Indomethacin	PEG, HPC	[29]
Extrusion-based	FDM	Oral films	Aripiprazole	PVA	[30]
		Caplets	Theophylline	HPC, Eudragit, PEG	[31]
		Bilayer tablets	Metformin, Glimepiride	Eudragit, PVA	[32]
Photopolymerization	SLA	Microneedle patch	Insulin	Dental SG resin	[33]
		Microneedle	Cisplatin	Class I biocompatible resin	[34]
	DLP	Microneedle	Diclofenac sodium	PEGDA	[35]
		Microneedle in hydrogel system	Rhodamine B	PEG450-DA, Irgacure 819	[36]
	CLIP	Drug-loaded spacers	Docetaxel, Dexamethasone	HEMA, PEG550-DMA	[37]
		Microneedle patch	Bovine serum albumin	PEG350-DMA, TPO	[38]

HPC hydroxypropyl cellulose, *HEMA* 2-hydroxyethyl methacrylate, *TPO* thermoplastic polyolefin

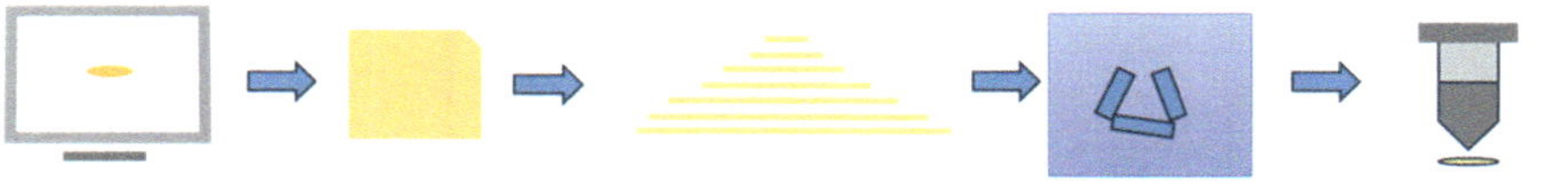

Fig. 1.3 Fundamental steps of 3D printing

1.4.2 Powder-Based Materials

The binder-jet 3D printing method applies the concept of droplets to create pharmaceutical products. A thin powder layer is spread on a build platform, and binder droplets are added dropwise onto the powder bed, binding the powdered particles in contact with the binder droplet. The roller will continuously spread new powder layers on top of the bound powder as droplets continue to be sprayed from the printhead, similar to the concept of layer-by-layer FDM, but powderwise until the complete product is formed [40]. Although this technique is relatively well researched, it is being replaced by more popularized AM 3D printing methods in the pharmaceutical industry, such as FDM, due to its complex postprocessing.

1.4.3 Fused Deposition Modelling (FDM)

FDM is an extrusion-based 3D printing method that relies on the heating of the filaments into hot melts and deposition of the thermoplastic drug-incorporated filaments on top of a build platform as shown in Fig. 1.4, which moves in a way that allows the drug to be formed layer-by-layer, moving in the x–y plane [41]. The incorporation of active pharmaceutical ingredients (APIs) into filaments can be achieved by the dipping method, hot melt extrusion (HME)-based FDM method, or filling-forming method, which produces a filament coil that is sent through the extrusion nozzle head [7]. AM is considered additive manufacturing due to the nature of layering or adding materials to build the product rather than removing fragments of a workpiece to form the end product [31]. For FDM, the material added is molten drug-plastic filaments, which are built layer-by-layer according to predetermined CAD paths.

FDM is capable of tailoring customized dosage forms with specified drug release profiles according to the individual needs of a patient, which is especially useful in conditions where the pharmacokinetics profile differs in certain specialized populations. A unique feature of FDM is its use of drug-loaded filaments containing small amounts of API combined with polymers and other excipients that make up the filament coil. Controlled drug release in pharmaceutical formulations is generally harder to achieve in conventional manufacturing practices due to complex downstream processing procedures [7]. In FDM, the layer-by-layer fabrication concept can alter specific drug concentrations and release modifiers and additives precisely to fix specific quantities of ingredients in each layer of the product. Adjusting the filament

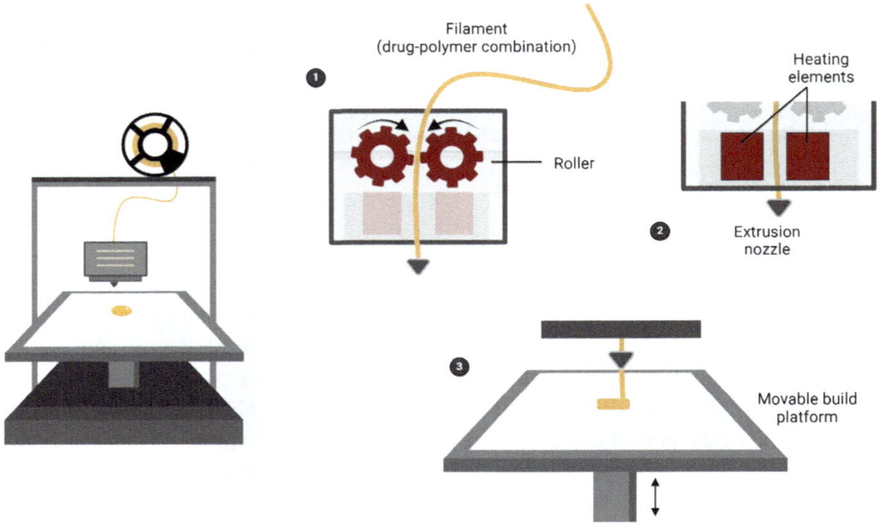

Fig. 1.4 Formation of products through the FDM method

composition and printing parameters, altering the infill density, and shifting the nozzle temperature allow for controlled drug release and drug dissolution [32].

Despite its many benefits, FDM has certain challenges that require special attention, such as uncertainty in ensuring uniform drug distribution within the filament, potential drug degradation problems during the printing process, and a lack of standards for validating the quality and performance of 3D-printed dosage forms.

1.4.4 Photopolymerization Method

3D printing through photopolymerization is currently a new trend in pharmaceutical 3D printing. It applies the concept of liquid photoactive monomers or oligomers that solidify and undergo photopolymerization reactions to form complex polymers upon exposure to light sources of different wavelengths in the electromagnetic region. Photoinitiators are crucial in this process to create chemically active free radicals, cations, or anions when in contact with lights such as UV rays, visible light, or even near-infrared (NIR) light for the solidification of products [42].

Here, VAT polymerization applies the concept of photopolymerization, in which the process occurs in a tank filled with resin material (resin vat) that is exposed to UV rays. It is by far the widest photopolymerization method studied in the pharmaceutical AM process, encompassing various techniques such as SLA, CLIP, DLP, and liquid crystal display (LCD) [43]. The resin vat used includes a formulation of monomers, additives, photoinitiators, and fillers that solidify the product layer after each layer as UV light strikes the surface of the resin. To gain a better grasp of the properties of the product, the formulation must be developed with consideration of

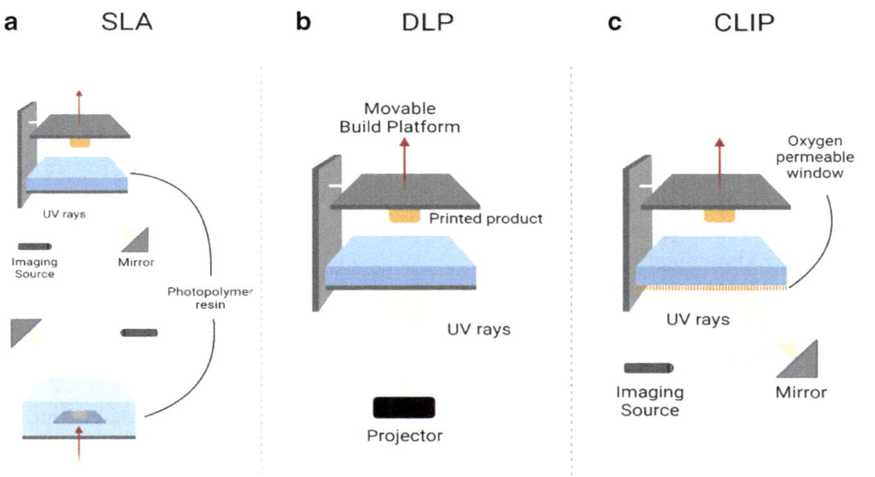

Fig. 1.5 VAT polymerization techniques in 3D printing. (**a**) Bottom-up and top-down SLA methods. (**b**) DLP technique. (**c**) CLIP technique

the use of photoinitiators and other components to control the photonic parameters, such as depth of penetration [44] and the critical energy (Ec) [45].

As with other 3D printing methods, VAT polymerization has challenges that need to be addressed, especially because of the importance of resin chemistry in the whole process [46]. The printing parameters need to be controlled to provide better control of the properties of the printed materials to ensure a safe and desirable end product. This includes changing certain conventional polymers that are incorporated with photosensitive initiators with redshifted absorption. SLA provides a high resolution and production speed with printing of a thickness of 1 μm for microstereolithography, allowing for intricate detail in the fabrication process. There are two types of SLAs, bottom-up and top-down SLAs, depending on the laser position. The UV rays are refracted by a mirror and shone into the resin to form layers of solid. Compared with DLP, DLP incorporates a projector as its light source, significantly increasing the speed of production. CLIP is the newest technique out of the three, with its main feature being the oxygen-permeable membrane and dead zone that is created between the membrane and the cured product. Here, polymerization is inhibited to allow the product to be pulled out from the resin continuously, as shown in Fig. 1.5 [46].

1.5 3D-Printed Pharmaceutical Compounding

The process of creating 3D-printed tablets, capsules, and implants involves selecting drugs based on therapeutic requirements and stability, using suitable polymers as excipients, and preparing filaments through processes such as hot melt extrusion. Physiochemical characterization of the filaments was conducted using various methods. A 3D model of the desired dosage form was designed using CAD software and saved in standard tessellation language (.stl) format for printing. The 3D printer settings are adjusted to ensure successful printing. The filament is loaded into the printer and printed according to the model design and settings. The printed product is then assessed and optimized to meet specific specifications, including targeted release pattern, geometry and accuracy, mechanical properties, and drug release profile and uniformity. The optimized final product should have tailored release patterns, customized geometry for patient-specific needs, and enhanced potential for personalized medication [47].

In vitro evaluation methods for 3D-printed drugs include breaking pressure measurements, and the pressure sensitivity of capsules is tested using a modified stress test device. This involved measuring the pressure required to break the capsules, imitating the conditions in the gastrointestinal tract. In addition, dissolution testing of the drug was performed in simulated gastric fluid without pepsin to determine the drug release profile under controlled conditions. In vivo evaluation methods use animal studies, such as studies on dogs, particularly beagle breeds, to evaluate the efficacy of 3D-printed drugs. Moreover, bioavailability testing of drugs is also performed on a dog subject by comparing traditional and 3D-printed drug levels in the blood stream [48].

1.5.1 3D Printing of Customized Tablets

3D printing technology has revolutionized the design of oral pharmaceutical dosage forms, including immediate-release tablets. These tablets allow precise customization of shape, size, infill density, and drug content, enabling adjustments in the surface-to-volume ratio to control drug dosage and dissolution rates. Comparing 3D-printed tablets, milled extrudate HME tablets, and directly compressed tablets containing itraconazole, it was found that itraconazole had the highest solubility in 3D-printed tablets (29.3 μg/mL), followed by extrudate (22.2 μg/mL) and direct compression (5.8 μg/mL). The dissolution profiles showed that 75.8% of the 3D-printed tablets released the most drug after 2 hours, which was attributed to molecular rearrangement of the API structure within the polymer matrix and increased surface area. Additionally, supersaturation of the 3D-printed tablets was maintained throughout the dissolution test, indicating enhanced drug release. Different infill densities, such as 20%, 35%, and 60%, influenced the dissolution of itraconazole from the 3D-printed tablets [49].

1.5.1.1 3D-Printed Modified-Release Tablets

In addition, in modified-release tablets, 3D printing enables controlled drug release over time. Complex geometries can be designed to achieve specific release profiles [50]. Medications with tailored doses and modified release characteristics can be manufactured by combining hot-melt extraction and FDM 3D printing. Figure 1.6 shows an illustration of the FDM process. 3D-printed dual-compartment dosing units with sealable compartments are used to compartmentalize drugs into dosing

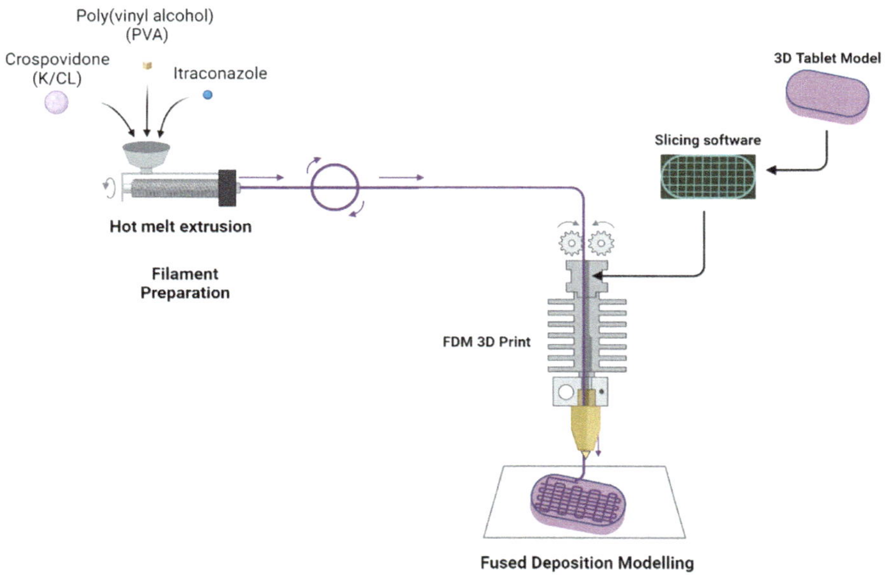

Fig. 1.6 FDM of tablets

units for tuberculosis treatment. This method prevents interactions between drugs, such as rifampicin and isoniazid. FDM can produce tablets with zero-order release kinetics, allowing constant drug release over time. The shape of the tablets can modify their dissolution profile, allowing for the development of novel dosage forms with targeted pharmacokinetic properties for different gastrointestinal tract sites. 3D printing combined with fluid bed coating can produce modified release formulations, such as budesonide tablets coated with an enteric polymer, for targeted release in the intestines. These modified-release tablets enhance drug stability, bioavailability, targeted delivery, and coadministration of chemically incompatible drugs [51].

1.5.1.2 3D-Printed Orodispersible Tablets

Orodispersible tablets (ODTs) are tablets that dissolve quickly in the mouth without water. 3D printing allows for porous structures and rapid disintegration [52]. The first 3D-printed ODT to be authorized by the US Food and Drug Administration in August 2015 was the anti-epileptic medicine Spritam® (levetiracetam), made by Aprecia Pharmaceuticals using ZipDose technology [53, 54]. This revolutionary, 3D-printed anti-epileptic medication provides a substitute for mass-producing Spritam® tablet. At very high dosages, Spritam® is an oral disintegrating tablet with a rapid disintegration rate (11 sec.), which is difficult to achieve with conventional direct compression methods [53, 54]. The binder jetting technology used in this process is suitable for creating highly porous tablets with high drug loading and low mechanical strength, which are ideal for immediate-release, fast-dissolving, and orodispersible forms. Since the mechanical strength is low when manufactured by this method, excipients such as binders are important to ensure that the physical characteristics are suitable. The hardness and binding strength can be increased by humectants with high water content, fillers with high water solubility and binders with high viscosity in solution [54].

1.5.1.3 3D-Printed Orodispersible Films

Moreover, in orodispersible films (ODFs), which are thin, flexible films that disintegrate in the oral cavity, 3D printing facilitates precise layering and drug distribution. Selective laser sintering is a 3D technology that allows precise control over the layer-by-layer deposition of materials. This is important in ODFs since each layer may fulfil a specific function. Porogens are incorporated into the films to introduce porosity while maintaining the required mechanical properties. The top layers that contain porogens ensure sufficient porosity, while the bottom layers that are free of porogens provide appropriate mechanical support. The ability to precisely control the porosity and mechanical properties of ODFs is important for drug delivery applications where rapid disintegration is needed. By adjusting the porogen content and hence the porosity, the disintegration time can be optimized within 30 seconds based on the FDA guidelines [55].

1.5.2 3D-Printed Capsule Technology

A study developed a 3D-printed capsule (3D-RECAL) to prevent opioid abuse. The capsules are filled with an aversion liquid, preventing manipulation for misuse. The drug used was metformin hydrochloride (MT). The capsule shell was created using a single-nozzle FDM 3D printer. The aversion liquid is a solution of sodium polyacrylamide starch and Sudan black dissolved in an oil base. The capsule's gelling when solvents are used to extract the drug results in large black nonsnortable particles, making it difficult to abuse. Drug release starts immediately upon ingestion, with more than 85% of MT released in 45 minutes in 1.0 N HCl (stomach condition). This study suggested that 3D printing technology can contribute to public health by creating safer drug delivery systems with a low risk of abuse [56].

1.5.2.1 3D-Printed Delayed-Release Capsules

Delayed-release capsules are capsules designed to resist stomach acid and dissolve in the intestine, making them useful for drugs that destroy stomach acid or irritate the stomach lining. This study explored the design and 3D printing of compartmental capsular devices with pharmaceuticals requiring a delayed release mechanism. PVA capsular devices were created using FDM 3D printing technology and CAD software. The material flow rate, layer thickness, and printing speed of the capsules were optimized using simple G code modifications. The design and manufacture of PVA 3D printing capsules could improve artisanal procedures in compounding pharmacies, as compounding medications takes time and prevent the creation of controlled-release dosage forms. This study has potential for improving the manufacturing process for pharmaceuticals [57].

1.5.2.2 3D-Printed Sustained-Release Gastric Floating Capsules

A study on FDM 3D-printed sustained-release gastric-floating verapamil hydrochloride has shown that 3D printing can precisely control the shape, size, and internal structure of formulations, enhancing the therapeutic efficacy of drugs. The shape of the formulation affects its floating behaviour, with cylinder-shaped formulations exhibiting longer floating times than capsules and hemisphere-shaped formulations. This decreases the complexity of traditional manufacturing procedures, such as optimizing formulation composition and production processes to prevent floating lag time. The geometry of shapes affects how gastric fluids interact with the surface, with flat surfaces providing more resistance to fluid penetration. Infill density also influences mechanical strength and drug release, with higher infill percentages resulting in greater mechanical strength and slower drug release due to a more solid barrier to drug diffusion [58].

1.5.2.3 3D-Printed Immediate and Delayed Release Capsules

Next, capsules containing two types of beads—one for immediate release and the other for delayed or extended release—called dual release capsules allow for a quick initial dose followed by a steady release of medication. The capsule design was composed of two hollow halves joined by a middle partition, creating separate compartments. The compartments can be customized in terms of wall thickness and composition, which allows controlled and varied drug release kinetics. As shown in Fig. 1.7b, i.e., Fig. 1.7a is a two-compartment model, while Fig. 1.7b is a two-compartment model with the lower compartment having a thicker wall. FDM is a 3D printing technique that involves the extrusion of thermoplastic polymers to create detailed, customized capsule parts. The results showed that two-pulse release patterns were achieved as intended, validating the design and manufacturing

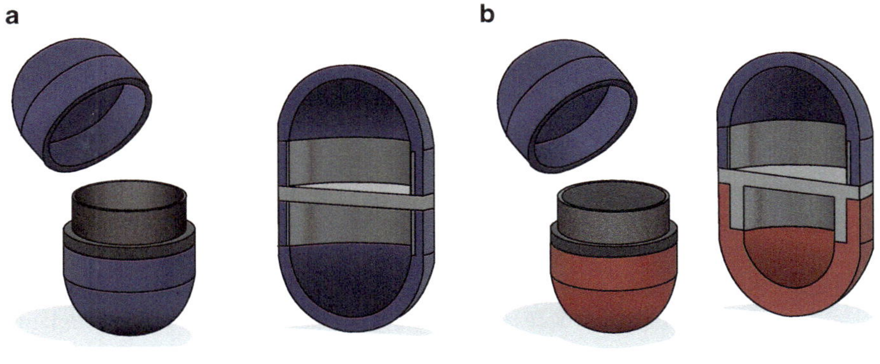

Fig. 1.7 (**a**) Two comparison capsules. (**b**) Two-compartment capsule with a thicker lower compartment wall

method. By tailoring the drug release profile in a single capsule, personalized medicines can be developed, and therapeutic outcomes and patient compliance can be improved. This technology allows complex dosing regimens to be made easy and can combine drugs that have negative interactions [59].

1.5.2.4 3D-Printed Enteric-Coated Capsules

3D printing has been used to create enteric-coated capsules that pass through the stomach without dissolving and only dissolve in the alkaline environment of the intestine. A prototype of capsules containing aqueous suspensions for colonic delivery was designed using 3D printing, adjusting the shape, thickness, and size of the capsules. Capsules with various shapes and characteristics can be rapidly screened using 3D printing. The capsules consist of an insoluble body and lid, an enteric outer lock cap, and an insoluble body and lid. They have been successfully delivered to the colon in both in vitro and in vivo tests. A benchtop FDM printer was used to 3D print the locking caps using PVA filaments and Eudragit S100, an enteric polymer that dissolves at pH values higher than pH 7. In vitro tests showed that the capsules were released after 5–6.5 hours in simulated intestinal fluid, while in vivo studies showed that the capsules remained intact in the stomach and opened in the distal small intestine or colon, indicating potential for targeted delivery [60].

1.5.3 3D-Printed Pharmaceutical Implants

3D printing has also enhanced the design of pharmaceutical implant dosage forms. 3D printing allows for the on-demand manufacture of implants that are tailored to individual patient needs. This provides an opportunity for better patient compliance and treatment outcomes. Inkjet-based 3D printing allows macroscopic control over release and personalization, as it makes it possible to create intricate geometries on demand to meet specific individual needs, and its multiple material features allow for the customization of the material spatial distribution down to the voxel level. An example is ibuprofen-loaded implants. Ibuprofen was attached to 2-hydroxyethyl acrylate by a cleavable ester bond, formulated for inkjet 3D printing, and successfully printed into solid dosage forms [56–61]. This approach showed a high drug loading capacity (up to 58 wt%) and the ability to tune the drug release profile by adjusting the formulation and printing parameters [61].

1.5.3.1 3D-Printed Dental Implants

Moreover, complex geometries are difficult for traditional manufacturing methods, but 3D printing can create porous structures, lattice designs, and internal channels, enhancing implant functionality. Compared with conventional machining methods, selective laser melting has been studied in the production of dental implants. Increased surface roughness and porous features achievable by 3D-printed implants are needed to improve osseointegration through improved cell attachment and

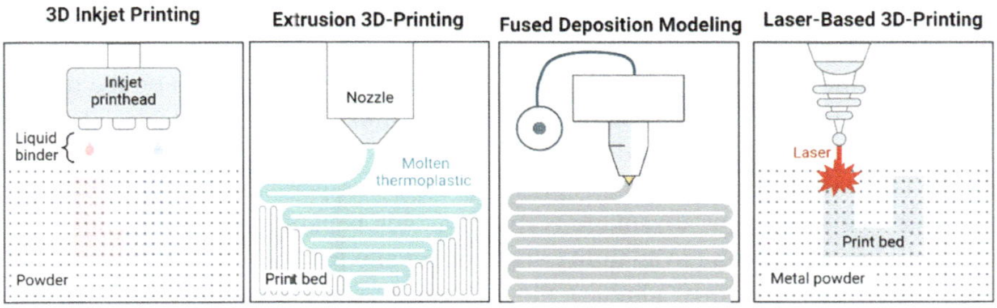

Fig. 1.8 Types of 3D printing methods

proliferation, especially for osteoblasts (hOBs) and mesenchymal stem cells (hAD-MSCs). The reactions of many oral implantology-relevant cell types, such as monocytes, hOBs, hGFs, and hAD-MSCs, to these implants were examined; the results showed increased osteogenic marker expression and proliferation on 3D-printed surfaces [62].

1.5.3.2 3D-Printed Drug-Eluting Implants

Furthermore, 3D implants can be used for the manufacture of drug-eluting implants; by incorporating drugs into the implant material, 3D-printed implants can provide localized drug release. Drug-eluting implants are medical devices that are designed to deliver therapeutic agents directly to a targeted area in the body, which allows for high concentrations at disease sites with few side effects. 3D-printed drug-eluting implants are used in a few medical fields, such as in producing stents and catheters for cardiovascular and urological applications, in gynaecological devices for delivering hormones and treating infections, in devices for bone treatment and surgical stents, in antitumoral devices for localized chemotherapy, and in surgical meshes to prevent hernia recurrence or delivery of antibiotics. The 3D printing methods that can be used are inkjet printing, FDM, extrusion 3D printing and laser-based printing [63]. Figure 1.8 shows the methods used for 3D printing.

1.5.3.3 Materials for 3D-Printed Implants

3D printing also allows the use of biocompatible materials such as titanium alloys, PEEK, and bioresorbable polymers. These materials promote tissue integration and minimize adverse reactions. Titanium alloys are used in implants because of their good mechanical properties, excellent corrosion resistance and biocompatibility. PEEK is also often used for implants because of its mechanical properties and biocompatibility. It is used for applications such as replacing ribs and as a vertebral stabilizer in the spine. However, printing with PEEK is demanding and requires printers with advanced abilities. Bioresorbable polymers, such as polylactide, are known for their biodegradability and biocompatibility. These materials are suitable for biodegradable implants [64].

1.5.4 3D-Printed Transdermal Dosage Forms

Aside from the oral and injectable routes, the skin is the largest organ on the human body and the most accessible location for drug administration. Transdermal delivery of drugs provides controlled drug release while achieving the desired systemic effect. The transdermal approach is primarily based on percutaneous drug penetration, and one significant advantage is that it avoids hepatic first-pass metabolism, improving medication bioavailability at the target site [65].

Nonetheless, transdermal administration is limited for a variety of reasons, including variable permeability at different skin sites, skin diseases, and the nature of both the skin and the medication. These constraints make the objective of tailored medications more challenging to achieve. As a result, the use of 3D printing or AM techniques in transdermal product design has considerably increased the ability to improve the efficiency of transdermal delivery systems in terms of individualized treatment.

There are various techniques used in 3D printing, one of which is the material extrusion approach, which can be differentiated into direct powder extrusion (DPE) (Fig. 1.9) and FDM (Fig. 1.10) [66]. DPE extrudes powder material through a printer nozzle and is extremely practical due to its simplicity, as it is a one-step process, resulting in a low production cost while also providing high flexibility as well as an accessible printer and supplies. For example, ethylene vinyl acetate (EVA)-based patches were loaded with ibuprofen, a model medicine. Ibuprofen is a nonsteroidal anti-inflammatory medicine that is generally used to treat pain and inflammation [67]. The preparation requires a micronized EVA copolymer (grade 4030 AC) and ibuprofen. The raw materials were weighed, mixed with a mortar and pestle, and then blended to produce a homogeneous powder mixture. The powder combination is then transported to the DPE printer, which has a nozzle with a diameter of 0.1 mm. The printer is tuned so that the speed, temperature, and layer height are optimal [67]. This method is particularly useful for preparing formulations with relatively low amounts of drug and excipients [66].

FDM is another common process used in 3D printing. This form of printing makes use of a hot melting extrusion process. This approach is often employed using a thermoplastic polymer in the form of a filament. The polymer is injected into the heated nozzle, where it softens to a molten state before being placed on an assembly plate and hardens again upon cooling. Layers of molten polymer are placed on top of the previous layer, building layer by layer and eventually resulting in the final product [66]. In terms of pharmaceutical products, the filament can be loaded with the drug in two ways: by soaking it in a drug solution or by combining the active ingredient with the polymer. PLA is a suitable polymer for this FDM method since it is inexpensive, nontoxic, and very biodegradable [68].

3D printing has substantially influenced the design of pharmaceutical transdermal delivery methods. The use of 3D printing enables the customization of transdermal products because it offers the patient's desired customized dose simply by changing the size, form, and drug release profile using a computer CAD program. Furthermore, this approach allows for the incorporation of several active components in a single patch; for example, FDM printers feature many print heads, which

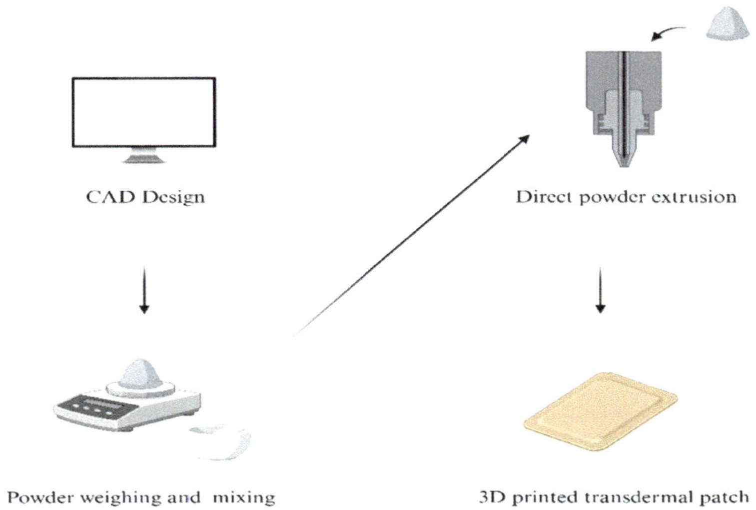

Fig. 1.9 General steps of DPE for producing transdermal patches

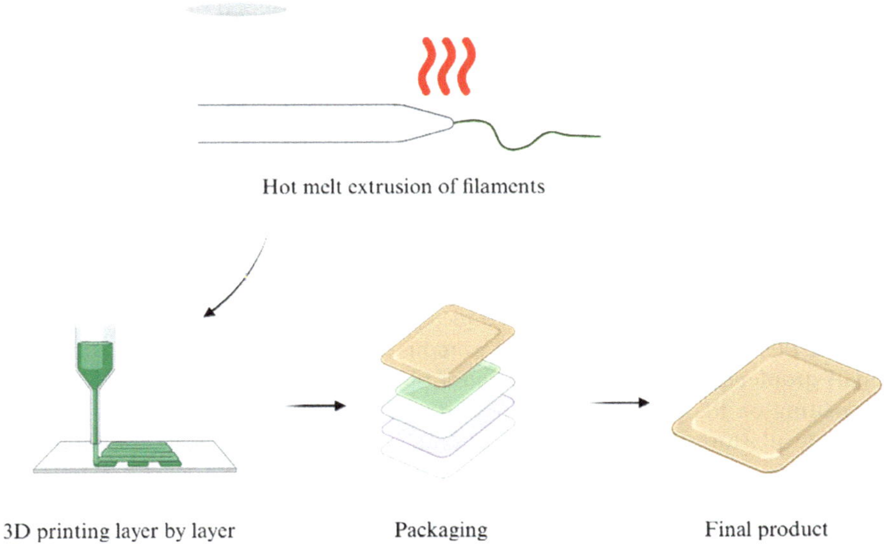

Fig. 1.10 General steps of FDM for producing transdermal patches

allows for the combination of different drugs with different polymers [68]. In brief, 3D printing can generate a single transdermal dosage form with high drug content, can release it at the desired rate, can be particularly beneficial for treating patients with multiple chronic diseases, and can gradually improve patient adherence [3].

The quality of 3D-printed transdermal patches can be assessed using a variety of control procedures, including weight uniformity, morphology, in vitro drug release, and in vitro drug permeation investigations. Weight homogeneity is vital in managing a constant amount of medicine released into the body from each of the patches. Morphological tests evaluate the reliability of 3D printing technology by determining the average weight and thickness of the finished product. In-vitro drug release is a crucial quality control process for determining content consistency within patches, as well as a secondary means of assessing medication absorption in vivo [67].

1.5.5 3D-Printed Microneedle-Based Transdermal Dosage Form

Microneedles (MNs) are an arrangement of micron-sized needles that penetrate the skin to provide an alternate path for skin permeation at the microscale, allowing them to skip the stratum corneum, the toughest skin layer [3]. It is an improved version of the traditional transdermal patch that allows for increased drug distribution and, as a result, better drug delivery to the target site.

MN works by creating a grip on the skin via the puncture of a needle with a height of 25 to 2000 microns and a diameter of 50 to 250 microns, allowing them to stay unchanged after application. It should also be emphasized that the application of MNs is painless and hence causes no patient discomfort, increasing patient compliance because it is very simple to apply. Like transdermal patches, MNs can be used to deliver various drugs. Polymers, silicon, and metals are common materials employed for the manufacture of MNs [65].

MNs can be made utilizing a variety of current processes, including laser cutting, lithography, and electrochemical and photochemical etching. Existing approaches often require more sophisticated and expensive equipment, as well as intricate processes. Therefore, the introduction of 3D printing can improve the manufacturing of MN patches [65]. Inkjet printing is one of the most commonly utilized 3D printing techniques for producing coated MN patches (Fig. 1.11). To define, it is the continuous or drop-on-demand deposition of small droplets onto a powder bed via a piezoelectric or thermal device. After depositing on the powder bed, they preferentially harden and create a layer. A movable platform is then lowered to create a new powder bed for sequential layer creation, ultimately forming the final product [65].

One good example is the creation of insulin MNs for transdermal delivery, in which an insulin polymeric layer is ink blasted onto metal MNs for coating. Insulin is primarily used to treat diabetes, and while it is frequently available as an injection pen, transdermal patches provide a simpler and quicker method of self-administration, improving patient adherence and reducing anxiety associated with self-injection [69]. Insulin is a protein; hence, it has the potential to hydrolyse and denature through the transdermal route. To solve this issue, a surfactant is used to stabilize the formulation. However, the presence of a surfactant reduces the rate of disintegration and absorption, resulting in a longer time for insulin to reach the site of

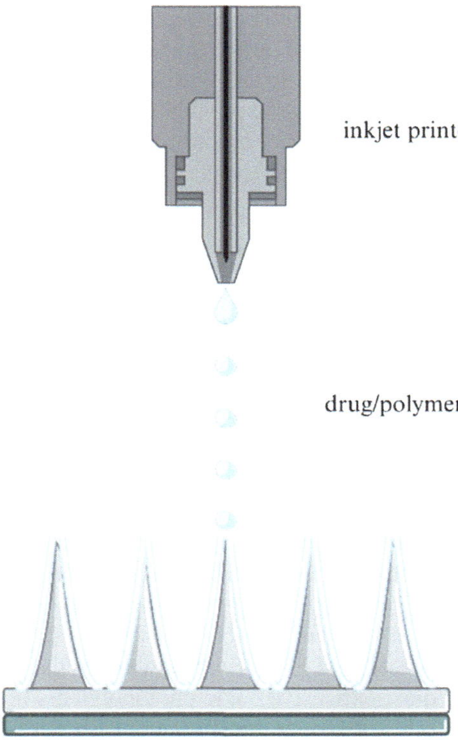

Fig. 1.11 Inkjet printing for the production of coated MN-based transdermal patches

action in the bloodstream. This promotes the development of insulin-polymer solutions that have the highest drug absorption onto the microneedle and deliver the maximum amount of medicine at the fastest rate [69].

Gelatin is an excellent candidate polymer for insulin because of its biocompatibility, biodegradability, and chemical inertness. The MNs were created by cutting 75 mm thick stainless-steel sheets with an infrared laser. The polymer was dissolved in deionized water before being mixed with bovine pancreas-derived insulin to generate the coating. The insulin/polymer droplets are subsequently inked onto the MN arrays using a piezoelectric inkjet printer at a drop-on-demand rate of 1–5 m/s [69].

Using 3D printing to manufacture coated MNs-based transdermal patches allows dose and frequency customization that meets the needs of the patient. This is because all MN patches are initially created using computer-aided design tools [70]. Furthermore, while coated MN systems have a quick drug release profile, the amount of medicine they can transport is quite limited. However, it can be converted into a different form of microneedle system known as hollow MNs by simply changing the microneedle geometries using software to boost the drug's bioavailability at the systemic level for greater efficiency [65].

Similar to 3D-printed transdermal patches, 3D-printed MNs-based patches must pass a variety of quality control tests. One of these methods is in vitro skin testing of MNs to determine their ability to penetrate the skin. A Franz diffusion cell was also used to investigate drug permeability in vitro. To ensure that the same amount of insulin is released to the receptor, chromatography is used to monitor the insulin concentration quantitatively [69].

1.6 Challenges

3D printing technology offers numerous benefits but also faces challenges. Although 3D printing is a potential method for personalizing medical therapy, there are still obstacles to its use in the pharmaceutical sector. The challenges are frequently classified into three categories: material, operation, and machinery. First, the materials used in production must be compatible with printing technology, which is strongly reliant on their physicochemical qualities. Incompatible raw materials can reduce content consistency and printing repeatability. As a result, one of the most limiting constraints in incorporating 3D printing into the sector is the availability of materials [71].

One of the main issues is the need for excipients, who must meet specific requirements based on the printing technology used. SLA, FDM, and SLS are some of the technologies used, but FDM is unsuitable for thermally unstable drugs, while SLA and SLS require expensive, toxic photopolymers [43]. Limited dedicated programs in 3D printing software and instruments also pose challenges. Continuous updates in modelling and slicing software are needed to meet higher standards. Printing instruments face issues such as nozzle clogging, material migration, and leakage, which affect print quality. Mechanical properties are crucial for quality control, but layer stacking can result in rough surfaces and low mechanical strength. Additionally, regulatory challenges include the need for specific guidelines for 3D-printed medicines, which are still in development [1].

Due to compatibility and toxicity issues, 3D printing technology requires careful selection of excipients, particularly for unique dosage forms. Different printing technologies have specific requirements for excipient properties, such as FDM technology, which requires suitable drug carriers, and SSE and DOP technologies, which require temperature control. The mechanical characteristics of dosage forms can also pose challenges, with distinctive layering of polymers or powders forming rough surfaces. Quality depends on factors such as surface tension, nozzle precision, and adhesive viscosity. Regular software updates are crucial for complex structure fabrication, while frequent stoppages and restarts increase the stability of the strain print head. Monitoring mechanical equipment, 3D printer instrumentation, operating procedures, and driving control systems is necessary to ensure that the 3D printing process is optimized and upgraded. Incorrect binder migration and nozzle clogging can influence the formulation produced [1].

1.6.1 Challenges of 3D Printing Applications in Transdermal Patches and MNs

Moreover, both transdermal patches and MNs require materials with high mechanical strength. The former ensures their durability, while the latter ensures that the microneedle is sufficiently sturdy to pierce the skin without breaking or bending. In addition to MNs, drug solubility and degradability are important limiting factors [69].

Furthermore, individuals with sophisticated operational skills are required since processing factors such as printer speed and temperature must be closely monitored throughout the process to ensure consistent product quality and eliminate batch variance. To ensure product reproducibility, a highly precise machine is needed. Furthermore, maintenance costs are greater than those of conventional equipment. Improper machine maintenance can lead to errors in the manufacturing process and, ultimately, in the product, lowering drug delivery efficiency. On the other hand, small-scale manufacturing equipment, such as FDM machines, is not suitable for large-scale production, restricting the application of this approach in industry [71].

1.7 Conclusion

This chapter covers the 3D printing technology utilized to create medication delivery systems, as well as the formulation, materials, and processing parameters to be considered. The ability to create 3D printing equipment capable of producing personalized doses to fit the needs of specific patients will determine the future of this technology. In summary, the 3D approach has the potential to revolutionize pharmaceutical delivery systems, but it will take some time to perfect. In the future, compounding and dispensing pharmacists will need to focus on developing customized 3D-printed dosage forms that are tailored to patient needs, materials, and processes.

Acknowledgement This work was supported by a Research Excellence and Innovation Grant (Project Code: REIG-FPS-2023/042) from the Centre of Excellence in Research, Value Innovation and Entrepreneurship (CERVIE), UCSI University, Malaysia. Every figure in the book chapter was created using BioRender.com.

References

1. Cui M, Pan H, Su Y, Fang D, Qiao S, Ding P, et al. Opportunities and challenges of three-dimensional printing technology in pharmaceutical formulation development. Acta Pharm Sin B. 2021;11(8):2488–504.
2. Basit AW, Trenfield SJ. 3D printing of pharmaceuticals and the role of pharmacy. Pharm J. 2022;308:7959.
3. Jain V, Haider N, Jain K. 3D printing in personalized drug delivery. Curr Pharm Des. 2018;24(42):5062–71.

4. Elbadawi M, McCoubrey LE, Gavins FK, Ong JJ, Goyanes A, Gaisford S, et al. Harnessing artificial intelligence for the next generation of 3D printed medicines. Adv Drug Deliv Rev. 2021;175:113805.
5. Tracy T, Wu L, Liu X, Cheng S, Li X. 3D printing: innovative solutions for patients and pharmaceutical industry. Int J Pharm. 2023;631:122480.
6. Huanbutta K, Burapapadh K, Sriamornsak P, Sangnim T. Practical application of 3D printing for pharmaceuticals in hospitals and pharmacies. Pharmaceutics. 2023;15(7):1877.
7. Wang S, Chen X, Han X, Hong X, Li X, Zhang H, et al. A review of 3D printing technology in pharmaceutics: technology and applications, now and future. Pharmaceutics. 2023;15(2):416.
8. King MFL, Singh GR, Gopichand A, Srinivasan V. Additive manufacturing for Industry 4.0. Hybrid metal additive manufacturing. CRC Press. p. 173–95.
9. Giuffrida S, Ventimiglia G, Petralia S, Conoci S, Sortino S. Facile light-triggered one-step synthesis of small and stable platinum nanoparticles in an aqueous medium from a β-Cyclodextrin host– guest inclusion complex. Inorg Chem. 2006;45(2):508–10.
10. Hellman S, Frisch P, Platzman A, Booth P. 3D printing in a hospital: centralized clinical implementation and applications for comprehensive care. Digital Health. 2023;9:20552076231221899.
11. Seoane-Viaño I, Trenfield SJ, Basit AW, Goyanes A. Translating 3D printed pharmaceuticals: from hype to real-world clinical applications. Adv Drug Deliv Rev. 2021;174:553–75.
12. Ahlfeld T, Guduric V, Duin S, Akkineni A, Schütz K, Kilian D, et al. Methylcellulose–a versatile printing material that enables biofabrication of tissue equivalents with high shape fidelity. Biomater Sci. 2020;8(8):2102–10.
13. Kiran ASK, Veluru JB, Merum S, Radhamani A, Doble M, Kumar TS, et al. Additive manufacturing technologies: an overview of challenges and perspective of using electrospraying. Nanocomposites. 2018;4(4):190–214.
14. Li J, Liang D, Chen X, Sun W, Shen X. Applications of 3D printing in tumor treatment. Biomed Technol. 2024;5:1–13.
15. Guo N, Leu MC. Additive manufacturing: technology, applications and research needs. Front Mech Eng. 2013;8:215–43.
16. Muehlenfeld C, Duffy P, Yang F, Zermeño-Pérez D, Durig T. Polymers for pharmaceutical 3D printing: printability and critical insight into material properties. In: 3D printing: emerging technologies and functionality of polymeric excipients in drug product development. Springer; 2023. p. 97–137.
17. Matijašić G, Gretić M, Vinčić J, Poropat A, Cuculić L, Rahelić T. Design and 3D printing of multi-compartmental PVA capsules for drug delivery. J Drug Deliv Sci Technol. 2019;52:677–86.
18. Pawar R, Pawar A. 3D printing of pharmaceuticals: approach from bench scale to commercial development. Future J Pharma Sci. 2022;8(1):48.
19. Katseli V, Economou A, Kokkinos C. A novel all-3D-printed cell-on-a-chip device as a useful electroanalytical tool: application to the simultaneous voltammetric determination of caffeine and paracetamol. Talanta. 2020;208:120388.
20. Bianchi M, Pegoretti A, Fredi G. An overview of poly (vinyl alcohol) and poly (vinyl pyrrolidone) in pharmaceutical additive manufacturing. J Vinyl Additive Technol. 2023;29(2):223–39.
21. Aguilar-de-Leyva Á, Linares V, Domínguez-Robles J, Casas M, Caraballo I. Extrusion-based technologies for 3D printing: a comparative study of the processability of thermoplastic polyurethane-based formulations. Pharm Dev Technol. 2023;28(10):939–47.
22. Agrawal A, Hussain CM. 3D-Printed hydrogel for diverse applications: a review. Gels. 2023;9(12):960.
23. Sohl J, Dias J. 3D printing of ceramics for modern medical engineering. In: Additive manufacturing in multidisciplinary cooperation and production. Springer; 2023. p. 235–43.
24. Meng M, Wang J, Huang H, Liu X, Zhang J, Li Z. 3D printing metal implants in orthopedic surgery: methods, applications and future prospects. J Orthop Transl. 2023;42:94–112.
25. Mantihal S, Kobun R, Lee B-B. 3D food printing of as the new way of preparing food: a review. Int J Gastron Food Sci. 2020;22:100260.

26. Vazquez-Martel C, Martins LF, Genthner E, Almeida C, Quintana AM, Bastmeyer M, et al. Printing green: microalgae-based materials for 3D printing with light. Adv Mater. 2024;36:2402786.
27. Vithani K, Goyanes A, Jannin V, Basit AW, Gaisford S, Boyd BJ. An overview of 3D printing technologies for soft materials and potential opportunities for lipid-based drug delivery systems. Pharm Res. 2019;36:1–20.
28. Park BJ, Choi HJ, Moon SJ, Kim SJ, Bajracharya R, Min JY, et al. Pharmaceutical applications of 3D printing technology: current understanding and future perspectives. J Pharm Investig. 2019;49:575–85.
29. Chang S-Y, Li SW, Kowsari K, Shetty A, Sorrells L, Sen K, et al. Binder-jet 3D printing of indomethacin-laden pharmaceutical dosage forms. J Pharm Sci. 2020;109(10):3054–63.
30. Jamróz W, Kurek M, Czech A, Szafraniec J, Gawlak K, Jachowicz R. 3D printing of tablets containing amorphous aripiprazole by filaments co-extrusion. Eur J Pharm Biopharm. 2018;131:44–7.
31. Tan DK, Maniruzzaman M, Nokhodchi A. Development and optimisation of novel polymeric compositions for sustained release theophylline caplets (PrintCap) via FDM 3D printing. Polymers. 2019;12(1):27.
32. Gioumouxouzis CI, Baklavaridis A, Katsamenis OL, Markopoulou CK, Bouropoulos N, Tzetzis D, et al. A 3D printed bilayer oral solid dosage form combining metformin for prolonged and glimepiride for immediate drug delivery. Eur J Pharm Sci. 2018;120:40–52.
33. Economidou SN, Pere CPP, Reid A, Uddin MJ, Windmill JF, Lamprou DA, et al. 3D printed microneedle patches using stereolithography (SLA) for intradermal insulin delivery. Mater Sci Eng C. 2019;102:743–55.
34. Uddin MJ, Scoutaris N, Economidou SN, Giraud C, Chowdhry BZ, Donnelly RF, et al. 3D printed microneedles for anticancer therapy of skin tumours. Mater Sci Eng C. 2020;107:110248.
35. Kundu A, Arnett P, Bagde A, Azim N, Kouagou E, Singh M, et al. DLP 3D printed “intelligent” microneedle array (iμNA) for stimuli responsive release of drugs and its in vitro and ex vivo characterization. J Microelectromech Syst. 2020;29(5):685–91.
36. Wang F, Chong Y, Wang F, He C. Photopolymer resins for luminescent three-dimensional printing. J Appl Polym Sci. 2017;134(32):44988.
37. Bloomquist CJ, Mecham MB, Paradzinsky MD, Janusziewicz R, Warner SB, Luft JC, et al. Controlling release from 3D printed medical devices using CLIP and drug-loaded liquid resins. J Control Release. 2018;278:9–23.
38. Sun X, Li D, Yang Y, Ren Y, Li J, Wang Z, et al. Microtubule-binding protein CLIP-170 is a mediator of paclitaxel sensitivity. J Pathol. 2012;226(4):666–73.
39. Englezos K, Wang L, Tan EC, Kang L. 3D printing for personalised medicines: implications for policy and practice. Int J Pharm. 2023;635:122785.
40. Mostafaei A, Elliott AM, Barnes JE, Li F, Tan W, Cramer CL, et al. Binder jet 3D printing—Process parameters, materials, properties, modeling, and challenges. Prog Mater Sci. 2021;119:100707.
41. Aho J, Bøtker JP, Genina N, Edinger M, Arnfast L, Rantanen J. Roadmap to 3D-printed oral pharmaceutical dosage forms: feedstock filament properties and characterization for fused deposition modeling. J Pharm Sci. 2019;108(1):26–35.
42. Bagheri A, Jin J. Photopolymerization in 3D printing. ACS Appl Polym Mater. 2019;1(4):593–611.
43. Franiak-Pietryga I, Ziemba B, Sikorska H, Jander M, Kuncman W, Danilewicz M, et al. Maltotriose-modified poly (propylene imine) Glycodendrimers as a potential novel platform in the treatment of chronic lymphocytic Leukemia. A proof-of-concept pilot study in the animal model of CLL. Toxicol Appl Pharmacol. 2020;403:115139.
44. Shabaninejad Z, Yousefi F, Movahedpour A, Ghasemi Y, Dokanehiifard S, Rezaei S, et al. Electrochemical-based biosensors for microRNA detection: nanotechnology comes into view. Anal Biochem. 2019;581:113349.

45. Allonas X, Hammouda B, Métral B, Goldbach E, Schuller AS, Ley C, et al. Controlling photopolymerization reaction in layer-by-layer photopolymerization in 3D printing. Appl Res. 3(4):e202400004.
46. Xu X, Awad A, Robles-Martinez P, Gaisford S, Goyanes A, Basit AW. Vat photopolymerization 3D printing for advanced drug delivery and medical device applications. J Control Release. 2021;329:743–57.
47. Pawar R, Pawar A. 3D printing of pharmaceuticals: approach from bench scale to commercial development. Future J Pharm Sci. 2022;8(1):48.
48. Berg S, Krause J, Björkbom A, Walter K, Harun S, Granfeldt A, et al. In vitro and in vivo evaluation of 3D printed capsules with pressure triggered release mechanism for oral peptide delivery. J Pharm Sci. 2021;110(1):228–38.
49. Jamróz W, Pyteraf J, Kurek M, Knapik-Kowalczuk J, Szafraniec-Szczęsny J, Jurkiewicz K, et al. Multivariate design of 3D printed immediate-release tablets with liquid crystal-forming drug—itraconazole. Materials. 2020;13(21):4961.
50. Pan S, Ding S, Zhou X, Zheng N, Zheng M, Wang J, et al. 3D-printed dosage forms for oral administration: a review. Drug Deliv Transl Res. 2024;14(2):312–28.
51. Angeliki S, Eleni T, Rekkas DM, Vlachou M. 3D-printed modified-release tablets: a review of the recent advances. In: Molecular pharmacology. IntechOpen; 2020.
52. Kim JH, Kim K, Jin H-E. Three-dimensional printing for oral pharmaceutical dosage forms. J Pharm Investig. 2022;52(3):293–317.
53. Milliken RL, Quinten T, Andersen SK, Lamprou DA. Application of 3D printing in early phase development of pharmaceutical solid dosage forms. Int J Pharm. 2024;653:123902.
54. Karalia D, Siamidi A, Karalis V, Vlachou M. 3D-printed oral dosage forms: mechanical properties, computational approaches and applications. Pharmaceutics. 2021;13(9):1401.
55. Elbl J, Veselý M, Blaháčková D, Ondruš J, Kulich P, Mašková E, et al. Development of 3D printed multi-layered orodispersible films with porous structure applicable as a substrate for inkjet printing. Pharmaceutics. 2023;15(2):714.
56. Palekar S, Nukala PK, Patel K. Aversion liquid-filled drug releasing capsule (3D-RECAL): a novel technology for the development of immediate release abuse deterrent formulations using a fused deposition modelling (FDM) 3D printer. Int J Pharm. 2022;621:121804.
57. Cotabarren I, Gallo L. 3D printing of PVA capsular devices for modified drug delivery: design and in vitro dissolution studies. Drug Dev Ind Pharm. 2020;46(9):1416–26.
58. Qian H, Chen D, Xu X, Li R, Yan G, Fan T. FDM 3D-printed sustained-release gastric-floating verapamil hydrochloride formulations with cylinder, capsule and hemisphere shapes, and low infill percentage. Pharmaceutics. 2022;14(2):281.
59. Maroni A, Melocchi A, Parietti F, Foppoli A, Zema L, Gazzaniga A. 3D printed multi-compartment capsular devices for two-pulse oral drug delivery. J Control Release. 2017;268:10–8.
60. Green Buzhor M, Abdi F, Luo Z, Leroux JC. Colonic delivery of aqueous suspensions using 3D printed capsules. Adv Mater Technol. 2024;9(9):2301975.
61. He Y, Foralosso R, Trindade GF, Ilchev A, Ruiz-Cantu L, Clark EA, et al. A reactive prodrug ink formulation strategy for inkjet 3D printing of controlled release dosage forms and implants. Adv Therap. 2020;3(6):1900187.
62. Iezzi G, Zavan B, Petrini M, Ferroni L, Pierfelice TV, D'Amora U, et al. 3D printed dental implants with a porous structure: the in vitro response of osteoblasts, fibroblasts, mesenchymal stem cells, and monocytes. J Dent. 2024;140:104778.
63. Domsta V, Seidlitz A. 3D-Printing of drug-eluting implants: an overview of the current developments described in the literature. Molecules. 2021;26(13):4066.
64. Grygier D, Kujawa M, Kowalewski P. Deposition of biocompatible polymers by 3D Printing (FDM) on titanium alloy. Polymers. 2022;14(2):235.
65. Economidou SN, Lamprou DA, Douroumis D. 3D printing applications for transdermal drug delivery. Int J Pharm. 2018;544(2):415–24.
66. Seoane-Viaño I, Otero-Espinar FJ, Goyanes Á. 3D printing of pharmaceutical products. In: Additive manufacturing. Elsevier; 2021. p. 569–97.

67. Maurizii G, Moroni S, Khorshid S, Aluigi A, Tiboni M, Casettari L. 3D-printed EVA-based patches manufactured by direct powder extrusion for personalized transdermal therapies. Int J Pharm. 2023;635:122720.
68. Azizoğlu E, Özer Ö. Fabrication of Montelukast sodium loaded filaments and 3D printing transdermal patches onto packaging material. Int J Pharm. 2020;587:119588.
69. Ross S, Scoutaris N, Lamprou D, Mallinson D, Douroumis D. Inkjet printing of insulin microneedles for transdermal delivery. Drug Deliv Transl Res. 2015;5:451–61.
70. Villota I, Calvo PC, Campo OI, Villarreal-Gómez LJ, Fonthal F. Manufacturing of a transdermal patch in 3D printing. Micromachines. 2022;13(12):2190.
71. Parulski C, Jennotte O, Lechanteur A, Evrard B. Challenges of fused deposition modeling 3D printing in pharmaceutical applications: where are we now? Adv Drug Deliv Rev. 2021;175:113810.

Fundamental Principles of Fused Deposition Modelling (FDM) Technology

2

Rajni Tanwar, Dinesh Kumar, Shivani, Kavita Bahmani, and Puja Gulati

Abstract

Fused deposition modelling (FDM), also known as fused filament fabrication (FFF), has emerged as a groundbreaking 3D printing technology due to its accessibility, cost-effectiveness, and versatility. This review provides a comprehensive overview of the FDM process, focusing on its advantages and limitations. FDM utilizes material extrusion to construct 3D objects based on computer-aided design (CAD) models. It is commonly employed in the fabrication of thermoplastic parts and prototypes, as well as in the prototyping of ceramics, metals, concretes, polymers, and their composites. However, FDM printing is process parameter-dependent, leading to potential issues with surface quality and the layer-wise appearance of printed parts. Additionally, the range of materials suitable for FDM printing is limited primarily to thermoplastic polymers such as PLA (polylactic acid) or ABS (acrylonitrile butadiene styrene). Post-processing steps, such as sanding, painting, or chemical smoothing, are often necessary to enhance surface finish and mechanical properties. By optimizing process parameters and considering post-processing techniques, users can improve the accuracy, strength, and surface finish of FDM-printed objects.

Keywords

Fused deposition modelling · Computer-aided design · Fused filament fabrication · Polylactic acid · Acrylonitrile butadiene styrene

R. Tanwar (✉) · D. Kumar · Shivani · P. Gulati
School of Pharmacy, Desh Bhagat University, Mandi Gobindgarh, Punjab, India

K. Bahmani
Department of Pharmaceutical Sciences, Guru Jambeshwar University of Science and Technology, Hisar, Haryana, India

K. Vinchurkar, S. Mane (eds.), *Innovations in Drug Manufacturing*,
https://doi.org/10.1007/978-981-96-9075-6_2

2.1 Introduction

A mainstay of additive manufacturing, fused deposition modeling (FDM) is recognized for its affordability, adaptability, and ease of usage. From being a cutting-edge prototype technique developed by S. Scott Crump in the late 1980s, FDM has become a widely used manufacturing technology in a variety of industries. The core ideas of FDM center on the layer-by-layer deposition of thermoplastic materials, which allows for the direct creation of intricate three-dimensional objects from digital models. This introduction seeks to give a thorough overview of FDM technology, examining its historical evolution, fundamental working principles, essential elements, and noteworthy recent developments [1].

2.1.1 Historical Development

In 1989, S. Scott Crump, a co-founder of Stratasys Inc., established the procedure that would lead to the development of FDM technology. FDM was first marketed in the early 1990s, and because of its ease of use and the wide range of applications for thermoplastic materials, it gained popularity very fast. FDM has made great strides in the last 30 years, including the creation of new materials, enhanced hardware, and sophisticated software, solidifying its place in the manufacturing and fast prototyping industries [15].

2.1.2 Basic Operating Principles

Material extrusion is the simple yet brilliant principle of FDM. A build platform is covered in layers of thermoplastic filament that is fed via a heated nozzle, melted, and deposited. Digital instructions obtained from a 3D model that is divided into horizontal layers with the aid of specialist software control the procedure. In order to precisely construct the thing from the bottom-up, the printer adheres to these instructions [2].

The essential components of an FDM printer include:

- *Filament Spool*: Supplies the thermoplastic material.
- *Extruder*: Feeds the filament into the hot end.
- *Hot End*: Melts the filament and extrudes it through a nozzle.
- *Print Bed*: Provides a surface for layer-by-layer construction.
- *Stepper Motors*: Control the precise movements of the print head and print bed in the X, Y, and Z axes.
- *Cooling System*: Solidifies the extruded material quickly to maintain structural integrity.

2.1.2.1 Key Components and Their Functions

Every one of an FDM printer's main parts is essential to the printing procedure. The raw material, which is usually thermoplastics like PLA, ABS, or PETG, is provided by the filament spool. The filament is forced into the hot end by the extruder mechanism, where it is heated to a precise temperature to provide the required viscosity. After the filament has melted, it is extruded via a tiny nozzle and placed onto the print bed, which could be heated to promote good adherence and avoid warping.

Building the object layer by layer, the print bed and print head move precisely in accordance with the instructions provided by the digital model. Stepper motors play a crucial role in regulating these motions, guaranteeing exceptional accuracy and consistency. The extruded material is nearly immediately solidified by the cooling system, which frequently consists of fans, preventing deformation when the next layer is deposited [3].

2.1.3 Recent Advancements and Applications

There have been notable developments in FDM technology in recent years. With the advent of composite filaments, which include fiber- and particle-reinforced materials, the variety of mechanical qualities that may be achieved with FDM has increased. Furthermore, new avenues for the development of parts with improved mechanical, thermal, and electrical properties have been made possible by the introduction of nanomaterials into filaments.

Rapid prototyping to functional end-use parts in consumer goods, automotive, aerospace, and healthcare industries are just a few of the many industries where FDM is now widely used. The possibilities of FDM technology are constantly expanding thanks to developments like improved cooling systems, adaptive slicing algorithms, and multi-material printing [4, 25].

Combined Deposition Modeling, which provides unmatched flexibility and efficiency, has completely changed the way we approach design and manufacturing. Though its core concepts are still based upon the material extrusion process, its capabilities are constantly being expanded by ongoing developments in hardware, software, and materials. This chapter explores the core ideas of FDM in greater detail, offering a comprehensive grasp of its workings, applications, and current advancements [6].

2.1.4 Steps to Manufacture a Product with FDM

1. *Design Phase*:
   - *CAD Modeling*: With computer-aided design (CAD) software, create a three-dimensional (3D) model of the item. The actual object's blueprint is found in this digital model [7].

2. *Preparation for Printing*:
   - Slicing: To make the 3D model into layers (slices) that the FDM printer can comprehend, use slicing software.
   - Orientation and Support Structures: Establish the model's ideal orientation for printing in order to reduce supports and obtain the required mechanical qualities [8].
3. *Printing Process*:
   1. Material Selection: Select the proper thermoplastic filament based on requirements for mechanical, thermal, and aesthetics [5].
   2. Printer Setup: Set up the temperature, layer height, and print speed of the FDM printer [9].
   3. Printing Execution: Begin the printing process by allowing the extruder to melt the filament and deposit it layer by layer in accordance with the sliced model [6].
4. *Post-Processing*:
   - Support Removal: Depending on the material being utilized, remove support structures with mechanical tools or soluble supports.
   - Surface Finishing: To attain the appropriate surface quality, use post-processing methods such chemical smoothing, sanding, or polishing [10].
5. *Quality Control*:
   (a) Dimensional Accuracy: Verify the dimensional accuracy of the printed part by comparing its measurements to the CAD model.
   (b) Mechanical Testing: To confirm the part's mechanical qualities, perform mechanical testing (tensile, flexural, impact, etc.) [11].

2.1.5 Key Process Parameters in FDM [12]

1. Nozzle Temperature: The nozzle's temperature has an impact on the filament material's viscosity, which in turn impacts surface finish and layer adhesion. Achieving the ideal nozzle temperature is essential to guaranteeing appropriate flow and layer bonding.
2. Bed Temperature: The temperature of the print bed influences the first layer's initial adhesion and helps to keep the bed from warping when printing. In order to maximize adhesion and reduce thermal stress, different materials need varied bed temperatures.
3. Print Speed: The nozzle's speed during material extrusion is determined by the print speed. Increased speeds can shorten the printing process, but they may also have an impact on the end part's mechanical qualities and print quality.
4. Infill Density: The quantity of material used inside a printed product is referred to as infill density. Greater infill densities consume more material and take longer to print, but they also make the item stronger and heavier.

5. Cooling Rate: The mechanical characteristics and crystallinity of the printed part might be impacted by the cooling rate. Sufficient cooling is required to promptly harden the extruded filament and preserve the intended geometry.
6. Extrusion Multiplier: This setting regulates how much filament the nozzle extrudes. Accurate dimensions and strong layer adhesion can be achieved with the extrusion multiplier adjusted.

2.1.6 Impact of Process Parameters on 3D Printing [13]

1. Mechanical Properties: Nozzle temperature, layer height, and infill density are a few examples of the variables that affect the printed items' mechanical strength, stiffness, and durability. Achieving optimal optimization of these factors can improve the printed products' mechanical performance.
2. Dimensional Accuracy: To achieve precise dimensions, variables such as print speed, extrusion multiplier, and nozzle temperature are important. Variations in these parameters may result in print flaws and dimensional errors.
3. Surface Finish: Layer height, print speed, and cooling rate all have an impact on the surface finish's smoothness and quality. Reducing the need for post-processing and improving surface aesthetics can be achieved by fine-tuning these settings.
4. Material Properties: The way that various thermoplastic materials react to process variables varies. For example, in order to maximize printing performance, certain settings are needed for PLA, ABS, PETG, and nylon. Achieving prints of excellent quality requires an understanding of the needs specific to each material.
5. Print Time and Efficiency: You may make big changes to the overall print time and material utilization by adjusting parameters like print speed, layer height, and infill density. For printing to be both economical and effective, these aspects must be balanced.

2.1.7 Recent Trends [14]

Improvements in print quality, material characteristics, and overall efficiency have been the main emphasis of recent developments in FDM technology and process parameter optimization. Among the noteworthy trends are:

1. Adaptive Slicing Techniques: These algorithms dynamically modify layer height according to the part geometry, improving surface quality and cutting down on print time.
2. Multi-material Printing: Advances in FDM printing allow for the combination of flexible and stiff materials in a single print, for example, to create complicated pieces with different qualities.

3. Improved Cooling Systems: Better cooling techniques, like liquid cooling systems and active cooling fans, aid in preserving ideal temperatures and improving print quality.
4. Advanced Filaments: The variety of applications for FDM technology is increased by the development of new filament materials, such as composites and high-performance polymers [4, 25].

2.1.8 Working Principle of FDM Printers

An application of additive manufacturing based on the extrusion of materials is fused deposition modeling, or FDM. It builds pieces with a thermoplastic filament, layer by layer, from the bottom up. This is a thorough explanation of how FDM printers operate [3]:

2.1.8.1 Components of an FDM Printer

1. Filament Spool: The raw material's source; typically a thermoplastic filament made of nylon, PLA, ABS, or PETG.
2. The device that feeds the filament into the hot end is called an extruder. Usually, it has a gear system and a motor.
3. Hot End: The area where the filament melts within the printer. It is made up of a nozzle and a heating element.
4. Print Bed: The base upon which the item is constructed. Heating it can help with adherence and keep it from warping.
5. Stepper Motors: These are the motors in the X, Y, and Z axes that move the print head and print bed.
6. Cooling System: To rapidly solidify the extruded filament, use fans or other cooling techniques.
7. Control System: The software and electronic parts that control printing [15].

2.1.8.2 Step-by-Step Working Principle

1. Design Creation: Using computer-aided design (CAD) software, a 3D model is first created to begin the process. After that, this model is transformed into a file type that the printer can read, usually an STL file.
2. Slicing: After importing the STL file into the program, the 3D model is divided into multiple layers, and G-code is produced. The G-code is a set of instructions that regulates the heating elements, the printer's movement, and the filament's extrusion.
3. Feeding the Filament: The thermoplastic filament is fed into the extruder by the filament spool. The filament is forced into the hot end by the extruder motor.
4. Heating and Extrusion: The filament is heated by the hot end to its melting point, which causes it to become semi-liquid. The G-code-defined route is followed by the nozzle as it extrudes the molten filament onto the print bed.
5. Layer-by-Layer Construction: The filament is deposited one layer at a time by the printer. The print bed descends (or the print head elevates) by the layer height

after a layer is finished, and the procedure is repeated for the subsequent layer. Almost instantly after extrusion, the filament cools and solidifies, joining with the layer underneath.

6. Cooling and Solidification: The cooling system helps the extruded filament solidify quickly, preventing distortion and ensuring that the layers attach correctly.
7. Completion: The print head goes away and the finished product is taken out of the print bed once all of the layers have been deposited. It can be necessary to perform post-processing procedures including surface polishing and the removal of support components [2, 16].

2.1.9 Materials Used in FDM

Thermoplastic polymers are the main material used in FDM technology since they can be melted and resolidified. The variety of materials utilized in FDM has recently increased thanks to developments in material science. These materials now include nanomaterials, fiber-reinforced polymers, and particle-reinforced polymers. The mechanical, thermal, and functional qualities of 3D printed parts are improved by these materials [17].

2.1.9.1 Particle Reinforced Polymer Materials

Small particles are incorporated into the thermoplastic matrix of particle-reinforced polymers to enhance characteristics including strength, stiffness, and wear resistance. Frequently utilized particles include metals, ceramics, and further inorganic substances.

- Metal Particles: Filaments packed with metal, including copper or aluminum particles, improve the printed objects' electrical and thermal conductivity. They are frequently employed in applications that call for enhanced EMI shielding or heat dissipation.
- Ceramic Particles: Wear resistance and thermal stability are enhanced by filters containing ceramic particles, such as silica or alumina. These materials are appropriate for parts that are subjected to abrasive conditions and high temperatures.
- Carbon Black: To enhance filaments' mechanical, electrical conductivity, and UV resistance, carbon black particles are added [18].

2.1.9.2 Fiber Reinforced Polymer Materials

In order to improve mechanical qualities like tensile strength, modulus, and impact resistance, fibers are placed into a polymer matrix to create composites known as fiber reinforced polymers, or FRPs. Short or continuous fibers are used in FDM filaments [19].

- Carbon Fiber: Filaments reinforced with carbon fiber have a high tensile strength and rigidity while being lightweight. They are perfect for uses like aerospace and automotive components, where strong yet lightweight materials are needed.
- Glass Fiber: Compared to carbon fiber, glass fiber reinforced filaments offer better strength, rigidity, and thermal stability at a cheaper cost. These materials are employed in load-bearing and structural applications.
- Kevlar Fiber: Suitable for protective gear and impact-resistant components, Kevlar reinforced filaments offer exceptional toughness and impact resistance [20].

2.1.9.3 Nanomaterials for FDM

Because of their huge surface area and special mechanical, electrical, and thermal properties, nanomaterials included into FDM filaments can greatly improve the printed items' qualities [21].

- Carbon Nanotubes (CNTs): Filaments reinforced with CNTs have better thermal, electrical, and mechanical conductivity. High-strength structural elements, sensors, and electrical components all use them.
- Improved filaments using graphene offer better mechanical strength, electrical and thermal conductivity, and barrier qualities. High-performance applications in electronics, aircraft, and medical devices can benefit from these materials.
- Nano clay: The mechanical strength, thermal stability, and barrier qualities of printed items are enhanced by filaments reinforced with nano-clay. Applications needing increased resistance to environmental conditions and durability can use them [22].

2.1.10 Advantages and Limitations of FDM Technology

Popular 3D printing technology fused deposition modeling (FDM) is renowned for its adaptability and affordability. Like every technology, it does have benefits and drawbacks. Comprehending these might aid in choosing the suitable applications and streamlining the procedure [15, 23].

2.1.10.1 Advantages of FDM Technology

1. *Cost-Effectiveness*:
   - Inexpensive Equipment: FDM printers often cost less than other 3D printing technologies like SLS or SLA. This opens them up to small enterprises, educational organizations, and hobbyists alike.
   - Low Material Cost: The cost of printing is further decreased by the comparatively low cost of the thermoplastic filaments used in FDM.
2. *Material Variety*:
   - Broad Variety of Thermoplastics: FDM is compatible with TPU, polycarbonate, composites, and a number of specialty materials in addition to thermo-

plastics like PLA, ABS, and PETG. This makes a wide variety of applications with various material qualities possible.
   - Composite Filaments: The mechanical and functional qualities of printed objects can be extended by the availability of particle and fiber reinforced filaments.
3. *Ease of Use*:
   - User-Friendly Software: FDM printers have user-friendly software that makes slicing easier and makes it simple for users to change printing parameters.
   - Minimal Setup: In comparison to other 3D printing technologies, routine maintenance is reasonably easy to perform and the setup process is uncomplicated.
4. *Scalability and Flexibility*:
   - Personalized Print Size: FDM printers are available in multiple dimensions, enabling the creation of both tiny and huge items.
   - Fast Prototyping: FDM's speed and capacity to generate workable prototypes in a timely manner make it the perfect material for fast prototyping.
5. *Environmental Benefits*:
   - Recyclable Materials: FDM is a more environmentally responsible solution because many of its materials, particularly PLA, are recyclable or biodegradable
   - Less Material Waste: FDM generates less material waste than subtractive manufacturing techniques.

2.1.10.2 Limitations of FDM Technology [4, 24, 25]

1. *Surface Finish and Resolution*:
   - Layer Lines: On the surface of printed objects, visible layer lines are a product of the layer-by-layer deposition process, which may have an impact on surface finish and aesthetics.
   - Resolution Constraints: The degree of precision and detail in produced objects is generally limited by FDM's lesser resolution when compared to other 3D printing technologies like SLA or PolyJet.
2. *Mechanical Properties*:
   - Anisotropy: Depending on the print orientation, parts made using fused deposition modelling (FDM) have different mechanical and strength characteristics. For applications that support loads, this might be a constraint.
   - Bonding Strength: Under stress, delamination may occur because the intra-layer strength in FDM is stronger than the inter-layer bonding.
3. *Print Speed*:
   - Time-Consuming: Printing intricate, high-resolution components can take a while, particularly when layer heights are reduced.
   - Post-Processing: To improve surface quality and eliminate support structures, post-processing procedures like sanding, painting, or chemical smoothing frequently take longer than expected.

4. *Material Limitations*:
   - Limited High-Performance Materials: Although thermoplastics come in a wide range, FDM is less appropriate for high-performance engineering materials that need to withstand harsh chemicals or high temperatures.
   - Support Structures: Support structures are frequently needed for complex geometries, and they can be challenging to remove and might leave markings on the printed item.
5. *Dimensional Accuracy*:
   - Warpage and Shrinkage: As thermoplastic materials cool, they may warp or shrink, resulting in dimensional errors that require adjustment and fine-tuning.
   - Tolerance Issues: It might be difficult to achieve precise tolerances, which may call for repeated tweaks and improvements.

2.2 Conclusion

Fused deposition modelling (FDM) is a revolutionary technology in additive manufacturing that revolutionizes design, prototyping, and production. Its principles include layer-by-layer material deposition, thermoplastic filament use, and precise control over the extrusion process. This allows for complex geometries, customization of parts, and rapid iteration, making it a preferred choice in industries like automotive and healthcare. Key aspects of FDM include material extrusion, layer-by-layer building, support structures, and computer-aided design (CAD) integration. FDM can use a wide range of materials, including ABS, PLA, and advanced composites, and continues to evolve with advancements in printer technology, software, and materials. The fundamental principles of FDM technology drive innovation, reduce lead times, and lower costs, and it promises to continue expanding its influence across various sectors, driving the future of manufacturing.

References

1. Crump SS. Apparatus and method for creating three-dimensional objects. US Patent No 5,121,329. 1992.
2. Ngo TD, Kashani A, Imbalzano G, Nguyen KTQ, Hui D. Additive manufacturing (3D printing): a review of materials, methods, applications and challenges. Compos Part B. 2018;143:172–96.
3. Turner N, Brian RS, Gold SA. A review of melt extrusion additive manufacturing processes: I. Process design and modeling. Rapid Prototyp J. 2014;20(3):192–204.
4. Hossain MS, et al. Impact of process parameters on tensile strength of FDM printed specimens. J Manufac Mat Process. 2018a;2(3):52.
5. Jones P, et al. Material properties and selection criteria for fused deposition modelling. Mat Today: Proceed. 2023;20(Part 2):1306–11.
6. Lee S, Kim J. Process parameters optimization in fused deposition modelling. Int J Precis Eng Manuf-Green Technol. 2022;9(1):177–88.
7. Li W, et al. CAD modeling techniques for fused deposition modelling. Comput Aided Des. 2020;121:102955.

8. Singh V, Gupta MK. Slicing algorithms for fused deposition modelling: a review. Rapid Prototyp J. 2019;25(1):158–76.
9. Smith J, Brown A. Fused deposition modelling printer setup and optimization. J Manuf Sci Eng. 2018;140(7):071010.
10. Wang H, Zhang Y. Surface finishing methods in fused deposition modelling. J Manuf Process. 2023;75:479–88.
11. Garzon-Hernandez S, Garcia-Gonzalez D, Jérusalem A, Arias A. Design of FDM 3D printed polymers: an experimental-modelling methodology for the prediction of mechanical properties. Mater Des. 2020;188:108414.
12. Panda BN, et al. Optimization of process parameters for fused deposition modeling. Mat Today: Proceed. 2021;45:5768–72.
13. Kumar R, et al. Influence of process parameters on the mechanical properties of 3D printed structures. J Manuf Process. 2020;49:398–407.
14. Chohan JS, et al. Effect of process parameters on mechanical properties of 3D printed parts: a review. Mater Sci Eng A. 2019;755:19–33.
15. Gibson I, Rosen DW, Stucker B. Additive manufacturing technologies: 3D printing, rapid prototyping, and direct digital manufacturing. Springer; 2015.
16. Galantucci LM, Lavecchia F, Percoco G. Experimental study aiming to enhance the surface finish of fused deposition modeled parts. CIRP Ann. 2009;58(1):189–92.
17. Hwang S, et al. Investigation of the mechanical properties of metal-polymer composites for 3D printing applications. J Mater Res. 2015;30(23):3436–43.
18. Zhong W, et al. Short fiber reinforced composites for fused deposition modeling. Mater Sci Eng A. 2001;301(2):125–30.
19. Tekinalp HL, et al. Highly oriented carbon fiber–polymer composites via additive manufacturing. Compos Sci Technol. 2014;105:144–50.
20. Li N, et al. 3D printing of continuous fiber reinforced thermoplastic composites: development, manufacture, microstructure, and properties. Compos Sci Technol. 2016;137:189–204.
21. Spitalsky Z, et al. Carbon nanotube–polymer composites: chemistry, processing, mechanical and electrical properties. Prog Polym Sci. 2010;35(3):357–401.
22. Kuang X, et al. Grayscale digital light processing 3D printing for highly functionally graded materials. Sci Adv. 2019;5(5):eaav5790.
23. Chua CK, Leong KF, Lim CS. Rapid prototyping: principles and applications. World Scientific; 2010.
24. Wong KV, Hernandez A. A review of additive manufacturing. ISRN Mech Eng. 2012;2012:208760.
25. Hossain MS, et al. Impact of process parameters on tensile strength of FDM printed specimens. J Manuf Mater Process. 2018b;2(3):52.

Materials for Fused Deposition Modelling (FDM) 3D Printing Technology

3

Rupal Dubey, Dinesh Kumar Mishra, Neeraj Upmanyu, and Kuldeep Vinchurkar

Abstract

Fused deposition modelling (FDM) has emerged as a transformative 3D printing technology in the pharmaceutical industry, offering unprecedented opportunities for personalized drug delivery systems, precise dosage control, and innovative therapeutic designs. This chapter provides a comprehensive overview of the materials utilized in FDM for drug manufacturing, emphasizing the critical role of material properties in determining the success of pharmaceutical applications. Key considerations include biocompatibility, process ability, stability under thermal conditions, and their influence on drug release profiles. The chapter categorizes materials into polymers, drug-loaded filaments, composites, and emerging smart materials, highlighting their unique attributes and applications.

Moreover, the challenges in developing suitable materials, such as thermal degradation of active pharmaceutical ingredients (APIs) and achieving uniform drug distribution, are explored. Advanced strategies for material optimization, including polymer modifications, additive blending, and innovative filament extrusion techniques, are discussed to address these hurdles. Case studies illustrate real-world applications, such as personalized tablets, multi-drug systems,

R. Dubey (✉)
Vidhyapeeth Institute of Pharmacy, Bhopal, MP, India

D. K. Mishra
Department of Pharmacy, Guru Ghasidas Vishwavidyalaya (A Central University), Bilaspur, Chhattisgarh, India

N. Upmanyu
SAGE University, Bhopal, MP, India

K. Vinchurkar
Department of Pharmaceutics, Sandip Institute of Pharmaceutical Sciences (SIPS), Affiliated To Savitribai Phule Pune University (SPPU, Pune), Nashik, Maharashtra, India

K. Vinchurkar, S. Mane (eds.), *Innovations in Drug Manufacturing*,
https://doi.org/10.1007/978-981-96-9075-6_3

and implants, demonstrating the potential of FDM to revolutionize drug manufacturing. Finally, the chapter identifies future trends in materials development, including bioinks, biodegradable polymers, and sustainable practices, positioning FDM as a cornerstone technology in modern pharmaceuticals.

Keywords

Fused deposition modelling · 3D printing · Drug manufacturing · Pharmaceutical materials · Polymers · Personalized medicine

Abbreviations

3DMF	3D manufacturing format
ABS	Acrylonitrile butadiene styrene
AM	Additive manufacturing
APIs	Active pharmaceutical ingredients
CAB	Cellulose acetate butyrate
CAD	Computer-aided design
CMC	Carboxymethyl cellulose
DSC	Differential scanning calorimetry
EVA	Ethylene vinyl acetate
FDM	Fused diffusion modelling
FFF	Fused filament fabrication
FTIR	Fourier-transform infrared spectroscopy
HIPS	High-impact polystyrene
HME	Hot melt extrusion
HPMC	Hydroxypropyl methylcellulose
ISO	International Standard Organization
PCL	Polycaprolactone
PEG	Polyethylene glycol
PET-G	Polyethylene terephthalate glycol-modified
PLA	Polylactic acid
PU	Polyurethane
STL	Stereolithographic
TPEs	Thermoplastic elastomers

3.1 Introduction

3.1.1 Overview of FDM 3D Printing in Drug Manufacturing

Fused deposition modelling (FDM) is an additive manufacturing technique increasingly gaining attention in pharmaceutical drug manufacturing. Its potential lies in the ability to produce personalized, on-demand dosage forms with precise control over drug release profiles, shape, and composition. Before discussing the FDM process, it is important to note that it is also known as fused filament fabrication (FFF). The term "FDM" is trademarked by Stratasys Inc., prompting some users to adopt "FFF" as an alternative to avoid trademark conflicts. Both terms refer to the same technology and are often used interchangeably.

Over the last 10 years, 3D printing (additive manufacturing) has shown great promise for revolutionizing how medicines, particularly oral and semi-solid dosage forms, are designed, manufactured, and used. 3D printing, a rapidly evolving field impacting technology, art, and science, involves building objects by depositing material layer by layer using a print head, nozzle, or similar method, based on a 3D model. This additive approach contrasts with traditional subtractive and formative manufacturing. The 2015 FDA approval of the first 3D-printed orodispersible tablet underscores the growing collaboration between scientists and the pharmaceutical industry to apply this technology to pharmaceutical science. This partnership highlights the importance of pharmaceutical technology in digital health and modern patient management.

The vast amount of research published in the last decade clearly demonstrates the immense potential of 3D printing in healthcare [1]. While various 3D printing technologies can be used for personalized medicine, fused deposition modelling (FDM) seems to be the most widely adopted [2].

3.1.2 Advantages of Using FDM in Pharmaceutical Applications

FDM offers numerous advantages for pharmaceutical applications, particularly in the creation of personalized and innovative drug dosage forms. One of its most significant benefits is the ability to tailor medications to individual patient needs, allowing for customized dosages, shapes, and drug combinations [3]. This is particularly useful in creating polypills, which combine multiple active pharmaceutical ingredients (APIs) in a single tablet, reducing the pill burden for patients with complex medication regimens. The technology also facilitates precise control over drug release profiles, enabling the production of tablets with immediate, sustained, or delayed-release characteristics through complex geometries and internal structures.

- FDM is well suited for on-demand manufacturing, making it ideal for small-batch production of rare or experimental medications. It accelerates drug development by enabling rapid prototyping of tablet designs for research and clinical trials, while its potential for point-of-care production in pharmacies or hospitals reduces lead times significantly. The process is cost-effective, as it minimizes material waste and eliminates the need for molds or extensive manufacturing setups, making it particularly appealing for small-scale or niche applications.
- Another key advantage of FDM is its versatility in materials. It works well with biocompatible and biodegradable polymers like PVA and PLA, which can be tailored for solubility, mechanical properties, and drug release. Additionally, the technology allows for the embedding of both hydrophilic and hydrophobic drugs

within the same matrix, offering flexibility in formulation. FDM also supports the creation of multilayer tablets, which can separate incompatible drugs or achieve dual-release profiles in a single dosage form.
- The precision and reproducibility of FDM ensure accurate dosing and even distribution of APIs throughout the dosage form. This level of control enhances patient compliance, as tablets can be designed in customized sizes, shapes, and even flavors, catering to specific age groups such as paediatric or geriatric populations. Moreover, its ability to produce visually appealing designs may improve adherence, especially in children.
- FDM is also environmentally sustainable, as it uses only the necessary number of materials, reducing waste. Localized production options further decrease transportation emissions, aligning with global sustainability goals.
- The technology's flexibility and precision make it an excellent tool for developing complex drug profiles, such as multi-drug therapies or advanced release mechanisms. With these advantages, FDM has the potential to revolutionize pharmaceutical manufacturing, particularly in personalized medicine and small-scale production.

3.1.3 Importance of Material Selection in FDM for Drug Formulation

Material selection is crucial in FDM for pharmaceutical applications as it directly impacts the safety, stability, and performance of the drug formulation. Polymers used must be biocompatible, thermally stable, and capable of encapsulating active pharmaceutical ingredients (APIs) without degradation. The material's properties, such as solubility, flexibility, and degradation rate, influence the drug release profile, allowing for tailored formulations like immediate, sustained, or delayed release. Additionally, consistent filament quality is essential for precise dosing and structural integrity. Proper material selection ensures the successful application of FDM in creating effective and safe drug products.

3.2 Fundamentals of FDM Technology in Pharmaceuticals

3.2.1 Working Principles of FDM

FDM operates on the principle of additive manufacturing, where objects are created layer-by-layer from a thermoplastic filament. The process begins with a digital 3D model of the desired object (Fig. 3.1), typically designed using computer-aided design (CAD) software. This model is sliced into thin horizontal layers by specialized software, generating instructions for the printer.

During printing, the thermoplastic filament is fed into a heated nozzle, where it is melted and extruded as a semi-liquid material. The nozzle moves in the X and Y directions, depositing the molten material onto the build platform

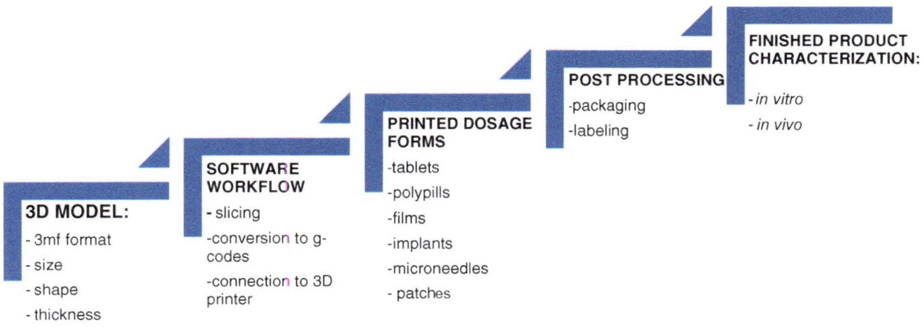

Fig. 3.1 Step up illustration of the additive manufacturing process for pharmaceutical products. (Reproduced from [4], IntechOpen, 2021)

according to the layer's design. Once a layer is deposited, the build platform or nozzle moves vertically in the Z direction to accommodate the next layer. As each layer cools and solidifies, it fuses with the previous layer, forming a cohesive structure. The process continues until the entire object is built. The printability and printout quality of equipment lacking a controlled printing chamber may be affected by the surrounding environment [4]. Therefore, in order to achieve the best output, the FDA's additive printing recommendations list important factors based on the size of the compartment, the type of orifice or nozzle, and other factors. The dose of loaded API is defined by the pre-designed dimensions based on the demands of each patient. Following the conversion of the design to a digital file, the software transforms the 3D manufacturing format (3DMF) or stereolithographic (STL) file to create g-code (computer numerical control programming language), which necessitates file compatibility between the various software programs and 3D printers. Post-processing (packaging and labelling) of the constructed dosage form occurs after printing is finished [4]. Depending on its nature, the completed dosage form is now prepared for both in vitro and in vivo characterizations.

The precision of FDM allows for intricate geometries and complex internal structures, making it suitable for applications ranging from prototyping to manufacturing. The technique's simplicity, material versatility, and cost-effectiveness have made it one of the most widely used 3D printing methods.

3.2.2 Key Components of an FDM Printer

As mentioned earlier, during printing, each layer cools, solidifies, and fuses with the previous one to create a cohesive structure. However, some 3D designs include overhangs that require additional support during the printing process. There are two primary methods for creating these support structures. The first involves printing the support in a more fragile state, allowing it to be easily clipped away after the print is complete. Alternatively, some printers are equipped with a second nozzle that

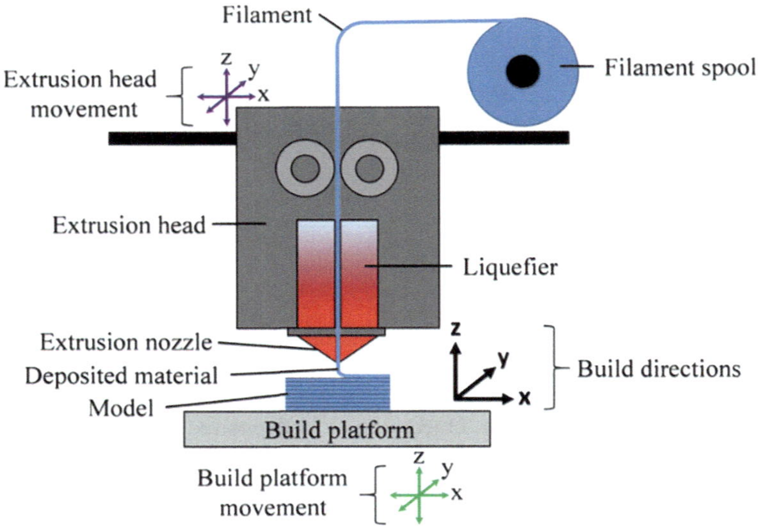

Fig. 3.2 Key components of an FDM printer [5] include mechanisms that enable movement in the x, y, and z directions. This movement can be achieved through the motion of the extrusion head (indicated by purple arrows), the build platform (indicated by green arrows), or a combination of both. For example, movement in the x and y directions is typically achieved by the extrusion head, while the z direction is managed by the movement of the build platform

uses a different material to build the support structure alongside the main component. Once printing is finished, this support material can be removed.

An FDM printer consists of several key components (Fig. 3.2) that work together to produce 3D-printed objects. These components include:

Filament Feed System

- Supplies the thermoplastic filament to the printer.
- Includes a spool holder and a stepper motor that controls the filament's movement into the extruder.

Extruder and Hotend

- The extruder drives the filament into the hotend, where it is melted for deposition.
- The hotend consists of a heating element and a nozzle, which melts the filament and extrudes it as a thin thread.

Nozzle

- A fine-tipped component in the hotend that controls the flow of melted filament, determining the layer's precision and thickness.

Build Platform (Print Bed)

- The surface on which the object is built.
- It can be heated to enhance adhesion of the first layer and prevent warping.

Stepper Motors

- Control the movement of the extruder and the build platform in X, Y, and Z axes, ensuring precise layer placement.

Frame

- Provides structural support and stability to the printer.
- Houses other components and ensures consistent printing performance.

Control System

- Comprises a microcontroller and associated electronics that interpret the 3D model instructions (G-code) and coordinate the printer's movements and temperatures.

Cooling Fans

- Help cool the extruded material quickly to solidify and maintain the object's shape.
- Also prevent overheating of the printer components.

Filament Material

- Thermoplastic filaments like PLA, ABS, PETG, or specialty materials that serve as the printing medium.

User Interface

- Includes a display screen, buttons, or a touch interface for adjusting printer settings and monitoring progress.
- Some printers feature remote control via software or mobile apps. These components work in harmony to achieve accurate and reliable 3D printing using the FDM process.

3.2.3 Type and Printing Technique of 3D Printers Used in Pharmaceutical Applications

Various types of 3D printing techniques are utilized in the pharmaceutical industry, with the choice of technique depending on the specific application and the nature of the product being manufactured. Despite the wide range of available 3D printing technologies, only a select few have been adopted for pharmaceutical applications. The selection of a suitable technique is influenced by the unique requirements of the product and the materials used. Below are examples of 3D printing techniques that have been implemented in this field.

3.2.3.1 Powder-Based 3D Printing

It is a technique where a binder solution or laser is applied to a powder bed to bind the particles together, forming a 3D structure [6, 7]. This system typically consists of a binder or ink reservoir, a powder reservoir, and a build platform. It has been used to create various pharmaceutical products, including fast-dissolving tablets [9], complex medications with zero-order release profiles [10], and uniquely shaped tablets [8].

3.2.3.2 Extrusion-Based 3D Printing

It involves the use of a heated nozzle to extrude a continuous strand of molten polymer, which is layered and cooled to create a 3D object [11]. This technique includes two primary methods: semi-solid extrusion and fused deposition modelling (FDM) [12]. Its simplicity and ease of parameter control have made it widely used in pharmaceutical research. This method has been employed to produce various pharmaceutical products, such as immediate-release tablets [13], floating tablets [14, 15], colonic drug delivery systems [16], and modified-release tablets [17]. However, there are challenges associated with its application. The active pharmaceutical ingredient (API) must remain stable at high temperatures due to the heated nozzle, and the medications must first be prepared as filaments before printing.

3.2.3.3 Inkjet-Based 3D Printing

Also known as digital inkjet printing, encompasses two primary technologies: continuous inkjet printing and drop-on-demand printing. Continuous inkjet printing uses a high-pressure pump to generate a steady flow of ink through an orifice with a diameter of 50–80 microns. In contrast, drop-on-demand printing creates droplets ranging from 10 to 50 microns in size, with volumes between 1 and 70 picolitres [18]. This technique utilizes an inkjet printhead to deposit layers of a photopolymer resin, which are then cured with a UV light source to form a 3D structure, inkjet-based printing is particularly suitable for labile drugs or heat-sensitive materials [19]. It has been employed to fabricate various pharmaceutical dosage forms, including tablets [19], implants [20], and orodispersible films [21].

3.2.3.4 Laser-Based 3D Printing

It, also referred to as selective laser sintering (SLS), laser beam melting, or stereolithography (SLA), involves the controlled fabrication of 3D objects. SLA, in particular, operates by solidifying a liquid resin through photopolymerization [22]. This method offers exceptional accuracy and precision, making it suitable for producing pharmaceutical products that demand high precision, such as microneedles [31].

In FDM 3D printing, the choice and type of materials used are significantly influenced not only by the printing methods but also by the techniques employed for drug incorporation into the printed 3D objects. These factors collectively determine the material's suitability for specific pharmaceutical applications, ensuring optimal performance and drug delivery characteristics.

3.2.4 Approaches to Incorporate the Active Pharmaceutical Ingredient (API) into the 3D-Printed Object

In FDM 3D printing, three primary strategies for incorporating active pharmaceutical ingredients (APIs) into filaments have been developed:

3.2.4.1 Impregnation-FDM

This method involves soaking a filament in a solution or dispersion of an API for several hours to days. After impregnation, the filament is dried in an oven until a stable weight is achieved and then stored in a vacuum desiccator. The API-loaded filament is subsequently used as raw material in the printer to produce oral dosage forms. First reported in 2014 [23], this approach is considered low cost and time efficient. However, it achieves relatively low API loading, typically ranging from 0.063% to 2.07% w/w [24, 25]. Higher drug loading is challenging due to limitations in solvent selection and the potential alteration of the filament's surface, which can compromise its printability [25, 26].

3.2.4.2 Print and Fill

In this strategy, an empty shell is printed and then filled with the API in either powder or liquid form. The shell, made from thermoplastic filaments, is designed to control the dissolution kinetics of the final dosage form. The filling step can occur either during or after the shell's printing process. Once filled, the device is sealed by resuming the shell's printing [27, 28].

3.2.4.3 HME-FDM (Hot Melt Extrusion with FDM)

Introduced in 2015 [29], this method quickly became the most widely used, accounting for 70.8% of studies. It involves mixing the API and excipients in the form of powder or pellets, which are then coextruded using a single or twin-screw conveyor to produce an API-loaded filament. This filament is subsequently used in the FDM printer for fabricating dosage forms.

Each strategy offers unique advantages and challenges, with the choice depending on the desired API loading, material properties, and application.

3.2.5 Role of Materials in FDM Printing Performance and Drug Delivery Applications

The choice of materials in FDM printing is crucial to both the performance of the printing process and the efficacy of drug delivery applications. Typically, thermoplastic filaments are used, and their properties determine not only the mechanical characteristics of the printed object but also its pharmaceutical suitability, including drug delivery capabilities. Materials must exhibit thermal stability to endure the heating process during extrusion without degrading, especially when active pharmaceutical ingredients (APIs) are incorporated, to prevent drug decomposition. Mechanical properties such as flexibility and strength are essential to ensure smooth extrusion, precise layer-by-layer deposition, and structural integrity of the printed object, particularly for intricate designs. Additionally, good adhesion and layer fusion are critical for creating cohesive dosage forms with consistent drug release profiles, while consistent filament diameter and smoothness enhance processability, minimizing defects and ensuring reproducibility.

Materials also play a key role in drug loading and compatibility. They act as carriers for APIs, requiring compatibility to maintain API stability and bioactivity throughout the printing process. The choice of material significantly influences drug release mechanisms; for instance, hydrophilic polymers like polyethylene glycol (PEG) enable rapid drug release, whereas hydrophobic polymers such as polylactic acid (PLA) or polycaprolactone (PCL) support sustained or delayed release. Moreover, materials can enable the incorporation of multiple APIs, facilitating the development of polypills for complex treatments. Biocompatibility and safety are paramount, with materials needing to avoid adverse biological responses. Biodegradable polymers like PLA and PCL are often preferred as they break down into non-toxic byproducts, reducing long-term side effects.

Material properties also enable customization and personalization in drug delivery. Filaments with tunable properties can produce tailored dosage forms, allowing for multi-layered designs with different drugs or release characteristics in each layer. Advanced FDM systems that use multiple materials simultaneously enable the fabrication of complex structures, such as dual-release tablets or devices with removable supports. Sustainability and cost-effectiveness are additional advantages, as biodegradable polymers support environmentally friendly practices, while easily processable materials reduce waste and production costs. Furthermore, materials have enabled novel applications, including biodegradable implants for extended drug release, rapid-release films for fast-acting medication, and tablets with intricate geometries for specific release profiles. Overall, the selection of appropriate materials is fundamental to advancing FDM printing in pharmaceuticals.

3.3 Criteria for Material Selection in FDM for Drug Manufacturing

Selecting suitable materials for FDM in drug manufacturing is a critical step that influences both the 3D printing process and the performance of the final pharmaceutical product. The following criteria are considered essential:

Thermal Properties

- The material must exhibit adequate thermal stability to withstand the high temperatures required for extrusion without degrading.
- For drug-loaded filaments, the material should protect the APIs from heat-induced decomposition.

Mechanical Properties

- Materials must have sufficient strength and flexibility for smooth extrusion and precise layer deposition.
- High mechanical integrity ensures the structural stability of intricate designs and minimizes defects during and after printing.

Drug Compatibility

- The polymer should be chemically compatible with the incorporated API to maintain drug stability and bioactivity during the extrusion and printing process.
- Interaction between the material and drug should not alter the drug's therapeutic properties.

Drug Loading Capacity

- The material must allow for adequate API incorporation, whether through direct embedding during filament preparation (e.g., hot-melt extrusion) or post-processing methods like impregnation.

Controlled Drug Release Potential

- Materials should support the desired release profile—rapid release for immediate effects (e.g., hydrophilic materials like PEG) or sustained/controlled release for prolonged effects (e.g., hydrophobic polymers like PLA and PCL).
- Multilayer or composite materials may be required for combination therapies with different release rates.

Biocompatibility and Safety

- Materials must be non-toxic, biocompatible, and suitable for human use without eliciting adverse biological responses.
- For implants or biodegradable dosage forms, the material should break down into safe byproducts after administration.

Processability

- The filament must have a uniform diameter, smooth surface, and consistent quality to ensure reliable feeding through the printer.
- The material should exhibit good adhesion between layers for strong and cohesive final structures.

Regulatory Compliance

- Materials must comply with pharmaceutical regulations and standards, including approval by bodies like the FDA or EMA for use in drug delivery systems.

Customizability

- Materials with adjustable properties (e.g., melting point, flexibility, or drug-loading capacity) allow for tailored dosage forms to meet individual patient needs.
- Advanced materials should support multi-material printing for complex dosage forms.

Environmental Sustainability

- Biodegradable materials are preferred to minimize environmental impact. Sustainable production practices and minimal waste generation are additional considerations.

Cost-Effectiveness

- Materials should be cost-efficient while maintaining high performance to support scalable production in pharmaceutical applications.
- Careful consideration of these criteria ensures the optimal performance of the FDM process and the creation of effective, safe, and tailored drug delivery systems.

3.4 Categories of Materials for FDM in Drug Manufacturing

Materials play a crucial role in FDM for drug manufacturing, influencing both the printing process and the functionality of pharmaceutical products. Materials used in FDM for drug delivery must meet specific criteria, including biocompatibility, thermal stability, mechanical integrity, and the ability to incorporate active pharmaceutical ingredients (APIs). Below is an exhaustive discussion of the types of materials (Table 3.1) commonly used in FDM for drug manufacturing:

3.4.1 Polymers as FDM Filament Base

In pharmaceutical 3D printing using FDM, the choice of polymer is crucial as it serves as the primary filament material. Polymers not only provide the mechanical structure for the printed object but also influence drug release profiles, compatibility with active pharmaceutical ingredients (APIs), and patient outcomes. FDM operates on the principle of extruding molten thermoplastic material to create 3D structures. Filaments with diameters ranging between 1.75 mm and 2.85–3 mm are commonly used to match the specifications of standard commercially available print heads. Typical filament materials include thermoplastic polymers like acrylonitrile butadiene styrene (ABS), polylactic acid (PLA), high-impact polystyrene (HIPS), polyethylene terephthalate glycol-modified (PET-G), and nylon. While high-quality filaments made from medical-grade polymers such as PLA and PVA are commercially available [30], filaments specifically prepared from pharmaceutical-grade polymers and embedded with active pharmaceutical ingredients (APIs) have yet to enter the commercial market.

3.4.1.1 Polylactic Acid (PLA)

Polylactic Acid (PLA) is a widely used polymer in FDM due to its biodegradable and biocompatible nature. With a low melting temperature of around 180–220 °C, PLA is particularly suited for formulating heat-sensitive drugs, ensuring their stability during the printing process. Its rigid structure and excellent printability make it

Table 3.1 Types of materials commonly used in FDM for drug manufacturing

Categories of FDM 3D printing materials		Examples	Properties	Application
Polymer-based materials	*Biodegradable polymers*	*Polylactic acid (PLA)*	Widely used due to its biocompatibility and ease of processing. Suitable for sustained or delayed drug release systems	Implants, tablets, and polypills
		Polycaprolactone (PCL)	Exhibits slow degradation, ideal for long-term drug delivery	Microspheres, implants, and scaffolds
		Polyglycolic acid (PGA)	Known for rapid degradation and high mechanical strength	Biodegradable sutures and implants
	Non-biodegradable polymers	*Polyethylene terephthalate (PET)*	Strong and durable	Implants and structural applications
		Polyvinyl alcohol (PVA)	Water-soluble and biocompatible	Rapid drug release films and soluble supports
	Thermoplastic elastomers	*Thermoplastic polyurethane (TPU)*	Combine flexibility with strength	Flexible drug delivery devices
Functionalized polymers	*Hydrophilic polymers*	*Polyethylene glycol (PEG)*	Enhances drug release in aqueous environments	Rapid-release dosage forms
		Hydroxypropyl methylcellulose (HPMC)	Used for controlled and sustained drug release	Oral tablets and mucoadhesive systems
	Hydrophobic polymers	*Polylactic-co-glycolic acid (PLGA)*	Degradable and suitable for controlled release	Injectable microspheres and scaffolds
		Ethylene vinyl acetate (EVA)	Provides sustained drug release by limiting water penetration	Transdermal patches and implants

(continued)

Table 3.1 (continued)

Categories of FDM 3D printing materials		Examples	Properties	Application
Composite materials	*Drug-polymer composites*	For example, ibuprofen-polylactic acid (PLA) composite, theophylline-polycaprolactone (PCL) composite, etc.	Combine active pharmaceutical ingredients (APIs) directly with polymers	Personalized dosage forms and polypills
	Polymer-ceramic composites	For example, hydroxyapatite (HA)-poly(lactic acid) (PLA) composite, calcium phosphate (CaP)-polycaprolactone (PCL) composite	Additives like hydroxyapatite for enhanced mechanical properties	Bone repair scaffolds and drug-loaded implants
Natural polymers	*Derived from natural sources, offering biocompatibility and bioactivity*	*Chitosan*	Antimicrobial properties and biodegradability	Wound healing and localized drug delivery
		Alginate	Forms hydrogels for encapsulating drugs	Oral dosage forms and tissue scaffolds
API-loaded materials	*Direct API integration*	Ibuprofen-loaded PLA filament Paracetamol-loaded PVA filament	Active drugs are blended with thermoplastics to create filaments	Controlled release formulation
	Impregnation method	Ibuprofen-loaded PLA filament using the impregnation method	APIs infused into pre-formed filaments for printing	Localized delivery, production of orodispersible
Multi-material combinations		Hydroxypropyl methylcellulose (HPMC) and PEG (polyethylene glycol) combination PCL and PLA (polycaprolactone and polylactic acid) combination	Used for printing complex drug delivery systems	Core-shell structures for dual-release profiles Multi-layered tablets with different APIs in each layer

Additives	*Plasticizers*	Glycerol, triethyl citrate	Improve filament flexibility and reduce brittleness	Reduce the brittleness of polymers by lowering their glass transition temperature (Tg)
	Stabilizers	Antioxidants like butylated hydroxytoluene (BHT)	Protect APIs from degradation during printing	Protect the filament and its drug content from degradation due to heat
	Fillers	Silica, calcium carbonate	Enhance mechanical properties or modify drug release	Added to polymers to improve mechanical strength, modify drug release
Novel materials	*Conductive polymrs*	Polyaniline (PANI), polypyrrole	Enable the integration of sensors or responsive systems in drug delivery devices	Electrically stimulated drug delivery devices
	Photopolymerizable materials	UV-curable resins combined with APIs	Used in hybrid FDM-SLA systems for added precision	Precision microneedles for drug delivery
	Smart polymers	Poly(N-isopropylacrylamide) (PNIPAAm)	Respond to external stimuli like pH, temperature, or light	Temperature-responsive implants
Customizable filaments	*Drug-free filaments*	Polylactic acid (PLA)–polyethylene glycol (PEG) blended filament	Used to create empty drug-delivery systems	Capsule
	API-embedded filaments	PVA filaments loaded with ibuprofen	Pre-loaded with active ingredients for direct printing	Create personalized films for pain management

ideal for creating precise dosage forms and implants. PLA has been effectively utilized in developing sustained-release drug delivery systems. For instance, PLA-based implants have been used to deliver antibiotics for localized infection treatment, where the implant gradually releases the drug over time to maintain therapeutic levels. However, PLA's limited flexibility and moderate hydrophobicity can restrict its use in rapid-release formulations, necessitating the combination with other materials for broader applications.

3.4.1.2 Polycaprolactone (PCL)

Polycaprolactone is a versatile polymer commonly used in FDM for pharmaceutical applications due to its unique properties. It is biodegradable and has a low melting point of around 60 °C, making it highly suitable for the processing of heat-sensitive drugs. Its flexibility and elasticity enable the creation of soft, adaptable structures, while its hydrophobic nature supports prolonged drug release, making it ideal for sustained delivery applications. Despite its advantages, PCL has relatively poor mechanical strength compared to materials like polylactic acid (PLA), which may limit its use in load-bearing or high-stress applications.

PCL has been effectively employed in the development of long-term drug delivery implants. For example, PCL-based implants have been used for the controlled release of contraceptive agents over extended periods, providing a reliable and patient-friendly alternative to traditional delivery methods. Additionally, PCL is widely utilized in fabricating microneedles for transdermal drug delivery [31]. A notable case involves the use of PCL microneedles to deliver vaccines and therapeutic agents painlessly through the skin, achieving precise dosage control and improved patient compliance. These practical applications highlight PCL's potential in advancing personalized and sustained-release pharmaceutical systems.

3.4.1.3 Polyethylene Glycol (PEG)

PEG is a widely used polymer in FDM for pharmaceutical applications due to its hydrophilic and water-soluble nature. It is biocompatible, making it suitable for oral drug delivery systems, and is available in a range of molecular weights, which allows customization of its physical and chemical properties. PEG is particularly effective in creating rapid-release dosage forms, as its water-soluble nature ensures quick disintegration and drug release upon contact with aqueous environments. However, PEG alone lacks sufficient mechanical strength, which often necessitates blending with other polymers such as PLA or PCL to enhance its printability and structural stability.

One practical application of PEG is in the fabrication of orodispersible tablets designed for patients with swallowing difficulties. For example, PEG-based filaments loaded with paracetamol have been used to print tablets that dissolve quickly in the mouth, providing rapid relief. Another significant application is the development of filaments for drugs requiring fast dissolution. A case study demonstrated the use of PEG in creating personalized 3D-printed filaments containing ibuprofen, which showed a significantly enhanced dissolution rate compared to conventional formulations. These examples underscore PEG's potential in advancing patient-centric drug delivery solutions while addressing challenges related to its mechanical limitations.

3.4.1.4 Polyvinyl Alcohol (PVA)

PVA is a water-soluble and biodegradable polymer that plays a significant role in the development of 3D-printed pharmaceutical products. Due to its high biocompatibility and solubility in water, PVA is often used in the formulation of orodispersible films and water-soluble capsules. It is an ideal material for creating fast-dissolving dosage forms, which can be particularly useful for patients who have difficulty swallowing traditional tablets. PVA also exhibits excellent compatibility with APIs, making it a suitable choice for drug delivery systems that require quick dissolution or controlled release.

One of the key applications of PVA in pharmaceutical 3D printing is as a support material in the fabrication of complex drug structures. In FDM printing, PVA can be printed alongside other materials to create intricate geometries, such as multi-layered tablets or combination therapy devices. The PVA support structures can easily dissolve in water, leaving behind the intended drug delivery system without the need for mechanical removal of supports. This feature is especially valuable in the production of structures that would be difficult to manufacture with traditional methods.

For instance, PVA has been used in the development of 3D-printed orodispersible films that rapidly release drugs, such as in a study by Goyanes et al. [32], where PVA-based films were used to create personalized oral dosage forms. Another application is in the creation of drug-loaded capsules, where PVA serves as the capsule matrix that dissolves upon ingestion, ensuring quick drug absorption. Despite its advantages, PVA's sensitivity to humidity can pose a challenge, as exposure to moisture can affect its mechanical properties and the printing process. This requires careful handling and storage of PVA filaments to ensure consistent print quality.

3.4.1.5 Ethylene Vinyl Acetate (EVA)

EVA is a versatile copolymer that combines flexibility, durability, and good drug permeability, making it a promising material in pharmaceutical 3D printing. Its elasticity allows for the fabrication of dosage forms that require deformation without breaking, while its drug-permeable nature is beneficial for controlled-release applications [33]. EVA is primarily used in transdermal drug delivery systems and sustained-release drug formulations due to its ability to regulate the release rate of APIs.

One of the primary applications of EVA in 3D printing for pharmaceuticals is in the production of controlled-release transdermal patches. These patches can be designed to release the drug over an extended period, offering a consistent therapeutic effect. In a case study, EVA-based transdermal patches have been used for the controlled release of pain management drugs like fentanyl, where the polymer matrix ensures that the drug is delivered at a steady rate to the skin over time. This sustained release reduces the need for frequent dosing, enhancing patient compliance. EVA is also utilized in sustained-release oral dosage forms, where it acts as a matrix material that controls the dissolution rate of the drug.

Despite its numerous advantages, EVA does have limitations. Its precise formulation is critical for ensuring the stability of the drug, as improper ratios of ethylene and vinyl acetate can affect the permeability and release kinetics of the drug. Additionally, when used in drug delivery systems, careful consideration must be given to the compatibility between the drug and EVA to avoid degradation of the API over time.

3.4.1.6 Polyurethane (PU)

PU is a highly versatile and durable material used in 3D printing for pharmaceutical applications due to its exceptional elasticity and mechanical strength. It can be tailored for both hydrophilic and hydrophobic active pharmaceutical ingredients (APIs), making it suitable for a wide range of drug delivery systems. Its flexibility and resilience allow it to be used in applications where the device needs to withstand mechanical stress or deformation while maintaining its structural integrity. This makes PU an ideal material for drug-eluting stents, flexible implants, and localized drug delivery systems.

One notable application of polyurethane in pharmaceuticals is in drug-eluting stents, which are used in vascular interventions. These stents are designed to release medication over an extended period directly to the site of the artery, preventing restenosis (re-narrowing of the artery). PU's elasticity ensures that the stent can maintain its shape and function, even under the stress of blood flow and artery movement, while the drug can be steadily released to prevent clot formation or inflammation. In a case study, PU-based drug-eluting stents have been used to release anti-inflammatory or anticoagulant drugs, helping to minimize complications post-surgery and improve patient outcomes [34].

Another significant application is in flexible, biodegradable implants for localized drug delivery. PU's mechanical properties and biocompatibility allow it to be used in the fabrication of implants that deliver drugs at a controlled rate directly to the targeted tissue. This approach is particularly beneficial in cancer therapy, where localized delivery of chemotherapeutic agents can reduce systemic side effects while maximizing the therapeutic impact at the site of the tumour.

However, despite its advantages, the use of polyurethane in 3D printing for drug delivery systems requires careful optimization of its thermal and mechanical properties. The material's melting point and elasticity must be fine-tuned during the printing process to ensure the final product performs as intended without compromising the stability or efficacy of the API.

3.4.1.7 Acrylonitrile Butadiene Styrene (ABS)

ABS is a widely used thermoplastic polymer in FDM 3D printing, known for its strength, durability, and excellent mechanical properties. It has a higher melting point, typically around 230 °C, which makes it suitable for printing structural components that need to withstand mechanical stress or wear. ABS is a versatile material, commonly used for creating rigid, tough parts due to its resistance to impact and high tensile strength. In the pharmaceutical industry, ABS is particularly useful for manufacturing durable, functional components for drug delivery systems, such as housings, casings, or structural supports for medical devices.

However, ABS's high processing temperature can present challenges when incorporating sensitive APIs in the filament, as the heat may degrade the drugs during the printing process. This material's limited biocompatibility compared to other polymers, such as PLA or PCL, further limits its direct application in drug delivery systems where direct contact with the human body is required. Despite these limitations, ABS has found practical use in the creation of pharmaceutical devices where the primary function is structural support rather than direct drug delivery.

A practical example of ABS in pharmaceutical applications is the development of structural components for drug delivery devices, such as inhalers or auto-injection pens. For instance, ABS has been used to print the outer casing of an inhaler, which holds the drug reservoir and controls the aerosolization of the drug during administration [35]. The strength of ABS allows for the creation of durable, lightweight, and cost-effective inhalers that can withstand mechanical stress during use without compromising performance. However, these devices typically use ABS for non-API-contacting parts, and API incorporation is done through other materials like PLA or PCL to avoid degradation.

Another application involves using ABS to print complex devices that hold or encapsulate drugs in various delivery systems, such as controlled-release tablets or pumps for drug infusion. In these cases, ABS provides structural integrity and can be combined with biocompatible materials to ensure the safe delivery of the drug.

3.4.1.8 Cellulose-Based Polymers

Cellulose-based polymers are derived from natural sources, making them a popular choice in pharmaceutical applications due to their biocompatibility and biodegradability. As naturally occurring biopolymers, cellulose and its derivatives, such as hydroxypropyl methylcellulose (HPMC) and carboxymethyl cellulose (CMC), offer the advantage of being both environmentally friendly and non-toxic, making them ideal for drug delivery systems. These polymers can be hydrophilic or hydrophobic depending on the specific chemical modifications (derivatization) they undergo, allowing for versatility in the design of controlled or sustained release formulations.

In FDM 3D printing, cellulose-based polymers are primarily used to fabricate tablets with tunable drug release profiles [36]. The hydrophilic nature of some cellulose derivatives allows for the creation of tablets that rapidly disintegrate in water, enabling fast drug release, while hydrophobic variants can be utilized for slow or controlled release. Additionally, cellulose-based materials are well-suited for water-soluble drug delivery systems, where the polymer matrix dissolves in contact with bodily fluids, providing a pathway for the controlled release of the API.

One practical application of cellulose-based polymers in FDM is the creation of oral dosage forms with customized release profiles. For example, cellulose acetate butyrate (CAB) and HPMC are used to design extended-release tablets that release the drug over a prolonged period [37]. These polymers help achieve a controlled release of the API, improving therapeutic outcomes by maintaining a stable drug concentration in the bloodstream. Studies have demonstrated the ability to 3D-print oral dosage forms with cellulose-based filaments to achieve zero-order drug release, where the drug is delivered at a constant rate, an ideal feature for treating chronic conditions requiring steady medication levels.

Another example involves the use of HPMC in the production of water-soluble films or tablets for drugs requiring rapid dissolution. For instance, a study by Melocchi et al. [38] showed that cellulose-based polymers could be used to print fast-dissolving tablets in the FDM process for quick therapeutic effect, such as in the case of pain relief medications or other drugs that require rapid onset of action. The tablets were designed to disintegrate in water, offering faster drug absorption compared to traditional solid forms.

Despite these advantages, cellulose-based polymers in FDM have some limitations. They exhibit moderate mechanical strength, which may restrict their use in load-bearing pharmaceutical devices, and they also have lower thermal stability compared to synthetic thermoplastics like PLA or PCL. As a result, careful formulation and optimization are required to improve their mechanical properties and thermal stability during the printing process.

3.4.1.9 Thermoplastic Elastomers (TPEs)

TPEs are a class of polymers that combine the processability of thermoplastics with the flexibility and elasticity of elastomers. These materials are highly valued in the pharmaceutical industry for their excellent durability, high elongation properties, and flexibility, making them ideal for applications that require both toughness and comfort. TPEs have a broad range of mechanical properties that can be tailored through various formulations, allowing for customization in drug delivery systems [39]. The versatility of TPEs in FDM 3D printing makes them an attractive choice for creating drug-loaded patches, implants, and other biomedical devices [40].

In the pharmaceutical field, TPEs are often used to develop customizable drug-loaded transdermal patches. These patches can deliver drugs at a controlled rate through the skin, offering a non-invasive method of drug administration. For instance, TPE-based transdermal patches can be designed for chronic pain management, delivering medications such as fentanyl or nicotine over extended periods. By incorporating the active pharmaceutical ingredients (APIs) into TPE matrices, the patches can achieve sustained release profiles, improving patient compliance and reducing side effects by avoiding the peaks and troughs typically seen with oral medications. The flexibility of TPEs also ensures that these patches remain comfortable on the skin for prolonged periods without causing irritation or discomfort.

One notable case study is the use of TPEs in the creation of flexible drug-eluting stents for localized drug delivery. In this application, TPEs are used to create stents that release a drug directly to the site of interest, typically within the cardiovascular system. These stents are printed using FDM and can be designed to release drugs such as sirolimus or paclitaxel, which prevent restenosis (the re-narrowing of blood vessels after stent placement). The flexibility and elasticity of TPEs make these stents adaptable to the complex geometry of blood vessels while maintaining the required drug release rates for therapeutic effectiveness.

Despite their advantages, TPEs do present challenges when used in FDM printing. One limitation is the need to optimize the polymer's compatibility with the drug being delivered. TPEs must be carefully chosen and processed to ensure that the drug remains stable and bioactive during the printing and delivery process. Additionally, TPEs can sometimes exhibit inconsistent drug release profiles, requiring careful formulation to balance the mechanical properties and the desired therapeutic outcomes.

3.4.2 Drug-Loaded Filaments as Printing Materials for FDM

Drug-loaded filaments are a key innovation in the field of pharmaceutical 3D printing, especially in FDM. These filaments are created by embedding APIs into a base polymer matrix, which can then be processed using 3D printing techniques. This method of incorporating drugs into filaments offers significant advantages in terms of personalized medicine, tailored dosage forms, and controlled drug release profiles. Drug-loaded filaments allow the creation of complex pharmaceutical structures, such as customized dosage forms, implantable devices, and bioresorbable drug delivery systems. These filaments can be designed with specific release rates, dose forms, and geometries, making them a powerful tool in pharmaceutical manufacturing.

The drug-loaded filaments are typically processed by HME or solvent casting methods to ensure uniform distribution of the API within the polymer matrix. The extruded filaments are then used in FDM printers to fabricate the desired drug delivery device or dosage form.

3.4.2.1 Applications of Drug-Loaded Filaments in FDM

- *Personalized Dosage Forms*: One of the most significant advantages of using drug-loaded filaments in FDM printing is the ability to create personalized medicine. This means that a patient's specific dosage and drug combination can be printed into customized dosage forms, such as tablets, capsules, or oral strips. FDM offers precise control over the size, shape, and drug content, which can be adjusted based on individual patient needs. Researchers have developed a system for printing tablets containing varying doses of acetaminophen based on individual patient needs [41].
- *Controlled Release Drug Delivery*: Drug-loaded filaments can be designed to offer specific controlled-release profiles. By selecting the right combination of polymer and API, manufacturers can create dosage forms that release the drug over an extended period. One promising application of drug-loaded filaments is in the production of long-acting injectable implants. These implants are made by loading drugs into filaments and using FDM printing to create implants that release drugs over a sustained period. For instance, levonorgestrel-loaded filaments have been used to print biodegradable implants for con-

traceptive delivery [42]. These implants can provide continuous drug release for several months, minimizing the need for daily administration and improving patient compliance.
- *Multilayered Drug Delivery Systems*: Drug-loaded filaments can also be used to create multilayered tablets or devices with multiple APIs incorporated into different layers [43]. This is particularly useful for combination therapies, where multiple drugs are required to be delivered simultaneously. An example of this is the development of polypills—tablets containing multiple drugs designed to treat cardiovascular diseases. By using FDM to print multilayered structures, researchers have successfully created combination pills that combine antihypertensives, lipid-lowering drugs, and antiplatelets in a single tablet, providing a single-dose solution for patients with multiple conditions. The layers can be designed to release the drugs at different rates, optimizing therapeutic efficacy and patient adherence.

3.4.3 Composite Materials Used in FDM Printing of Pharmaceuticals

In the context of FDM for pharmaceuticals, composite materials refer to materials that combine a polymer matrix with other substances such as APIs, ceramics, metals, or other polymers to enhance the performance of the printed product. Composite materials allow the creation of complex drug delivery systems with specific properties, such as controlled release, improved mechanical strength, and enhanced biocompatibility. These materials are integral to advancing the capabilities of 3D-printed pharmaceuticals, enabling the development of personalized medicines, implants, and devices for various drug delivery applications.

3.4.3.1 Types of Composite Materials Used in FDM Printing

3.4.3.1.1 Polymer-API Composites

Polymer-API composites are the most common composite materials used in FDM for pharmaceuticals. In these composites, the API is incorporated into a polymer matrix to control its release and stability. The polymer serves as the carrier for the drug, allowing for customized release profiles and precise dosing. Common polymers used in these composites include PLA [44], PCL, PEG, and HPMC. These composites are primarily used to create tablets, capsules, and implantable devices with precise and sustained release profiles.

3.4.3.1.2 Polymer-Ceramic Composites

Polymer-ceramic composites combine the biodegradability and printability of polymers with the mechanical strength and biocompatibility of ceramics. These composites are often used in the creation of implantable devices for drug delivery, particularly for controlled and localized release. The ceramic components in these composites are typically bioceramics like hydroxyapatite, bioactive glasses, or zirconia, which are known for their bone-compatibility and bioactivity [45]. The polymer-ceramic composites are used to print drug-eluting stents, bone implants, and scaffolds for localized drug delivery. For example, hydroxyapatite-filled PLA filaments have been used in 3D printing bone scaffolds for localized drug delivery.

3.4.3.1.3 Polymer-Metal Composites

Polymer-metal composites combine polymers with metal particles or metal alloys to enhance their mechanical properties, thermal conductivity, or bioactivity. These composites are used to print drug delivery devices or implants that require added strength, conductivity, or antibacterial properties [46]. The metals used in these composites can range from stainless steel and titanium to silver and copper. These metals are often incorporated into the polymer matrix to provide additional strength, as well as antimicrobial properties. Silver and copper, for instance, have known antibacterial properties, which can be useful in preventing infection in drug delivery devices or implants. For example, silver-loaded PLA filaments have been used in the creation of antimicrobial wound dressings [47]. The silver particles help to reduce infection, while the polymer base allows for controlled release of other drugs, such as antibiotics, to the wound site.

3.4.3.1.4 Polymer-Polymer Composites

Polymer-polymer composites are created by combining two or more polymers with different properties to achieve a balanced performance for drug delivery applications. These composites can be tailored to achieve desired properties such as flexibility, hydrophilicity, biodegradability, and controlled release. The blending of polymers allows for the design of drug delivery systems with multiple release profiles or physical properties [48]. This type of composite is often used to print bilayer or multilayered tablets, where each layer contains a different drug or has a different release rate.

3.4.3.1.5 Polymer-Carbon Composites

Polymer-carbon composites combine carbon-based materials, such as graphene oxide or carbon nanotubes, with polymers to enhance the electrical conductivity, mechanical strength, or drug delivery capabilities of the material.

These composites are useful for applications requiring conductivity or nanomaterial properties, such as in biosensors, stimuli-responsive drug delivery systems, or wound healing [49]. The addition of carbon materials can also improve the mechanical properties of the printed structure, making it stronger and more durable.

Graphene oxide-loaded PLA filaments have been explored for use in wound dressings with both antibacterial properties and electrical conductivity [50]. The conductive properties of the graphene oxide allow the wound dressing to be used as part of electrotherapy, which accelerates the healing process while simultaneously delivering drugs locally to the wound site.

Composite materials play a crucial role in advancing the capabilities of 3D printing in pharmaceuticals, particularly with FDM. By combining polymers with APIs, ceramics, metals, and other materials, composite filaments can be engineered to meet specific drug delivery requirements, from controlled-release formulations to personalized medicines.

3.4.4 Emerging Materials for FDM 3D Printing of Pharmaceuticals

As the field of 3D printing in pharmaceuticals continues to evolve, new materials are being developed to expand the possibilities of FDM. These emerging materials aim to address limitations of traditional FDM filaments, such as restricted drug release profiles, thermal stability, and compatibility with active pharmaceutical ingredients (APIs). Innovations in this space focus on enhancing the functionality, biocompatibility, and versatility of materials to meet the demands of advanced drug delivery systems and personalized medicine [2]. Table 3.2 highlights various emerging materials for FDM 3D printing in the pharmaceutical field, emphasizing their unique properties, potential applications, case study examples, and associated challenges.

Table 3.2 Types of emerging materials for FDM 3D printing of pharmaceuticals

Material type	Properties	Applications	Case study example	Challenges
Thermoresponsive polymers	Change properties with temperature Example: Poly(N-isopropylacrylamide) (PNIPAM)	Temperature-controlled drug release On-demand implants for cancer or localized infection	PNIPAM-based implants releasing drugs at elevated temperatures for cancer treatment	Limited thermal stability—Requires blending with other polymers for better printability
pH-responsive polymers	Alter solubility or swelling based on pH Example: Eudragit® polymers (S100, L100)	Colon-targeted drug delivery Tablets with pH-sensitive drug release	PLA/Eudragit composites for delayed-release anti-inflammatory tablets reducing gastric irritation	Limited thermal stability
Bioprintable polymers	Derived from biomaterials like alginate and Gelatin-methacryloyl (GelMA)	Tissue scaffolds with drug delivery Wound healing growth factor delivery	Alginate-GelMA scaffolds releasing growth factors for wound healing	Requires crosslinking mechanisms (e.g., UV light)

(continued)

Table 3.2 (continued)

Material type	Properties	Applications	Case study example	Challenges
Electrically conductive polymers	Examples: Polypyrrole (PPy), polyaniline (PANI) Allow stimuli-responsive behaviour	Smart drug delivery via electrical stimulus Biosensing applications	PLA-PPy composites for neural or cardiac implants with electrical drug release capabilities	Balancing conductivity and biocompatibility
Bioactive glass composites	Enhance bioactivity for bone regeneration Example: 45S5 bioactive glass with PLA or PCL	Bone healing implants Antibiotic-loaded scaffolds	Bioactive glass composites for infection-site bone regeneration with localized antibiotic release	Uniform dispersion of glass particles in polymer matrix
Nanomaterial-enhanced polymers	Use nanomaterials like graphene oxide and carbon nanotubes	Multi-functional implants Advanced drug delivery with electrical or mechanical benefits	PLA-graphene oxide composites for implants combining strength, biosensing, and controlled drug release	Avoiding aggregation of nanomaterials during processing
Polysaccharide-based materials	Examples: Chitosan, alginate, starch Biodegradable and natural origin	Orodispersible films and capsules Immediate drug release	Chitosan-PVA composites for fast-dissolving antibiotic-loaded capsules	Limited thermal stability and mechanical strength
Metal-organic frameworks (MOFs)	Porous materials with high drug-loading capacity Example: ZIF-8	Drug-eluting implants Sustained drug release systems	PLA-MOF composites for localized anticancer drug delivery implants	Maintaining MOF thermal stability during filament production

3.4.4.1 Advantages of Emerging Materials in FDM for Pharmaceuticals

Enhanced Functionality: New materials offer features like stimuli-responsiveness, multi-drug compatibility, and controlled degradation rates.

Personalized Medicine: Emerging materials enable the fabrication of patient-specific drug delivery systems.

Versatility: These materials allow for the creation of advanced dosage forms such as implants, patches, and multilayer tablets.

3.5 Material Optimization Strategies for FDM 3D Printing in Pharmaceuticals

Material optimization is critical to enhance the performance and applicability of FDM 3D printing in pharmaceuticals. Strategies involve improving polymer properties, understanding drug-polymer interactions, and advancing filament extrusion technologies to meet the unique demands of pharmaceutical manufacturing.

3.5.1 Adjusting Polymer Properties

Polymers form the foundation of FDM 3D printing, and their properties can be tailored to optimize performance:

- *Incorporating Plasticizers*: Plasticizers are added to reduce the glass transition temperature (Tg) of polymers, improving their flexibility and processability. For example, adding PEG to PLA enhances its ductility, making it suitable for printing complex geometries without cracks.
- *Copolymerization*: Copolymerization involves blending polymers to achieve a balance of properties, such as improving hydrophilicity or mechanical strength. A combination of PLA and polycaprolactone PCL can create filaments with enhanced flexibility and biodegradability.
- *Surface Modification*: Modifying polymer surfaces can improve drug loading and release characteristics, such as grafting hydrophilic groups onto hydrophobic polymers to enable controlled release.

3.5.2 Drug-Polymer Interaction Studies

Understanding drug-polymer interactions is vital to maintaining drug stability and efficacy during the printing and post-processing phases:

- *Stability Assessments*: Thermal and chemical compatibility between the drug and polymer must be evaluated to prevent degradation during the high-temperature

FDM process. Differential scanning calorimetry (DSC) and Fourier-transform infrared spectroscopy (FTIR) are commonly used techniques.
- *Drug Loading Efficiency*: Investigating how APIs interact with polymers at the molecular level can optimize drug loading and release. For example, hydrophobic drugs may require polymer modifications or blending with surfactants to improve solubility and distribution.
- *Controlled Release Mechanisms*: Material properties, such as hydrophobicity or crystallinity, are tailored to control drug release rates. This can enable rapid, sustained, or targeted drug delivery systems.

3.5.3 Advances in Filament Extrusion Technologies

Filament quality plays a significant role in FDM 3D printing performance, and advancements in extrusion technologies can significantly impact pharmaceutical applications:

- *Customized Filaments*: Novel extrusion techniques enable the incorporation of APIs directly into pharmaceutical-grade filaments with precise drug loading and homogeneity. Twin-screw extrusion, for instance, facilitates the uniform mixing of APIs and polymers.
- *Multilayer Filaments*: Extrusion technologies can now produce multilayer filaments, allowing for the simultaneous incorporation of multiple drugs or functionalities, such as a combination of immediate and sustained-release layers.
- *Processing Enhancements*: Improvements in extrusion processes ensure consistent filament diameter, smooth surfaces, and reduced defects, which are essential for reliable printing. This also minimizes waste and enhances the reproducibility of dosage forms.

3.6 Challenges in Material Development for FDM in Pharmaceuticals

The development of materials for FDM 3D printing in pharmaceuticals involves several challenges that must be addressed to achieve safe, effective, and reproducible drug delivery systems. These challenges include drug-material compatibility, thermal stability, dosage uniformity, and regulatory compliance.

3.6.1 Compatibility of Drugs with Filament Materials

One of the primary challenges is ensuring the compatibility of APIs with the filament material. Many drugs may not interact favourably with certain polymers, leading to issues like phase separation, reduced bioavailability, or instability during storage. Additionally, achieving a homogenous distribution of the drug within the polymer matrix is critical for consistent therapeutic effects. Material modifications or the development of specialized polymer blends are often required to address these issues.

3.6.2 Thermal Degradation of Drugs During the Printing Process

The high temperatures required for FDM printing can degrade heat-sensitive APIs, reducing their efficacy or creating toxic byproducts. For example, drugs with low thermal stability may not withstand the processing temperatures of common FDM filaments like PLA or ABS. To mitigate this, researchers are focusing on low-melting-point polymers, plasticizers, or advanced printing techniques that minimize thermal exposure.

3.6.3 Ensuring Uniformity and Reproducibility in Drug Dosage

Achieving uniform drug distribution within filaments is essential for consistent dosage in printed pharmaceuticals. Variations in filament composition or printing conditions can result in uneven drug release profiles, which pose significant risks in clinical applications. Advanced extrusion techniques, such as twin-screw extrusion, and rigorous quality control measures are necessary to ensure reproducibility and uniformity in drug-loaded filaments.

3.6.4 Regulatory and Quality Control Challenges

Material development for pharmaceutical FDM must adhere to stringent regulatory guidelines to ensure safety, efficacy, and quality. However, the lack of standardized protocols for assessing the performance of 3D-printed drug products poses a significant hurdle. Regulatory bodies need to establish clear frameworks for evaluating material properties, drug release profiles, and biocompatibility. Additionally, quality control of printed products must address variability in mechanical properties, drug content, and dissolution rates [51].

Overcoming these challenges requires interdisciplinary collaboration between materials scientists, pharmaceutical researchers, and regulatory authorities. Innovations in polymer chemistry, printing technologies, and process optimization will play a key role in addressing compatibility, stability, and quality issues. Establishing robust regulatory standards will further enable the safe and effective integration of FDM 3D printing into pharmaceutical manufacturing.

3.7 Future Trends in FDM Materials for Drug Manufacturing

The field of FDM 3D printing for pharmaceuticals is rapidly evolving, with advancements in materials playing a pivotal role in addressing current challenges and expanding application possibilities. Emerging trends focus on bioinks, digital innovation, and sustainability, each of which holds significant potential for transforming drug manufacturing.

3.7.1 Development of Bioinks for Hybrid FDM Applications

The future of FDM materials is expected to integrate bioinks—hydrogel-based materials enriched with biological components—for hybrid printing systems. These bioinks can combine the mechanical robustness of thermoplastic polymers with the biocompatibility and functional versatility of hydrogels, enabling applications such as cell-laden implants or tissue-engineered drug delivery systems [52]. For example, hybrid FDM setups could allow the creation of devices that simultaneously deliver drugs and support tissue regeneration, offering new possibilities for personalized medicine and regenerative therapies.

3.7.2 Integration of Digital Technologies for Material Innovation

Advances in digital technologies, such as machine learning and computational modelling, are set to revolutionize material development for FDM. These tools can predict polymer-drug interactions, optimize filament compositions, and simulate drug release kinetics, accelerating the design of materials tailored to specific pharmaceutical applications. Furthermore, real-time monitoring systems in FDM printers could enhance process control, ensuring consistent material properties and drug dosages during manufacturing.

3.7.3 Sustainable Materials for Eco-Friendly Pharmaceutical Printing

As the pharmaceutical industry faces increasing pressure to adopt environmentally sustainable practices, the development of green materials for FDM is gaining momentum. Biodegradable and renewable polymers, such as those derived from natural sources, are being explored to minimize environmental impact. Additionally, research is focused on creating materials that require lower processing temperatures, reducing energy consumption during printing. Sustainable filament production methods, such as using waste-derived feedstocks, also represent a growing trend.

The future of FDM materials in drug manufacturing is poised to embrace bioinks for complex biomedical applications, leverage digital innovation for precision and efficiency, and prioritize sustainability to align with global environmental goals. These trends collectively promise to enhance the versatility, safety, and eco-friendliness of 3D printing technologies, positioning FDM as a cornerstone of next-generation pharmaceutical manufacturing.

3.8 Conclusion

Advancements in materials for FDM 3D printing have significantly broadened the scope of its applications in drug manufacturing. From the development of biodegradable polymers to the incorporation of composite and emerging materials with tailored properties, these innovations are enabling the fabrication of personalized, multifunctional, and sustainable drug delivery systems. The ability to integrate APIs directly into 3D printing filaments and create complex dosage forms with controlled-release properties underscores the transformative potential of this technology.

The impact of FDM on the pharmaceutical industry extends beyond material innovation. By offering a scalable, efficient, and customizable approach to drug production, FDM can revolutionize traditional manufacturing processes, enabling on-demand production and personalized medicine. This can improve treatment outcomes while reducing waste and production costs.

However, realizing the full potential of FDM in pharmaceuticals requires interdisciplinary research and collaboration among material scientists, pharmacists, engineers, and regulatory bodies. Addressing challenges such as drug-material compatibility, thermal stability, and regulatory compliance will necessitate a concerted effort across disciplines. By fostering such collaborations, the pharmaceutical industry can leverage the full capabilities of FDM technology to advance patient care and drive innovation.

References

1. Mohammed A, Elshaer A, Sareh P, Elsayed M, Hassanin H. Additive manufacturing technologies for drug delivery applications. Int J Pharm. 2020;580:119245.
2. Cailleaux S, Sanchez-Ballester NM, Gueche YA, Bataille B, Soulairol I. Fused Deposition Modeling (FDM), the new asset for the production of tailored medicines. J Control Release. 2021;330:821–41.
3. Katstra WE, Palazzolo RD, Rowe CW, Giritlioglu B, Teung P, Cima MJ. Oral dosage forms fabricated by Three Dimensional Printing (TM). J Control Release. 2000;66:1–9.
4. Khalid GM, Selmin F. Applications of alginates in the design and preparation of orodispersible dosage forms. In: Deniz I, editor. Properties and applications of alginates. 1st ed. London: IntechOpen; 2021. p. 13. Available online: https://www.intechopen.com/online-first/77732. Accessed on 15 Feb 2022.
5. Gordelier T, Thies P, Turner L, Johanning L. Optimising the FDM additive manufacturing process to achieve maximum tensile strength: a state-of-the-art review. Rapid Prototyp J. ahead-of-print. 2019; https://doi.org/10.1108/RPJ-07-2018-0183.

6. Mostafaei A, Elliott AM, Barnes JE, Li F, Tan W, Cramer CL, Nandwana P, Chmielus M. Binder jet 3D printing—Process parameters, materials, properties, modeling, and challenges. Prog Mater Sci. 2021;119:100707. [CrossRef].
7. Sen K, Mehta T, Sansare S, Sharifi L, Ma AW, Chaudhuri B. Pharmaceutical applications of powder-based binder jet 3D printing process–a review. Adv Drug Deliv Rev. 2021;177:113943. [CrossRef].
8. Yu D-G, Shen X-X, Branford-White C, Zhu L-M, White K, Yang XL. Novel oral fast-disintegrating drug delivery devices with predefined inner structure fabricated by three-dimensional printing. J Pharm Pharmacol. 2009;61:323–9. [CrossRef] [PubMed].
9. Jacob J, Coyle N, West TG, Monkhouse DC, Surprenant HL, Jain NB. Rapid disperse dosage form containing levetiracetam. U.S. Patent US20140271862A1, 17 May 2016.
10. Yu DG, Yang XL, Huang WD, Liu J, Wang YG, Xu H. Tablets with material gradients fabricated by three-dimensional printing. J Pharm Sci. 2007;96:2446–56. [CrossRef] [PubMed].
11. Thanawuth K, Sutthapitaksakul L, Konthong S, Suttiruengwong S, Huanbutta K, Dass CR, Sriamornsak P. Impact of drug loading method on drug release from 3D-printed tablets made from filaments fabricated by hot-melt extrusion and impregnation processes. Pharmaceutics. 2021;13:1607.
12. Algahtani MS, Mohammed AA, Ahmad J. Extrusion-based 3D printing for pharmaceuticals: contemporary research and applications. Curr Pharm Des. 2018;24:4991–5008.
13. Jivraj M, Martini LG, Thomson CM. An overview of the different excipients useful for the direct compression of tablets. Pharm Sci Technol Today. 2000;3:58–63.
14. Sriamornsak P, Huanbutta K, Sangnim T. Recent advances in 3D printing for floating drug delivery platforms. Sci Eng Health Stud. 2022;16:22010001.
15. Huanbutta K, Sangnim T. Design and development of zero-order drug release gastroretentive floating tablets fabricated by 3D printing technology. J Drug Deliv Sci Technol. 2019;52:831–7.
16. Sangnim T, Tangpanithanon A, Khamtheantong M, Charoenwai J, Huanbutta K. Development of personalized colonic drug delivery systems prepared by 3D-printing technology. In: Key engineering materials. Bäch: Trans Tech Publications Ltd; 2021. p. 144–50.
17. Huanbutta K, Sriamornsak P, Kittanaphon T, Suwanpitak K, Klinkesorn N, Sangnim T. Development of a zero-order kinetics drug release floating tablet with anti–flip-up design fabricated by 3D-printing technique. J Pharm Investig. 2021;51:213–22.
18. Ahlfeld T, Akkineni AR, Förster Y, Köhler T, Knaack S, Gelinsky M, Lode A. Design and fabrication of complex scaffolds for bone defect healing: combined 3D plotting of a calcium phosphate cement and a growth factor-loaded hydrogel. Ann Biomed Eng. 2017;45:224–36. [CrossRef].
19. Sen K, Manchanda A, Mehta T, Ma AW, Chaudhuri B. Formulation design for inkjet-based 3D printed tablets. Int J Pharm. 2020;584:119430. [CrossRef].
20. Islam R, Sadhukhan P. An insight of 3d printing technology in pharmaceutical development and application: an updated review. Curr Trends Pharm Res. 2020;7:56–80.
21. Huanbutta K, Sriamornsak P, Singh I, Sangnim T. Manufacture of 2D-printed precision drug-loaded orodispersible film prepared from tamarind seed gum substrate. Appl Sci. 2021;11:5852.
22. Chia HN, Wu BM. Recent advances in 3D printing of biomaterials. J Biol Eng. 2015;9:4. [CrossRef] [PubMed].
23. Goyanes A, Buanz ABM, Basit AW, Gaisford S. Fused-filament 3D printing (3DP) for fabrication of tablets. Int J Pharma. 2014;476(1–2):88–92.
24. Goyanes A, Buanz ABM, Hatton GB, Gaisford S, Basit AW. 3D printing of modified-release aminosalicylate (4-ASA and 5-ASA) tablets. Eur J Pharm Biopharm. 2015;89:157–62.
25. Ibrahim M, Barnes M, McMillin R, Cook DW, Smith S, Halquist M, et al. 3D printing of metformin HCl PVA tablets by fused deposition modeling: drug loading, tablet design, and dissolution studies. AAPS Pharm Sci Tech. 2019;20(5):195.
26. Skowyra J, Pietrzak K, Alhnan MA. Fabrication of extended-release patient tailored prednisolone tablets via fused deposition modelling (FDM) 3D printing. Eur J Pharma Sci. 2015;68:11–7.

27. Okwuosa TC, Soares C, Gollwitzer V, Habashy R, Timmins P, Alhnan MA. On demand manufacturing of patient-specific liquid capsules via co-ordinated 3D printing and liquid dispensing. Eur J Pharma Sci. 2018;118:134–43.
28. Linares V, Casas M, Caraballo I. Printfills: 3D printed systems combining fused deposition modeling and injection volume filling. Application to colon-specific drug delivery. Eur J Pharm Biopharm. 2018;134:138–43.
29. Pietrzak K, Isreb A, Alhnan MA. A flexible-dose dispenser for immediate and extended release 3D printed tablets. Eur J Pharma Biopharma. 2015;96:380–7.
30. Jamróz W, Szafraniec J, Kurek M, Jachowicz R. 3D Printing in pharmaceutical and medical applications—recent achievements and challenges. Pharm Res. 2018;35:176. https://doi.org/10.1007/s11095-018-2454-x.
31. Ko P-T, I-Chi L, Chen M-C, Tsai S-W. Polymer microneedles fabricated from PCL and PCL/PEG blends for transdermal delivery of hydrophilic compounds. J Taiwan Inst Chem Eng. 2015; https://doi.org/10.1016/j.jtice.2015.01.0.
32. Goyanes A, et al. 3D printing of medicines: engineering novel oral devices with unique design and drug release characteristics. Mol Pharm. 2015;12(11):4077–84.
33. Schneider C, Langer R, Loveday D, Hair D. Applications of ethylene vinyl acetate copolymers (EVA) in drug delivery systems. J Control Release. 2017;262:284–95.
34. Seo EH, Na K. Polyurethane membrane with porous surface for controlled drug release in drug eluting stent. Biomater Res. 2014;18:15. https://doi.org/10.1186/2055-7124-18-15.
35. Czajka R, et al. Acrylonitrile Butadiene Styrene (ABS) and its applications in pharmaceutical device design. Pharma Technol. 2020;44(5):24–30.
36. Moohan J, Stewart SA, Espinosa E, Rosal A, Rodríguez A, Larrañeta E, Donnelly RF, DomínguezRobles J. Cellulose nanofibers and other biopolymers for biomedical applications. A review. Appl Sci. 2020;10(1):65. https://doi.org/10.3390/app10010065.
37. Giri B, Poudel S, Kim D. Cellulose and its derivatives for application in 3D printing of pharmaceuticals. J Pharm Investig. 2020;51:1–22. https://doi.org/10.1007/s40005-020-00498-5.
38. Melocchi A, Parietti F, Maroni A, Foppoli A, Gazzaniga A, Zema L. Hot-melt extruded filaments based on pharmaceutical grade polymers for 3D printing by fused deposition modeling. Int J Pharm. 2016;509:255–63.
39. Chen Q, Liang S, Thouas GA. Elastomeric biomaterials for tissue engineering. Prog Polym Sci. 2013;38(3–4):584–671. https://doi.org/10.1016/j.progpolymsci.2012.05.003.
40. Frick A, Rochman A. Characterization of TPU-elastomers by thermal analysis (DSC). Polym Test. 2004;23(4):413–7.
41. Liu B, Han X, Wang Z, Zhang H, Liu N, Gao X, Gao J, Zheng A. Three-dimensional printing personalized acetaminophen sustained-release tablets using hot melt extrusion. J Drug Deliv Sci Technol. 2021;66:102855. ISSN 1773-2247. https://doi.org/10.1016/j.jddst.2021.102855.
42. Manoukian OS, Arul MR, Sardashti N, Stedman T, James R, Rudraiah S, Kumbar SG. Biodegradable polymeric injectable implants for long-term delivery of contraceptive drugs. J Appl Polym Sci. 2018;135(14):46068. https://doi.org/10.1002/app.46068. Epub 2017 Nov 29. PMID: 29430061; PMCID: PMC5801541.
43. Patil H, Tiwari RV, Repka MA. Hot-melt extrusion: from theory to application in pharmaceutical formulation. AAPS PharmSciTech. 2016;17:20–42.
44. Banks J. Adding value in additive manufacturing: researchers in the United Kingdom and Europe Look to 3D printing for customization. IEEE Pulse. 2013;4:22–6.
45. Kumar R, Singh R, Hashmi MSJ. Polymer- Ceramic composites: a state of art review and future applications. Adv Mater Process Technol. 2020;8(1):895–908. https://doi.org/10.1080/2374068X.2020.1835013.
46. Yang L, Wang H, Zhang X. Recent progress in preparation process of ionic polymer-metal composites. Results Phys. 2021;29:104800. ISSN 2211-3797. https://doi.org/10.1016/j.rinp.2021.104800.
47. Astaneh ME, Fereydouni N. Silver nanoparticles in 3D printing: a new frontier in wound healing. ACS Omega. 2024;9(40):41107–29. https://doi.org/10.1021/acsomega.4c04961.

48. Bryll K, Piesowicz E, Szymański P, Slaczka W, Pijanowski M. Polymer composite manufacturing by FDM 3D printing technology. MATEC Web of Conferences. 2018;237:02006. https://doi.org/10.1051/matecconf/201823702006.
49. Díez-Pascual AM. Carbon-based polymer nanocomposites for high-performance applications II. Polymers (Basel). 2022;14(5):870. https://doi.org/10.3390/polym14050870. PMID: 35267693; PMCID: PMC8912748.
50. Maleki M, Zarezadeh R, Nouri M, Sadigh A, Pouremamali F, Asemi Z, Kafil H, Alemi F, Yousefi B. Graphene oxide: a promising material for regenerative medicine and tissue engineering. Biomol Concepts. 2020;11(1):182–200. https://doi.org/10.1515/bmc-2020-0017.
51. Gudeman J, Jozwiakowski M, Chollet J, Randell M. Potential risks of pharmacy compounding. Drugs R D. 2013;13(1):1–8. https://doi.org/10.1007/s40268-013-0005-9.
52. Mota C, Camarero-Espinosa S, Baker MB, Wieringa P, Moroni L. Bioprinting: from tissue and organ development to in vitro models. Chem Rev. 2020;120:10547–607.

Regulatory Challenges, Quality Standards, and Compliances for 3D Printed Pharmaceuticals

4

Swati Sharma, Kasangaki Wilberforce, and Shachi Patel

Abstract

Three-dimensional (3D) printing is an exponentially growing technology in pharmaceuticals. It is layer-by-layer deposition of polymer on a solid substrate, offering various opportunities for the development of personalized medicines, patient-specific dosing and safe solid dosage forms. This technology has been applied in several pharmaceutical and biomedical products like microchips, modified drug delivery, fast disintegrating tablets, and implants. Furthermore, the USFDA's approval to Spritam® (levetiracetam), a 3D printed tablet and a few medical devices approved by different regulatory agencies demonstrated great market potential. However, besides many benefits, 3D printing technology presents a number of regulatory challenges. These products cannot be tested using traditional quality-by-testing (QbT) methods, which are time-consuming, laborious, and destroying. Therefore, considering the limitations, the current chapter explores the application of quality-by-design (QbD) approach and process analytical technology (PAT) tool for the fabrication and testing of 3D printed medicines and devices. Effective QC strategies relating to material selection, process validation and consistency of the 3D printed medications are discussed. The chapter delves into the framework and process required for 3D printed product approval by various national medical regulatory agencies. Overall, it illustrates and delivers insights regarding the utilization of the 3D printed products considering the product quality, safety and efficacy.

S. Sharma · K. Wilberforce · S. Patel (✉)
Department of Pharmaceutics, Ramanbhai Patel College of Pharmacy, Charotar University of Science and Technology (CHARUSAT), Changa, Gujarat, India
e-mail: shachikapatel.ph@charusat.ac.in

K. Vinchurkar, S. Mane (eds.), *Innovations in Drug Manufacturing*,
https://doi.org/10.1007/978-981-96-9075-6_4

Keywords

3D printing · Quality-by-design (QbD) · Process analytical technology (PAT) Quality control (QC)

4.1 Introduction

Three-dimensional (3D) printing is an additive manufacturing technology which involves application of computer-aided design (CAD) model, followed by creating layered deposition of 3D printed product [1]. A 3D printing technique offers creation of complex geometries in a short time span. As a technology, 3D printing continues to evolve in medicine, from the first patent in 1986 to the first pharmaceutical product [2]. It provides several advantages in comparison to conventional pharmaceutical processes. The technology includes low material waste, minimal post-processing and organized manufacturing steps and makes it a feasible for future [3]. According to the American Society for Testing and Materials (ASTM), the 3D printing techniques are categorized as (a) jetting, (b) binder jetting, (c) powder bed fusion (PBF), (d) material extrusion, (e) vat photopolymerization, (f) energy deposition and (g) sheet lamination [4, 5].

A standard inkjet printing technology is a type of material jetting technique. It includes deposition of small liquid droplets through a nozzle which is further occurred in presence of some external stimuli. Thermoplastic and photoresist materials are widely used in this process. The inkjet printing is a developing technology through great potential in the field of pharmacy. Its precise, smooth material deposition and flexibility demonstrate fabrication of smart dosage forms with desired release profile [6]. Binder jetting is another type of inkjet printing method. The technique includes spraying of binder solution on a powder bed for developing a 3D printed structure. The printing system comprises of a binding solution tank, powder reservoir and a substrate for printing system. The technique includes rolling of powder on the printing platform, followed by spraying binder solution for developing a 3D printed product of desired geometry [7]. The USFDA approval to Spritam®, 3D printed tablets became a breakthrough in pharmaceutical industry for the treatment of epilepsy [8]. Spritam® was developed by the binder jetting-based printing, later named as "ZipDose technology." This method is specifically used for the development of fast disintegrating or mouth dissolving tablets [9].

In addition to this, powder bed fusion is another technology that fuses the powder particles together to develop a 3D printed objects. The PBF method is further classified to laser sintering, multi jet blending technique and electron beam melting [10]. The PBF is the process of spreading a layer of powder on the initial deposited layer. Material extrusion is a type of 3D printing method that includes deposition of material via a heated nozzle for development of 3D object. The technique is known as fused deposition remodelling [11].

Vat photopolymerization is a light-based 3D printing technique that uses photoresist for the development of a unique, stable geometry product. It includes methods like stereolithography, digital light processing, two-photon polymerization or continuous liquid polymerization [12]. Energy deposition and sheet lamination are other techniques used in 3D printing. Despite the significant advancement in the technique, this method is still new to the healthcare industry.

3D printing technique offers versatility in the creation of complex configurations, enabling alteration of drug doses, and the combination allows accurate regulation of drug release. The methodology has been applied in developing personalized medicine, tissue engineering or in creation of medical implants [14]. Oral dosage forms (ODF) are considered to be the most widely adapted pharmaceutical products, especially tablets. Conventional ODFs are formed in limited structure and shape. Binder jetting is a commonly explored method for designing immediate release or long acting solid ODFs [15]. The technique have been used in variety of medicinal products like fast disintegrating, controlled release, microneedles, implants or transdermal patches [16]. The 3D printing offers flexibility to produce formulation of varying geometries and structure by systematic deposition of the polymers in layer-by-layer fashion [17]. A study conducted by Feunmayor et al. compared the release profile of caffeine-containing tablet designed by direct compression, injection moulding and fused filament fabrication. The prepared tablets by direct compression demonstrated faster drug release while the injection moulding demonstrated the slow release of caffeine. However, the fused filament fabrication technique represented both the types of release profiles depending on the printing parameter [18]. Moreover, 3D printing has also revolutionized transdermal drug delivery of therapeutic molecules. The major limitation of drug to be delivered via this route is minimal drug loading, immediate release and an invasive procedure [19]. A group of researchers developed a 3D printed customized transdermal patches by applying powder extrusion technology [20]. The researchers developed ethylvinyl acetate-based transdermal patch for on-demand drug release. Ibuprofen and diclofenac sodium were used as model drugs in the study to understand the drug release behaviour.

Apart from pharmaceuticals, the technique has demonstrated remarkable advantages in the field of medical devices and healthcare. The 3D printed biomedical devices provide a cost-effective, safe, personalized solution with on-demand manufacturing of the product whenever required. The manufacturing of patient-centric orthopaedic implants using traditional approach is challenging. However, 3D printing is a systematic approach focussed on choice of materials and outline scheme of product. Hence, it is feasible to develop a customized patient-complaint implant [21]. In addition to it, researchers are also focussing on developing artificial organs as a part of regenerative medicine, surgical haemostat [22, 23] and surgical guides [24] for simplifying the medical procedure.

Since the approval of Spritam® in 2017, no other successful 3D printed medicines are available. This is due to the non-existence of regulation for 3D printed medicines. Despite the significant advancement in the technique, this method is still new to the healthcare industry. Streamlining regulatory structure and supporting robust quality standards in designing 3D-printed products are needed for these advanced techniques. Several regulatory agencies and non-government organizations have issued guidelines on the technical considerations of 3D-printed medical devices [25]. Although standard nomenclature is required for the better search and availability of literature for the upcoming researchers. The "ISO/ASTM52900" offers standard terminology for the additive manufacturing technologies [13]. The standard terminology will lead to improved clarity and ease of search in publication. The current chapter depicts the journey of the first approved 3D-printed drug product on the market from conceptualization to the clinical stage. It also explores the unique challenges of product testing and useful tools for QC methods of 3D-printed products. Moreover, unique discussions on regulatory frameworks designed by regulatory agencies and regulatory challenges pertaining to cutting-edge technology were addressed. Furthermore, it offers future insight into 3D printing technology and a list of approved 3D-printed products along with future-ready products in the pipeline.

4.2 "SPRITAM": The World's First 3D Printed Drug from Lab to Market—the Story of Pioneering ZipDose® Technology

New Drug Application (NDA) for Spritam® (levetiracetam) approved by the US Food and Drug Administration (FDA), setting benchmark of first regulatory-approved pharmaceutical product using 3D printing technology. The product was developed by Aprecia Pharmaceuticals (Aprecia) using a unique ZipDose® formulation technology [2].

4.2.1 Product Theory Visualization and Necessity of ZipDose®

Spritam®, a highly prescribed medicine in the management of several presentations of epilepsy, contains levetiracetam as therapeutic moiety. It is perceived to be a unique easy-to-ingest oral dosage form. Levetiracetam was approved by USFDA in 1999 as KEPPRA through NDA 21035 [2].

Traditionally, levetiracetam is supplied as film-coated tablets compressed in fixed doses ranging from 250 mg to 1000 mg in order to offer an immediate release mechanism after a whole tablet is swallowed intact [2].

Because of the large amount of drug that must be accommodated in each unit, the tablets are predisposed to be presented in large sizes, consequently leading to poor adherence due to difficulty in swallowing them. In fact, KEPPRA tablets are lengthened in nature with various lengths corresponding to the particular dosing strengths [2].

Difficulty in swallowing large intact tablets is a common phenomenon exhibited by extended release tablets as they do not offer any remedy for the challenge. As a result, there is limited commercial appeal for patients suffering from Dysphagia. Dysphagia is most commonly linked to children and the elderly [26].

Levetiracetam for paediatric patients is usually presented in form of oral solution making it easy to swallow. Whereas it is convenient to be swallowed by the paediatrics, there is a challenge of accurately measuring off the dose 12-hourly consistently. The fact that the solution is packed in bottles creates a limitation of transportability due to the bulk size of bottles [2].

Aprecia Pharmaceuticals addressed this issue by developing the world's first 3D printed tablet, Spritam®. The 3D printing process produces porous tablets that instantly dissolve in patients' mouths. Therefore, regardless of strength, patients can easily take Spritam®.

4.2.2 Regulatory Pathway

Right from the initial development phase, Spritam® was aimed at providing a unique dosage form regarding the strength, disintegration action, and dissolution rate, which collectively presented the required quality attributes to promote adherence to levetiracetam when administered in the paediatrics and those with swallowing difficulties.

These formulation modifications in the critical quality attributes of Spritam® favoured neither filing ANDA nor a full standalone NDA regulatory pathway. NDA would have dictated a repetition of conducting both preclinical and clinical studies of the reference product as had been earlier done by the innovator.

Given such situations, hybrid medicine authorization process is used by Aprecia Pharmaceuticals. Such hybrid approval pathway is the 505(b)(2) NDA. Moreover, this approval process in the USA applies to generic molecules that have a slight change from the reference medicine and can use published data, including previous FDA submissions and communications, to support their re-approval by the FDA [27].

505(b)(2) NDA regulatory pathway requires the applicant to submit the relevant data to connect the new drug candidate to the reference drug attributes in order to attain approval via hybrid regulatory pathway.

Comparable to traditional NDAs, where comprehensive reports of safety and efficacy investigations are given; however, the data needed for approval is derived from research that was not carried out by the applicant, or publicly available literature and the FDA's earlier conclusions regarding the safety and effectiveness of an RLD may be included in this submission.

4.2.3 Developing "Spritam®" Pioneering ZipDose® Medicine

Between 2013 and 2014, Aprecia Pharmaceuticals held several communications with FDA to introduce 3D printing and ZipDose technology. These formal meetings, especially type B, were aimed at seeking FDA's guidance and advice on the appropriate clinical development leading to Spritam® approval. The total product profile (TPP) for Spritam® was based on the predicted variation in labelling of the new 3D printed product compared to the reference listed drug tablet. ZipDose technology utilized generally recognized as safe (GRAS) materials rather depending on unfamiliar or new excipients.

ZipDose technology may be employed in clinical development and formulation of a wide range of products such as nutraceuticals and pharmaceuticals. The biggest advantage of ZipDose technology is the capacity to incorporate large quantities of the active ingredients and still achieve high disintegration profile in the mouth as demonstrated by the commercially viable 1000 mg loading dose of levetiracetam. Good manufacturing practice (GMP) regulations should be adhered to, ensure use of not toxic solvents and select a working environment such as temperature to escape any degradation of the API. The early development phases of Spritam® were executed by a special machine purposefully designed to create a conducive GMP formulation environment to encompass registration, verification, validation and product commercial launch undertakings. It is worth noting that ZipDose technology supports taste-masking operations such as use of flavours and sweetening agents. The technology also aids unit operations including coating to provide a physical barrier or chemical complexation processes.

4.2.4 Clinical Journey of "Spritam®"

The Aprecia filed an NDA application for Spritam® under 505(b)(2) using immediate-release tablets KEPPRA® (levetiracetam) as the reference listed drug (RLD). Primarily, BA/BE study connecting the test drug and the RLD as well as PK study evaluating levetiracetam PK following administration of "Spritam®" (without taking water) were conducted without efficacy trial. In single-dose crossover design, "Spritam®" was shown to have equal rate and extent of absorption to Keppra® IR tablets under fasted conditions [28].

A single dose, one treatment, one period, open-label PK study illustrates similarity in PK profile when clinical trial was conducted with the test product administered with water under fasted conditions the PK of levetiracetam 1000 milligrams (from Aprecia) exhibits similarities [28].

Based on study, "Spritam®" labelling mentioned it to take the tablet with sip of water to disintegrate in the mouth and swallow afterwards or add whole Spritam® tablet(s) in desired amount of water prior to consumption [29].

4.3 Conventional Quality Standards and Unique Need of 3D Printed Tablets

In contrast to traditional centralized factory-based manufacturing, research on individualized 3D printed medications has presented the concept of decentralized manufacturing of pharmaceuticals [30]. Traditional regulatory environment for the production of pharmaceuticals has been conditioned to accommodate large-scale batch manufacturing systems. Quality-by-testing (QbT) approach has been utilized in conventional dosage forms, which emphasizes specified pharmacopeial tests for final products. This methodology of testing is destructive, costly and time-consuming [31, 32].

The strength of conventional tablet dosage forms is usually tested using traditional hardness testing which may not be applicable for 3D printed dosage forms. This may be as a result of variation in mechanical strength and the formulation may also contain plastic raw materials. However, disintegration and friability tests are conducted as mandatory in order to conform to the quality attributes of solid dosage forms [33].

On the other hand, pharmaceutical 3DP for customized dosage forms entails small-scale, on-demand manufacturing with little to no lead time to conduct quality control testing. Furthermore, quality control tests usually differ based on the clinical development and formulation procedure employed to attain the finished 3D printed products.

Hence, in-line testing using process analytical technology (PAT) tools at point of care facilities facilitates product safety and efficacy with non-destructive measures.

4.3.1 Application of QbD and PAT in 3D Printed Medicine

In order to enable effective manufacturing development in flexible manner, incorporating patient expectations with the regulatory and industries perspective, a quality-by-design (QbD), quality management framework has been introduced in early phase development [34]. This would increase the acceptability of 3DP's incredibly creative technology and guarantee regulatory compliance [35].

4.3.2 QbD and PAT (Process Analytical Technology) Approaches for Quality Control (QC) of 3D Medicine

QbD emphasizes the significance of comprehending the interaction between materials and process for achieving anticipated product quality. Defining the quality target product profile (QTPP) is a mandatory step in the QbD step-by-step cycle. The key needs for the upcoming product are established from both the regulatory and patient perspectives, guaranteeing that the clinical standards are satisfied [35]. After establishing QTPP, based on scientific knowledge and risk management, the rationale for critical quality attributes (CQAs) of individual quality process and operation has been identified while considering product knowledge and regulatory necessities [30].

Linking CQAs with critical material attributes (CMAs) and critical process parameters (CPPs) is the next vital step in QbD process [30]. After establishing CPPs and CMAs, manufacturer can analyse those with PAT tools. There are several PAT techniques used including spectroscopic techniques such as near IR spectroscopy, nuclear magnetic resonance spectroscopy, Raman spectroscopy, and UV/vis spectroscopy, among others [36].

Both PAT and QbD employ real-time release testing (RTRT) in order to optimize the quality of 3D printed medicines without compromising the end-product testing [30].

4.3.3 Useful PAT Tools

(a) *Near-IR Spectroscopy (NIRS)*

With little to no sample preparation, together transmittance NIRS (tNIRS) and reflectance NIRS (rNIRS) enable quantitative and qualitative assessments of samples [30].

The NIR spectroscopy has been widely used as an in-line PAT technology in a variety of processes, including the prediction of solid state form, drug dissolution, blend uniformity, coating thickness, drug loading, tablet hardness and blend uniformity [32].

(b) *Raman Spectroscopy (RS)*

Raman spectroscopy and microscopy can be used in the pharmaceutical industry to see the constituents of a sample matrix. Raman spectroscopy has been widely used to quantify the amorphous/crystalline drug form within drug products and to monitor solid-state form transitions in real time. Besides these tools, researcher may utilize terahertz spectroscopy, chemometric analysis and X-ray microtomography to monitor or predict dosage form critical quality attributes in the arena of 3D printed pharmaceuticals [36, 37].

4.3.4 Actual Quality Control Measures for 3D Printed Solid Oral Dosage Form

To improve both quality control (QC) and quality assurance (QA), simulation techniques and process analytical technology (PAT) could be combined into a 3D printed medication [38, 39].

Newly established and validated methods used in measuring mechanical strength are required. Tools such as Instron tensile tester or texture analyser are desirable to quantify the 3DP medicine hardness, tensile strength, fracture strain, etc. [40].

The United States Pharmacopeia (USP) prescribes several disintegration tests with the corresponding disintegration times according to categories of tablets. Due to their porous structure, tablets made using specific 3DP processes, however, had an extremely short disintegration period. Since the disintegration apparatus does not have such a facility, USP disintegration tests are incapable to distinguish between pharmaceutical products created using various constituents and techniques [33, 41]. Most organoleptic parameter such as resolution, layer height, and surface porosities for such 3D printed drug can be analysed by scanning electron microscopy (SEM) to assess important quality attribute [39].

4.4 3D Printing for Medical Device and Additive Manufacturing

The 3D printed medical devices like surgical models, medical implants, surgical instruments, and personal protection equipment serve as equipment or tools in medical sciences to detect, manage, or cure medical conditions [42]. In response to the need for individualized devices for each patient, point of care (3D) printing was developed. This allows use of patient's imaging data for creating precise and smart 3D printed diagnostic tools, surgical instruments, or other medical devices. The devices can be created on-site at a facility owned by the health care organization, such as a hospital, or in a centrally located facility [43]. The 3D printing applied at easy-to-use diagnostics has potential to significantly improve public health by enabling the quick and flexible fabrication of devices and the incorporation of anatomical models for surgical planning [44].

Traditional manufacturing method is subtractive manufacturing technique that begins with a block of material and eliminates surplus using techniques like milling and machining to produce the desired end result [43]. Conversely, the method of manufacturing of 3D printed medical device is additive manufacturing, which allows complex device fabrication in a unit piece by layering and successively building two-dimensional (2D) structures and enables device manufacturers to rapidly create alternative designs without the need for retooling [45]. Typical phase of additive manufacturing-assisted fabrication of the medical device is depicted in Fig. 4.1 [46].

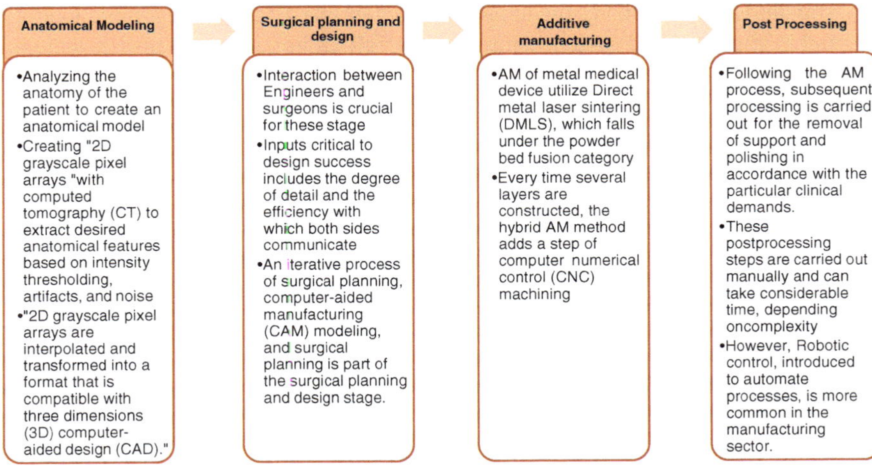

Fig. 4.1 Phases of additive manufacturing process

4.4.1 Regulation Overview

Acknowledging the rapid expansion of point-of-care 3D printing (3DP) and its application to healthcare facilities worldwide, countries such as China, the USA and the EU has been working extensively to develop its 3DP market and the regulations to govern it [47].

(a) China

First action plan was developed by China in the form of "Additive Manufacturing Industry Development Action Plan (2017–2020)" jointly by 12 departments, including the Ministry of Industry and Information Technology, with the goal of fostering the quick and sustainable growth of additive manufacturing sector and accelerating the creation of new forces for manufacturing development [48].

In February 2018, to strengthen additive manufacturing technology, the "Customize-Designed Additive Manufactured (3D Printed) Medical Device Technical Review Draft Guideline" was released by Centre of Medical Device Evaluation [49].

However, device classification is governed by risk level presented at rule "Regulations for the Supervision and Administration of Medical Devices (Decree NO. 650)" published on July 30, 2014, is still used for 3D-printed devices and depicted in Table 4.1 [50].

The China National Institutes for Food and Drug Control (NIFDC) under the National Medical Products Administration (NMPA) has actively applied since 2014 for the creation of a focal point for the 3D printed medical device industry standards after realizing the application potential of 3D printing in the medical field. This standard system addresses the full additive manufacturing technology process chain and covers five key areas: raw materials, equipment, data transfer, process verification methods and risk management [52].

The adoption of advanced standards set the groundwork for quality control in the sector.

(b) *USA*

Even the US government was keeping up with publishing direction on "Technical Considerations for Additive Manufactured Medical Devices" in December 2017, which offers the US Food and Drug Administration's (USFDA) primary views on technical issues exclusive to devices made with additive manufacturing and device testing with at least one step or part made using additive manufacturing [52]. The same manufacturing procedures and regulations apply to 3D printed medical devices as they do to conventional medical devices in terms of approval.

The National Centre for Devices and Radiological Health (CDRH) of the FDA oversees enterprises that produce, repack, relabel, and import medical devices that are traded in the USA [53].

Draft guideline mentioned in former paragraph comprises of two sections, mainly Design and Manufacturing Considerations (Section V) and Device

Table 4.1 Risk-based classification of devices as per CFDA and USFDA with regulatory requirements

Device classification terminology	CFDA [50]		USFDA [51]	
	Requirement	Type of application	Requirement	Type of application
Class-I Low risk level	Completely safe and effective	Filling	–	Exempt from Premarket Notification 510(k)
Class-II Moderate risk level	Strict administration is obligatory to guarantee their safety and effectiveness	Registration	"Substantially Equivalent" is established to a legally marketed device from Product Classification Database	510(k) clearance before device is officially marketed
Class-III Higher risk	Controlled via special measures in respect to safety and effectiveness	Registration	Clinical trial evidence of the device's safety and efficacy	Premarket approval (PMA) before device is officially marketed

Testing Considerations (Section VI). The technical reflections listed in the Design and Manufacturing Considerations section are necessary to fulfil the quality system (QS) requirements for 3D printed device. These requirements are determined by the classification of device according to applicable regulation [54]. Fundamentally, risk-based classification is applied to the 3DP devices, where control rises from Class I to Class III devices, and the type of premarket submission for AM device is determined by the regulatory classification of device (Table 4.1). The testing section incorporates information on premarket notification submissions (510(k)), premarket approval (PMA) applications, humanitarian device exemption (HDE) applications, de novo requests, and investigational device exemption (IDE) applications. The regulatory classification of AM device dictates the kind of premarket submission that is necessary [55].

The 510(k) approach has been used to approve the most of 3D printed medical devices by FDA. Through the "de novo" process, devices lacking a "substantial equivalent" but with a rational assurance of safety (based on certain FDA rules) might be designated as Class I or Class II devices [43].

Legislation also describes software workflow, material control, post-processing, process validation, device testing consideration, removing and sterilization aspect including labelling.

Aside from developing medical devices, AM too spurs invention in biologicals and tissue-engineered goods for regenerative medication, such as the bioprinting of living cell constructions and tissue scaffolds. Even though there are not any FDA-approved or cleared biologic products made by AM in the USA at the moment, the Centre for Biologics Evaluation and Research (CBER) at the

FDA has responded to a number of investigations regarding bio-printing, bio-printed (additive manufactured) cellular products, and tissue-engineered constructs, which has received customized feedback [54].

(c) *International Medical Device Regulators Forum (IMDRF)*

In order to shape the solid foundational work of the Global Harmonization Task Force on Medical Devices (GHTF), a volunteer group of medical device regulators from around the world formed the International Medical Device Harmonization and Convergence Forum (IMDRF), which seeks to fast-track international medical device regulatory harmonization and convergence [56].

The IMDRF published a personalized medical device guidance on September 14, 2023, with the goal of standardizing the ways in which various regulatory bodies monitor personalized devices. The guidance also addresses situations in which the regulatory body may require a different approach to handling a given device whereas IMDRF categorizes custom-made devices, patient-matched devices and adaptable medical devices under the aegis of personalized medical devices [57]. These device criterias, along with specifications, manufacturing requirements, and statement requirements, are illustrated in Table 4.2.

IMDRF strongly encouraged that local representatives or makers of all personalized medical devices register or notify the regulatory body in the jurisdiction where the products are delivered [58].

Jurisdictions may define and regulate a "medical device production system" (MDPS) based on the device counting the intended usage for the device validated by the maker of the medical device production system, if control over an additive manufacturing process is required outside of a regulated facility [59].

An MDPS comprises the final medical device that it is meant to create as well as the intended usage of the device that has been verified in compliance with the safety and performance standards of the applicable regulatory authority [59].

Custom-made device makers must evaluate and record their post-production experience and establish a method for reporting to authorities regarding their post-market vigilance. Manufacturers must specifically adhere to reporting regulations in the jurisdictions in which their devices are provided. These regulations may include disclosing adverse events connected to the device or field safety corrective action (such as a recall) [57].

(d) *Australia* [60]

The Therapeutic Goods Administration (TGA) of Australia in February 2019 held a talk for the "proposed regulatory scheme for personalized medical devices, including 3D printed devices." As a result, regulatory variations for custom-made medical devices Version 6.0 were enacted in December 2023 for personalized medical devices (including 3D printed devices).

Different four-tier classification system was proposed under TGA regulation (Table 4.3) based on risk posed by device.

Table 4.2 Personalized medical devices requirements under IMDRF [57]

Device	Specification	Manufacturing and record keeping	Statement requirements
Custom-made medical device	Intended for a use of a particular individual Made according to a specific request from an authorized professional Designed to address the unique anatomical or pathological conditions of the individual	The device's chemical, physical and biological attributes Infection and microbial contamination Sterilization technique; construction and environmental attributes Radiation protection Specifications for medical devices that are connected to or equipped with an energy source Information provided by the manufacturer, with labels	Information used to identify the device A declaration for specific patient and patient's name The name and address of the licensed healthcare The device's specific features as listed in the pertinent written request A declaration of device safety and performance requirements The rationale of device's safe use The manufacturer's name and address
Patient-matched medical device	Matched to a patient's anatomy within a design envelope Produced in a batch that can be validated and reproduced Design may be developed in consultation with a healthcare professional but remains under the manufacturer's responsibility	Worst-case configurations and device geometries in order to demonstrate safety and performance Validation and/or verification testing on physical samples Records for the design envelope validation procedure	–
Adaptable medical device	Mass-produced and adapted at the point of care Adjusted, assembled or shaped to suit an individual's specific features based on the manufacturer's instructions Typically involves thermoforming or intraoperative contouring	The manufacturer of the device must supply verified instructions that outline how to modify, assemble, shape or alter the device The validation process must guarantee that the device's performance and safety are not adversely affected by the allowed point-of-care modifications	–

Table 4.3 Four-tier classification of medical devices by Therapeutics Goods Administration [61, 62]

Medical device classification	Level of potential harm
Class I	Lowest Pose minimal risk to patients or users and are often simple in design and function
Class Is, Class Im	Sterile and intended for short-term use Not sterile and intended for long-term use
Class IIa	Low to moderate More regulatory control than Class I devices
Class IIb	Moderate to High Higher level of regulatory control than Class IIa
Class III	High High-risk devices that pose the greatest risk to patients or users

According to TGA guidelines, manufacturing the device within approved parameters of a certain design envelope is one of the regulatory concerns for creating patient-matched devices.

As suggested by the definitions, the specified design envelope is the lowest and extreme dimensions, performance limits, or other relevant factors that accurately describe a medical device for fabrication purposes and may be grounded on a standard device template.

Another prima-facie requirement as suggested by TGA includes robust manufacturing procedures that can be verified or validated and easily reproducible.

Similar to IMDRF, category like custom-made device, patient-matched device and adaptable medical devices exist under the aegis of personalized medical devices within TGA regulations.

4.4.2 Quality System of Medical Devices

Conventional products usually have a 2- to 3-year shelf life, which gives quality control testing a fair amount of time at the end of manufacture. Guidelines have been set by regulatory agencies such as the US Food and Drug Administration (FDA) to guarantee the safety and effectiveness of medical devices. But these rules were mostly created for conventional production techniques [34]. To adjust them to the intricacies of 3D printing, a more sophisticated strategy is needed. Making sure 3D printed medical gadgets adhere to the same safety regulations as conventionally manufactured ones is the primary concern. A quality control data will take different forms and amounts based on the device type, intended usage, risk profile, and classification and/or regulations. Quality control of 3D printed device starts from preprocessing step which end to post-processing stage [34] (Fig. 4.2).

Each component used in the fabrication of the device should be recognized because the additive manufacturing (AM) method either makes the end material or modifies the starting material during the process.

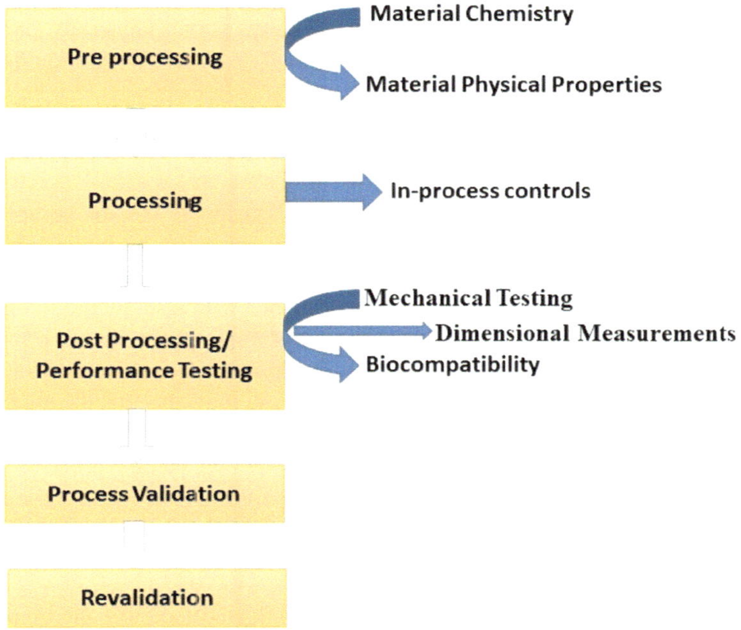

Fig. 4.2 Quality control of 3D printed device

Material chemistry and material physical properties play crucial role in defining final product characteristics; therefore, depending upon state of starting material employed, different tests need to be carried out.

Implementing real-time monitoring systems during the printing process allows for early detection of any anomalies. This helps prevent defective devices from reaching patients. Subsequent criteria need to be checked [54]:

- Manual or automated visual inspection with defined acceptance criteria
- Non-destructive evaluation
- Build-space environmental conditions (e.g., temperature, pressure, humidity)
- Status of mechanical elements of the printing system

Devices that have been manufactured and put through all post-processing, cleaning, and sterilizing procedures should have employed for performance testing. The completed gadget should be utilized, or an explanation should be given, as with any prescribed testing [63].

Production operations must be carefully planned, carried out, regulated and monitored to guarantee that devices or components are not negatively influenced by fabrication orientation, because the orientation and position of the device may have an impact on its mechanical qualities.

Given that some devices might not have distinct sizes, like small, medium and large, it is advisable to identify device's range of dimensions. Generally, parameters such as dimensional tolerances and dimensional measurements should be carried out.

It is advised that biocompatibility be assessed utilizing the completed device and taking into account the type of interaction in accordance with international standards like ISO 10993-1 [64].

After performance testing, when a process's outcomes cannot be completely confirmed by testing and inspection, the process must be highly validated and approved in accordance with established protocols. Additionally, software needs to be verified for its intended application in accordance with a set methodology. Once the product is successfully placed in market, it is important to identify and assess any modifications to the device, manufacturing process or process deviations for any potential risks they may present. This assessment indicates that the modification or departure might necessitate revalidating the procedure [54, 65].

4.5 Regulatory Challenges for 3D Printed Pharmaceuticals

(a) Decentralization [66]

3D printed medicinal products, especially devices, exhibit and demonstrate a decentralized feature of production that could easily bring in regulatory concerns such as evasion of regulations established for guiding the pharmaceutical manufacturing industry and they end up manufacturing 3D printed products that are non-compliant with the set safety and quality standards which compromises public health. Manufacturers using 3D printing technology, but are not traditional medical device manufacturers, may be ignorant of regulations applicable to the industry or may consider themselves exempted. This presents a strong challenge in an attempt to implement the existing regulations as it requires more resources for operative, monitoring and controlling of manufacturing activities outside of industry setting.

(b) Non-standard Terminology and Ambiguous Guideline [67]

Nearly all main authorities follow risk-based classification of medical devices with a few important exclusions, whereby some 3D printed devices may not be subjected to the usual applicable regulations in their respective risk category. The sole purpose of these exemptions is aimed at hastening access to technologies that are urgently required, hence the need for a special regulatory process. These exemptions differ with various authorities and are designed in order not to sidestep the traditional regulatory systems and contravene the risk-based regulatory approach as far as patient safety is concerned. Various jurisdictions have different terminologies for exemptions such as "personalized device," "custom-made device," among others, which causes an impasse to stakeholders.

(c) Integrating GMP Standards to 3D Printed Pharmaceuticals [68, 69]

ICH guidelines on quality, safety, and efficacy can be adapted for application in 3D printing technology for pharmaceutical products. But GMP standards are not clearly well-defined probably due to the diversity of 3D printers fabrication, different manufacturing processes, and the final product quality. Unless the cleaning concepts are definitely defined, verified and validated, 3D printers should be considered as specialized equipment by pharmaceutical firms. Solving cleaning validation concerns is vital to avoid cross-contamination

(d) Upholding Excipients Quality [70]

There is limited options for excipients used in 3D printing technology as compared to those used in conventional pharmaceutical processes. Whereas several non-pharmaceutical grade ingredients maybe used in printing processes, their use in 3D printing is considerably hindered by their undesirable side effects and compatibility issues. Therefore, this calls for a hasty research of nontoxic, biodegradable, biocompatible, and physicochemical stable excipients. ICH guideline Q3C (R5) prescribes a list of residual solvents with their respective minimum tolerable amounts. Consequently, establishing limits of exceptional residual solvents used in 3D printing technology of pharmaceuticals by scientific research can hasten the product approval.

(e) Quality Control Mechanism [71]

Distinct unit operations are used at every essential stage of the production process to assure quality during tablet manufacture using traditional pharmaceutical manufacturing techniques. This is attained by checking and controlling in-process quality before proceeding to the next stage of production. Such in-process checks and controls have proved difficult to apply during 3D printing since the process is a single step, which is dynamic and continuous in nature. It is therefore of paramount importance to establish regulations devoted to 3D printed pharmaceuticals in order to streamline and ease regulatory approval.

4.6 Conclusion and Future Prospects

The growth and expansion of 3D printing in the development of pharmaceuticals and medical devices hold great potential for precision medicine. It is a potential technique in the fabrication of on-demand manufacturing, creation of the personalized medicine and thereby improving patient compliance. Since the inception of 3D printed process, there is just one FDA-approved product available. In order to qualify for marketing, 3D printed product must satisfy current manufacturing practices along with control standards [8, 70, 72]. Despite a huge success of the first approved 3D printed pharmaceuticals "Spritam®," the regulatory agencies lack the basic framework in approval of this 3D printed pharmaceuticals. The Spritam® tablets commercialized by Aprecia Pharmaceuticals were approved via type of NDA known as a 505(b)(2) NDA, considering the intended uses and the concept of the product [2]. However, current regulatory landscape for 3D printed pharmaceutical product is opaque and ambiguous.

In this regard, FDA, in 2017, proposed a guidelines regarding the technical consideration in the development and use of a 3D printed medical devices. The document was designed to outline the concepts associated with design and manufacturing considerations and device testing considerations for 3D printed medical devices [54].

However, these considerations are not applicable to the 3D printed pharmaceuticals. Besides USFDA, regulatory agencies such as China Food and Drug Administration (CFDA), Therapeutic Goods Administration (TGA), European Medicines Agency (EMA) and Health Sciences Authority (HSA) with some non-government organizations like IMDRF had created initial framework for regulation of 3D printed devices.

Moreover, while a variety of 3D printed pharmaceuticals are under research, the designing of a GMP-compliant 3D printer was also a concern in its establishment [73, 74]. However, the reproducibility, quality and safety of the product remain challenging due to not fitting with current manufacturing practices. To match these standards, pharmaceutical companies participated in developing 3D printers that match the pharmaceutical requirement. A specialized 3D printer named M3DIMAKER™ was intended to design personalized medicine at the hospital settings. In addition to that, Good Manufacturing Practice (GMP)-based Pharma Inks have been introduced by CurifyLabs to enable pharmacies and hospitals to produce customized and patient-tailored medications on-site [75, 76].

Considering the numerous benefits in the pharmaceutical and medical industry, the technology has shown a remarkable potential in the development of personalized medicine. The on-demand manufacturing of the patient centric medicine improved the supply chain efficiency and reduced product waste. However, product liability issues, along with legal challenges by a supplier or software provider and intellectual property issues for this technology, remain outstanding, as multiple service providers were involved from product manufacturing to distribution [77].

Considering the market potential, global pharmaceutical firm Triastek has developed and filed applications for various 3D printed dosage forms. Portfolio product of Triastek are depicted in Table 4.4.

Table 4.4 3D printed product portfolio [78]

Product name	Technology	Pathway/ phase	Approval status	Technique	Company
Spritam (Levetiracetam)	Zip dose fast disintegrating tablet	NDA 505(b)(2)	USFDA approved	Powder-based binder jet 3D printing technique	Aprecia Pharmaceuticals
Promising 3D printed product world wide					
T19 RA, PsA, AS	3DμS-DR	IND	FDA and NMPA	Melt extrusion deposition (MED)	Triastek Inc.
T20 AF, VTE	3DμS-SE	IND	FDA		
T21 UC	3DμS®-CT	IND	FDA		
T22 PAH	3DμS®-GR	IND	FDA and NMPA		
D23 IgAN	3DμS®-MR	IND	China		

RA rheumatoid arthritis, *PsA* psoriatic arthritis, *AS* ankylosing spondylitis, *AF* atrial fibrillation, *VTE* venous thromboembolism, *UC* ulcerative colitis, *PAH* pulmonary arterial hypertension, 3DμS-DR/SE/CT/GR: 3D microstructure for delayed release/solubility enhancement/colon targeting/gastric retention

In a nutshell, to handle advanced pharmaceutical technology like 3D printing, a robust and harmonized regulatory framework for product lifecycle management needs to be conceptualized to provide quality medicines by ensuring safety and efficacy.

References

1. Wang S, Chen X, Han X, Hong X, Li X, Zhang H, et al. A review of 3D printing technology in pharmaceutics: technology and applications, now and future. Pharmaceutics. 2023;15(2):416.
2. West TG, Bradbury TJ. 3D printing: a case of ZipDose® technology—World's First 3D printing platform to obtain FDA approval for a pharmaceutical product. 3D 4D Print Biomed Appl. 2019;(1):53–79.
3. Jandyal A, Chaturvedi I, Wazir I, Raina A, Ul Haq MI. 3D printing—A review of processes, materials and applications in industry 4.0. Sustain Oper Comput [Internet]. 2022;3:33–42. Available from: https://doi.org/10.1016/j.susoc.2021.09.004
4. Alghamdi SS, John S, Choudhury NR, Dutta NK. Additive manufacturing of polymer materials: progress, promise and challenges. Polymers (Basel). 2021;13(5):1–39.
5. Peralta E, Elhadad AA, Rosa-sainz A, Ca R, Balbuena M, Alcudia A, et al. Applications and multidisciplinary perspective on 3D printing techniques: recent developments and future trends. Mater Sci Eng R. 2023;156 https://doi.org/10.1016/j.mser.2023.100760.
6. Carou-Senra P, Rodríguez-Pombo L, Awad A, Basit AW, Alvarez-Lorenzo C, Goyanes A. Inkjet printing of pharmaceuticals. Adv Mater. 2024;36(11):1–28.
7. Sen K, Mehta T, Sansare S, Sharifi L, Ma AWK, Chaudhuri B. Pharmaceutical applications of powder-based binder jet 3D printing process—A review. Adv Drug Deliv Rev [Internet]. 2021;177:113943. Available from: https://doi.org/10.1016/j.addr.2021.113943
8. Chen X, Wang S, Wu J, Duan S, Wang X, Hong X, et al. The application and challenge of binder jet 3D printing technology in pharmaceutical manufacturing. Pharmaceutics. 2022;14(12):2589.
9. Kaur SD, Kapoor DN. 3-D printing technology in pharmaceutical manufacturing. Pharma Times. 2023;55(11):15–6.
10. Awad A, Fina F, Goyanes A, Gaisford S, Basit AW. Advances in powder bed fusion 3D printing in drug delivery and healthcare. Adv Drug Deliv Rev [Internet]. 2021;174:406–24. Available from: https://doi.org/10.1016/j.addr.2021.04.025
11. Siddique SH, Hazell PJ, Wang H, Escobedo JP, Ameri AAH. Lessons from nature: 3D printed bio-inspired porous structures for impact energy absorption—a review. Addit Manuf [Internet]. 2022;58(April):103051. Available from: https://doi.org/10.1016/j.addma.2022.103051
12. Xu X, Awad A, Robles-Martinez P, Gaisford S, Goyanes A, Basit AW. Vat photopolymerization 3D printing for advanced drug delivery and medical device applications. J Control Release [Internet]. 2021;329:743–57. Available from: https://doi.org/10.1016/j.jconrel.2020.10.008
13. Alexander AE, Wake N, Chepelev L, Brantner P, Ryan J, Wang KC. A guideline for 3D printing terminology in biomedical research utilizing ISO/ASTM standards. 3D Print Med. 2021;7(1):4–9.
14. Serrano DR, Kara A, Luciano FC, Ongoren B, Anaya BJ, Molina G, et al. 3D printing technologies in personalized medicine, nanomedicines, and biopharmaceuticals. Pharmaceutics. 2023;15(2):313.
15. Tracy T, Wu L, Liu X, Cheng S, Li X. 3D printing: innovative solutions for patients and pharmaceutical industry. Int J Pharm [Internet]. 2023;631:122480. Available from: https://doi.org/10.1016/j.ijpharm.2022.122480
16. PK BG, Mehrotra S, Marques SM, Kumar L, Verma R. 3D printing in personalized medicines: a focus on applications of the technology. Mater Today Commun [Internet]. 2023;35(February):105875. Available from: https://doi.org/10.1016/j.mtcomm.2023.105875

17. Park S, Shou W, Makatura L, Matusik W, Fu KK. Review 3D printing of polymer composites: materials, processes, and applications. Mater [Internet]. 2022;5(1):43–76. Available from: https://doi.org/10.1016/j.matt.2021.10.018
18. Fuenmayor E, Forde M, Healy AV, Devine DM, Lyons JG, McConville C, et al. Comparison of fused-filament fabrication to direct compression and injection molding in the manufacture of oral tablets. Int J Pharm [Internet]. 2019;558(January):328–40. Available from: https://doi.org/10.1016/j.ijpharm.2019.01.013
19. Mahato R. Microneedles in drug delivery [Internet]. In: Emerging nanotechnologies for diagnostics, drug delivery and medical devices. Elsevier; 2017. p. 331–53. Available from: https://doi.org/10.1016/B978-0-323-42978-8.00013-9.
20. Maurizii G, Moroni S, Khorshid S, Aluigi A, Tiboni M, Casettari L. 3D-printed EVA-based patches manufactured by direct powder extrusion for personalized transdermal therapies. Int J Pharm [Internet]. 2023;635(February):122720. Available from: https://doi.org/10.1016/j.ijpharm.2023.122720
21. Wu Y, Liu J, Kang L, Tian J, Zhang X, Hu J, et al. An overview of 3D printed metal implants in orthopedic applications: present and future perspectives. Heliyon [Internet]. 2023;9(7):e17718. Available from: https://doi.org/10.1016/j.heliyon.2023.e17718
22. Yang X, Si X, Pan L, Li X, Ji Z, Shi C. Double-network structure sponge with enhanced mechanical properties, procoagulant potential, and 3D printability for acute hemorrhage. Chem Eng J [Internet]. 2024;487(March):150608. Available from: https://doi.org/10.1016/j.cej.2024.150608
23. Zhang X, Wang X, Yuan P, Ma C, Wang Y, Zhang Z, et al. A 3D-printed cuttlefish bone elastomeric sponge rapidly controlling noncompressible hemorrhage. Small. 2024;20(19):1–18.
24. Zaidi S, Naik P, Ahmed S. Three-dimensional printed instruments used in a septoplasty: a new paradigm in surgery. Laryngoscope Investig Otolaryngol. 2021;6(4):613–8.
25. Di Prima M, Coburn J, Hwang D, Kelly J, Khairuzzaman A, Ricles L. Additively manufactured medical products—the FDA perspective. 3D Print Med [Internet]. 2016;2(1):4–9. Available from: https://doi.org/10.1186/s41205-016-0005-9
26. Reddy CV, Balamuralidhara V, Venkatesh MP, Pramod Kumar TM. First FDA approved 3D printed drug paved new path for increased precision in patient care. Appl Clin Res Clin Trials Regul Aff. 2019;7(2):93–103.
27. Hybrid Medicines and 505(b)(2) NDA Approval Pathways [Internet]. [cited 2024 Jun 18]. Available from: https://www.altasciences.com/sites/default/files/202204/TheAltascientist_issue6_505B2_2022.pdf
28. Center for drug evaluation and research application number: 207958Orig1s000 [Internet]. [cited 2024 Jun 18]. Available from: https://www.accessdata.fda.gov/drugsatfda_docs/nda/2015/207958Orig1s000ClinPharmR.pdf
29. Highlights of prescribing information [Internet]. Available from: https://www.accessdata.fda.gov/drugsatfda_docs/label/2021/207958s019lbl.pdf
30. Jørgensen AK, Ong JJ, Parhizkar M, Goyanes A, Basit AW. Advancing non-destructive analysis of 3D printed medicines. Trends Pharmacol Sci [Internet]. 2023;44(6):379–93. Available from: https://doi.org/10.1016/j.tips.2023.03.006
31. Grangeia HB, Silva C, Simões SP, Reis MS. Quality by design in pharmaceutical manufacturing: a systematic review of current status, challenges and future perspectives. Eur J Pharm Biopharm [Internet]. 2020;147:19–37. Available from: https://doi.org/10.1016/j.ejpb.2019.12.007
32. Bendicho-Lavilla C, Rodríguez-Pombo L, Januskaite P, Rial C, Alvarez-Lorenzo C, Basit AW, et al. Ensuring the quality of 3D printed medicines: integrating a balance into a pharmaceutical printer for in-line uniformity of mass testing. J Drug Deliv Sci Technol [Internet]. 2024;92:105337. Available from: https://doi.org/10.1016/j.jddst.2024.105337
33. Yu DG, Shen XX, Branford-White C, Zhu LM, White K, Yang XL. Novel oral fast-disintegrating drug delivery devices with predefined inner structure fabricated by Three-Dimensional Printing. J Pharm Pharmacol. 2009;61(3):323–9.

34. Mohurle MSM, Asnani JA, Chaple RD, Kurian MJ, Bais GA. Quality by Design (QbD): an emerging trend in improving quality and development of pharmaceuticals. Saudi J Med Pharm Sci. 2019;05(12):1132–8.
35. Adalbert L, Kanti SPY, Jójárt-Laczkovich O, Akel H, Csóka I. Expanding quality by design principles to support 3D printed medical device development following the renewed regulatory framework in Europe. Biomedicines. 2022;10(11):2947.
36. Trenfield SJ. Quality control of 3D printed pharmaceuticals using process analytical technologies. [Doctoral dissertation, University College London]
37. Fanous M, Bitar M, Gold S, Sobczuk A, Hirsch S, Ogorka J, et al. Development of immediate release 3D-printed dosage forms for a poorly water-soluble drug by fused deposition modeling: Study of morphology, solid state and dissolution. Int J Pharm [Internet]. 2021;599:120417. Available from: https://doi.org/10.1016/j.ijpharm.2021.120417
38. Andreadis II, Gioumouxouzis CI, Eleftheriadis GK, Fatouros DG. Correction: the advent of a new era in digital healthcare: a role for 3D printing technologies in drug manufacturing? Pharmaceutics. 2022;14(12):609. https://doi.org/10.3390/pharmaceutics14030609.
39. Kreft K, Fanous M, Möckel V. The potential of three-dimensional printing for pediatric oral solid dosage forms. Acta Pharma. 2024;74(2):229–48.
40. Parhi R. A review of three-dimensional printing for pharmaceutical applications: quality control, risk assessment and future perspectives. J Drug Deliv Sci Technol [Internet]. 2021;64(February):102571. Available from: https://doi.org/10.1016/j.jddst.2021.102571
41. Rahman Z, Yang Y, Korang-Yeboah M, Siddiqui A, Xu X, Ashraf M, et al. Assessing impact of formulation and process variables on in-vitro performance of directly compressed abuse deterrent formulations [Internet]. Int J Pharma Elsevier BV. 2016;502:138–50. Available from: https://doi.org/10.1016/j.ijpharm.2016.02.029
42. Ng WL, An J, Chua CK. Process, material, and regulatory considerations for 3D printed medical devices and tissue constructs. Engineering. 2024;36:146–166
43. Beitler BG, Abraham PF, Glennon AR, Tommasini SM, Lattanza LL, Morris JM, et al. Interpretation of regulatory factors for 3D printing at hospitals and medical centers, or at the point of care. 3D Print Med. 2022;8(1):1–7.
44. Discussion Paper: 3D printing medical devices at the point of care.
45. Morrison RJ, Kashlan KN, Flanangan CL, Wright JK, Green GE, Hollister SJ, et al. Regulatory considerations in the design and manufacturing of implantable 3D-printed medical devices. Clin Transl Sci. 2015;8(5):594–600.
46. Hang Bob Yung C, Fung Tse L, Fung Edmond Yau W, Yi MS. Perspective chapter: additive manufacturing in customized medical device. In: Advanced additive manufacturing [Internet]; 2022. Available from: https://www.intechopen.com/chapters/79336#.
47. Khanna A. Gateway House. 2020. Regulations for 3D Printing.
48. Multiple departments jointly issued a document to support the development of additive manufacturing industry [Internet]. 2017 [cited 2024 May 19]. Available from: https://www.gov.cn/xinwen/2017-12/14/content_5246754.htm
49. Palma GF. Regulatory Open Forum-RAPS. [cited 2024 May 19]. NMPA focuses on 3D printed device: five guidelines issued in three months. Available from: https://connect.raps.org/communities/community-home/digestviewer/viewthread?GroupId=97&MessageKey=11bda3dc-7f64-43fe-b2d4-b8d729e40f65&CommunityKey=5af348a7-851e-4594-b467-d4d0983b6d89&hlmlt=VT. Accessed on 19/08/5/24.
50. CIRS [Internet]. [cited 2024 May 19]. Classification and category of medical devices in China. Available from: https://www.cirs-group.com/en/md/classification-and-category-of-medical-devices-in-china
51. Classify Your Medical Device [Internet]. Available from: https://www.fda.gov/medical-devices/overview-device-regulation/classify-your-medical-device
52. Jin Z, He C, Fu J, Han Q, He Y. Balancing the customization and standardization: exploration and layout surrounding the regulation of the growing field of 3D-printed medical devices in China. Bio-Design Manuf. 2022;5(3):580–606.

53. FDA's regulatory framework for 3D printing of medical devices at the point of care needs more clarity [Internet]. Available from: https://www.pewtrusts.org/en/research-and-analysis/issue-briefs/2022/07/fdas-regulatory-framework-for-3d-printing-of-medical-devices-needs-more-clarity
54. Administration F and D. Technical considerations for additive manufactured medical devices: guidance for industry and food and drug administration staff document. Center for Devices and Radiological Health; 2017. p. 1–30.
55. Bhise MG, Patel L, Patel K. 3D printed medical devices: regulatory standards and technological advancements in the USA, Canada and Singapore-A Cross-National Study. Int J Pharma Investig. 2024;14(3):888–902.
56. IMDRF/MDSAP WG and GTHF Documents [Internet]. Available from: https://www.fda.gov/medical-devices/medical-device-single-audit-program-mdsap/imdrfmdsap-wg-and-gthf-documents
57. IMDRF. Personalized Medical Devices Regulatory Pathways. Int Med Device Regul Forum [Internet]. 2019;2023(Edition 2):1–13. Available from: http://www.imdrf.org/docs/imdrf/final/consultations/imdrf-cons-pmd-rp.pdf
58. International Medical Device Regulators Forum. Definitions for personalized medical devices. Defin Pers Med Devices [Internet]. 2018;(October):10. Available from: http://www.imdrf.org/docs/imdrf/final/technical/imdrf-tech-181018-pmd-definitions-n49.pdf
59. IMDRF. Personalized medical devices regulatory pathways. Int Med Device Regul Forum [Internet]. 2023;2023(Edition 2):1–13. Available from: http://www.imdrf.org/docs/imdrf/final/consultations/imdrf-cons-pmd-rp.pdf
60. Therapeutic Goods Administration. Personalised medical devices (including 3D-printed devices) - Regulatory changes for custom-made medical devices. 2023;(December):Version 6.0.
61. What classification is my medical device? [Internet]. Available from: https://www.tga.gov.au/resources/what-classification-my-medical-device#node-554
62. A guide to TGA medical device classification [Internet]. Available from: https://vickipartridge.com/tga-medical-device-classification
63. Mohurle SM, Asnani AJ, Chaple DR, MAGB JK. Quality by Design (QbD): an emerging trend in improving quality & development of pharmaceuticals. Saudi J Med Pharm Sci. 2019;5(12):1132–8.
64. Use of International Standard ISO 10993-1, "Biological evaluation of medical devices - Part 1: evaluation and testing within a risk management process" [Internet]. [cited 2024 Jul 6]. Available from: https://www.fda.gov/regulatory-information/search-fda-guidance-documents/use-international-standard-iso-10993-1-biological-evaluation-medical-devices-part-1-evaluation-and
65. REGULATORY GUIDELINE FOR 3D PRINTED MEDICAL DEVICES. (2021). [Medical Devices Branch Medical Devices Cluster Health Products Regulation Group Health Sciences Authority].
66. Horst A, McDonald F. Uncertain but not unregulated: medical product regulation in the light of three-dimensional printed medical products. 3D Print Addit Manuf. 2020;7(5):248–57.
67. Therapeutic Goods Administration Department of Health. Consultation: proposed regulatory scheme for personalised medical devices, including 3D-printed devices. 2019;(February):1–23. Available from: https://www.tga.gov.au/sites/default/files/consultation-proposed-regulatory-scheme-personalised-medical-devices-including-3d-printed-devices.pdf
68. Ilias El Aita. Advantages and challenges of pharmaceutical 3D printing [Internet]. 2021. Available from: https://www.pharmaexcipients.com/news/advantages-challenges-pharmaceutical-3d-printing/
69. Ferraz C, Chaves M. 3D printing of medicines. Current challenges; 2021. p. 1–50.
70. Cui M, Pan H, Su Y, Fang D, Qiao S, Ding P, et al. Opportunities and challenges of three-dimensional printing technology in pharmaceutical formulation development. Acta Pharm Sin B [Internet]. 2021;11(8):2488–504. Available from: https://doi.org/10.1016/j.apsb.2021.03.015

71. Kar, N. (n.d.). 3D PRINTING IN PHARMACEUTICAL MANUFACTURING: AN OVERVIEW. World Journal of Pharmaceutical Research, 13(9):763–784.
72. Jamróz W, Szafraniec J, Kurek M, Jachowicz R. 3D printing in pharmaceutical and medical applications—recent achievements and challenges. Pharm Res. 2018;35(9):1–22.
73. Liu L, Fu K, Hong S, Wang Z, Mo M, Li S, et al. Improving the quality and clinical efficacy of subdivided levothyroxine sodium tablets by 3D printing technology. J Drug Deliv Sci Technol [Internet]. 2023;89(August):105008. Available from: https://doi.org/10.1016/j.jddst.2023.105008
74. González K, Larraza I, Berra G, Eceiza A, Gabilondo N. 3D printing of customized all-starch tablets with combined release kinetics. Int J Pharm. 2022;622:1–8.
75. Shaikhnag A. 2023. CurifyLabs launches GMP pharma inks for on-site 3D printing of personalized medicines. Available from: https://3dprintingindustry.com/news/curifylabs-launches-gmp-pharma-inks-for-on-site-3d-printing-of-personalized-medicines-225510/
76. abRx's pharmaceutical 3D printer for personalised medicines, M3DIMAKER™, is now available! [Internet] 2020. Available from: https://www.fabrx.co.uk/2020/04/06/fabrxs-pharmaceutical-3d-printer-for-personalised-medicines-m3dimaker-is-now-available
77. Bhuiyan SH. What are the legal issues related to 3D printing in medicine and healthcare [Internet]. 2021. Available from: https://blog.ipleaders.in/what-are-the-legal-issues-related-to-3d-printing-in-medicine-and-healthcare/
78. Hoffman DW. No 主観的健康感を中心とした在宅高齢者における 健康関連指標に関する共分散構造分析Title [Internet]. Available from: https://www.triastek.com/pipeline.html

Design and Development of 3D Printed Drug Formulations Using FDM Technique

5

Arti A. Bagada, Priya V. Patel, and Heena Bagada

Abstract

The growing need for customized pharmaceuticals and medical equipment has accelerated the influence of additive manufacturing in recent years. 3D printing has emerged as one of the most novel and powerful tools for precisely creating specifically designed dosage forms, tissue engineering, and disease modeling. The ability of 3D printing to generate pharmaceuticals with exact measurements tailored to particular patients' requirements has demonstrated the feasibility of manufacturing personalized medicines in innovative dosage forms. The discovery enables a clear vision of dose structures on various forms, sizes, and surfaces, as well as the obstacles connected with delivering them under such planned settings. The dissolving patterns of active pharmaceutical ingredients (APIs) in pharmaceutical formulations have a substantial impact on their pharmacokinetic behavior. Current successes include multifunctional drug delivery systems with faster release, customizable and personalized dose forms, implants and phantoms modeled after individual patient anatomy, and cell-based materials for regenerative medicine. Unlike traditional production processes, 3DP technology enables exact control of the geometry, internal structure, and surface area that influence dissolution kinetics. The current chapter summarizes all the advanced techniques in various 3D printed dosage forms with limitations and challenges.

Keywords

3D printed dosage form · FDM polymers · Approaches · Challenges

A. A. Bagada (✉) · P. V. Patel
Department of Pharmaceutical Sciences, Saurashtra University, Rajkot, Gujarat, India

H. Bagada
A. R. College of Pharmacy & G.H. Patel Institute of Pharmacy,
Vallabh Vidyanagar, Gujarat, India

K. Vinchurkar, S. Mane (eds.), *Innovations in Drug Manufacturing*,
https://doi.org/10.1007/978-981-96-9075-6_5

5.1 Introduction

Due to a fit-for-all methodology, conventional mass manufacture of dosage forms only achieves 30% effectiveness in attaining anticipated therapeutic objectives. Due to this deficiency, there is a growing interest in personalized therapy, which recognizes individuals' substantial genetic predispositions and the chromatin alterations that cause DNA epigenetic aberrations. By customizing therapy requirements to each patient's unique needs, this strategy seeks to improve outcomes and lessen the need for a one-size-fits-all approach [1].

Targeting, flexible drug administration, and effective diagnostic genetics are the main focuses of personalized medicine. Flexible dosage manufacturing techniques are used in patient-tailored formulations to provide precise and dynamic dose adjustments. This method is essential when a patient's therapy plan includes a variety of dosages or active pharmacological substances. The financial strain on healthcare systems drives the need for effective outpatient services, such as telehealth care, emphasizing the need for a digitally controlled, patient-tailored, safe, remote dose-controlling system [2].

Using computer-aided design (CAD) software, 3D printing is a 3D manufacturing process that includes building up layers of material to produce a 3D digital model. The pharmaceutical sector is using it more and more to provide individualized therapies. By adjusting API release, medication loading, size, shape, taste, and texture, 3DP approaches can improve patient forms' acceptance and customize them. Creating printed versions of novel pharmaceutical entities or creating polypills with many active ingredients are two further possible uses. Small, personalized batches of medications can also be produced in drug production facilities by utilizing 3D printers [3].

The creation of three-dimensional (3D) objects is achieved through the process of 3D printing, which involves the layer-by-layer deposition of materials using a computer-driven process based on a digital model. The pharmaceutical industry can benefit from this technology by delivering customized and on-demand medications to prevent unpredictable side effects and adverse reactions during drug therapy. Additionally, it can be used to formulate patient-centric fixed-dose combinations, which can reduce the need for multiple daily doses and consequently increase patient compliance. Various 3D printing techniques have been documented in the literature, including fused deposition modeling (FDM), binder deposition, pen-based 3D printing, molding, and inkjet printing [4].

The field of healthcare has shown great promise for 3D printing, especially in the area of customized medications. Because of its ease of use, fused deposition modeling, or FDM, is the most widely used method. FDM filaments are made of thermoplastic polymers impregnated with active pharmacological ingredients (APIs). 3D printing's physical characteristics are determined by extruder, process, and structural factors. FDM is a widely used 3D printing method because of its ease of use [5–8].

5.2 FDM Technologies for 3D Printed Drug Formulations

Using a rapid prototyping technique called three-dimensional (3D) printing, an object that has been previously created using computer software may be produced layer by layer. It is a form of additive manufacturing (AM) process [9, 10]. Active pharmaceutical ingredients (API) may be delivered to the body in a safe and regulated manner thanks to the widespread usage of 3D printing technology in medication delivery. Different formulas and geometries may be used to create tablets, giving exact control over the distribution of API in terms of both time and space. Tablet printing settings have an impact on the dissolving profile as well, which enhances patient compliance as well as safety and efficacy. Microneedles, implants, and oral dosage forms are the main applications for 3D printing, and the technology shows promise for transdermal medication administration [11].

Rapid prototyping, or 3D printing, is an additive manufacturing (AM) that entails three phases. Using computer-aided design (CAD) software, a medication formulation is designed in the first phase. The design is then exported with selected processing settings, such as printing temperature and speed, into a stereolitography file format for fast prototyping. After that, the printer produces sliced layers for production [11–14]. The creation of things by material deposition utilizing a print head, nozzle, or other printer technology is what the ISO refers to as three-dimensional printing [15]. There are six different types of 3D printing methods, each with unique difficulties: nozzle-based deposition systems, inkjet systems, and writing systems based on lasers [12, 13, 16]. Due to its low cost, compact equipment requirements, capacity for complicated prototype creation, and lack of organic solvent usage all of which facilitate the production of oral solid dosage forms and customized medication, FDM is a widely used 3D printing method in pharmaceutical research [13, 15, 17, 18]. The most widely used material extrusion-based additive manufacturing technique was developed in 1989 by Stratasys co-founder Scott Crump and is known as fused deposition modeling (FDM) [19].

FDM 3D printing involves the ejection of material from a nozzle, which is then distributed into successive layers on the build plate. The feed material is supplied as filaments, created by the physical combination of polymers and API melted extrusion [20]. A polymer-based intermediate product (IP) is melted and extruded during the FDM 3D printing process. A filament from a prior hot melt extrusion (HME) technique, employed in the pharmaceutical sector to create solid dispersions of the DDS type, can be utilized for the procedure. Feed hoppers are used to input the raw materials, which are then transferred to a screw assembly where temperature and energy are controlled to melt the materials. The process known as "fused filament fabrication" (FFF) 3DP begins when the filament emerges from the die as a filament and is heated by a printer's nozzle before deposition [3].

Thermoplastic polymers such as polylactic acid (PLA), polycarbonate (PC), and acrylonitrile butadiene styrene (ABS) are used in the material extrusion method known as FDM [19, 21]. The procedure comprises storing the filaments on a roller that is attached to a build platform in Z and an extrusion head that travels in X and Y directions. There is a 1.75–3.0 mm variance in the filament diameter. Three phases make up the FDM technique: pre-processing, manufacturing, and post-processing. CAD software is used to produce product designs, which are then saved in STL format for later pre-processing. Before slicing the file, important factors including machine temperature, building orientation, and slicing parameters are taken into account [22, 23]. Software such as Idea Maker or Quick Slice is used for the slicing, and the tool path is marked with G-code. After being heated to the semi-liquid state, the feedstock material forms two-dimensional layers on top of the build platform. Up until 3D things are formed, the layers form. The filament is printed with a dimensional precision of 100 μm and heated between 150 and 300 °C [24]. Initially, the support foundation is printed before the necessary item is produced. Post-processing is applied to the finished product to enhance surface quality [25, 26]. Chemical and mechanical post-processing procedures are available. Chemical techniques include painting, coating, heating, and vapor deposition, while mechanical processes include vibratory, machining, sanding, abrasive, and barrel finishing [24].

Feed mechanisms and heads are used to categorize various FDM techniques. With the single-head process, composite materials such as metals, fibers, wood, and polymers are produced using a single filament. This process can only be used to fabricate objects made of many types of material. Compared to the single-head approach, the dual-head method is quicker and allows for the creation of components with various materials by using two material filaments. This technique is applied to the creation of skeletal structures such as square cells and honeycombs. Because filaments are delivered directly into the nozzle head, mixed, and printed, the in-nozzle impregnation process is distinct [27, 28].

5.2.1 Excipients of FDM 3D Printing Techniques

5.2.1.1 Polymers

Polymers are the most often utilized materials in 3D printing to build a product or prototype. Acrylonitrile butadiene styrene (ABS), polylactic acid (PLA), polyethylene (PE), polypropylene (PP), nylon/polyamide (PA), and polycarbonates (PC) are among the materials that are often utilized in the FDM process [8, 29, 30].

Because of poor physical qualities, pure polymers like PLA, PA, and ABS are mostly utilized for prototypes. On the other hand, components that need better qualities are made of polystyrene (PS), polyethyleneimine (PEI), polyetherketoneketone (PEKK), and polyetheretherketone (PEEK). These materials possess high mechanical, thermal, and chemical resistance qualities. Since they have poor physical qualities, ABS, PLA, and PA are mostly used for prototypes. Other specific ABS materials, such as ABSi, ABS-M30, ABS-M30i, ABS-ESD7, and ABS Plus, are also utilized as the printing medium in FDM processors. In contrast, for components that need better quality, materials such as polyethyleneimine, polystyrene (PS), polyetheretherketone (PEEK), polyetherketoneketone (PEKK), and polyetherimide (PEI) are utilized. High mechanical, thermal, and chemical resistance qualities are possessed by these materials [31–33].

5.2.1.2 Composites

To make the composite fabrics, polymers, ceramic, fibers, and nanomaterials were added to the foundation polymers. Two primary categories of materials are employed with polymers: biodegradable and non-biodegradable materials.

5.2.1.2.1 Biodegradable Materials for FDM

A market for bio-based plastics has emerged as a result of the increased demand for eco-friendly polymers, especially in recyclable and medicinal items. Compared to non-biodegradable materials, biodegradable materials like PLA and ABS are less expensive, easier to find, and have better mechanical qualities. For these reasons, they are utilized in composites [34]. Because of their compatibility, PLA/PCL blends have been the subject of much recent research on polymer blends for biomedical purposes. Mechanical features of PCL/PLA composite combined with PEG, high impact strength, and elastic modulus values were observed in one investigation. The elongation of acetyl tributyl citrate was shown to be increased in another study that looked at the mechanical, thermal, and morphological properties of biodegradable blends of poly(3 hydroxybutyrate), poly (lactic acid), and plasticizer [35, 36].

Alumina, silica, zirconia, calcium phosphate, and bioactive glass ceramics are examples of biodegradable ceramic materials that are utilized to substitute human bone. PLA/ceramic composites have delivered a greater tensile modulus and strength in one investigation. Polyamide 12 was examined using β-TCP and zirconia in another investigation [37–39]. Natural fibers are very strong, reasonably priced, and biodegradable. When it comes to mechanical qualities, composites outperform PLA. Composites made of PLA with continuous flax fiber (CFF) exhibit improved stiffness and tensile strength. Composites made of PLA/jute and PLA/flax fibers exhibit higher stiffness and tensile strength. Additionally, different PLA/flax and PLA/bamboo l/d ratios enhance stiffness [40–44].

5.2.1.2.2 Non-biodegradable Materials for FDM

The reason non-biodegradable bioplastics are interesting is that their microbial degrading persistence strikes a compromise between the benefits of reduced carbon footprint during manufacturing and improved resource quality [45]. The study shows that blends of PA6 and PP have excellent mechanical and dimensional stability, with an appropriate SME deformation temperature of 175 °C. A PMMA and ABS polymer combination with a decreased impact strength of 14.9 kJ/m^2 was created. Comparing the mechanical characteristics of PolyFlexTM/ABS blend with other materials showed their potential for a range of uses [46, 47].

Powdered iron and aluminum are often used as fillers in PMC. The mechanical characteristics of PLA reinforced with bronze fill powder and magnetic iron were compared. The results showed lower mechanical strength than the original materials. ABS/copper composites' dynamic mechanical characteristics revealed increased tan delta, loss modulus, storage modulus, and glass transition temperature. A metal flow study of the ABS-iron polymer-metal composite was carried out in one of the investigations [48, 49].

Short and continuous fibers were mixed with polymers to improve the mechanical characteristics of 3D printed goods, providing stiffness, corrosion resistance, and lightweight [50]. Using compression molding and FDM printing, the microstructure, processability, and mechanical characteristics of an ABS/CF reinforced composite were investigated. Varied amounts of ABS were used to strengthen the composite, and varied temperatures were used to extrude the filament. The ABS filament that included 40% CF was unable to print because of nozzle blockage. Investigations into the anisotropic features of short carbon fiber-filled polypropylene revealed that 10-weight percent of CF combined with PLA had superior qualities [51, 52]. Separate filaments for CFR and thermoplastic are fed into the nozzle, fused therein, and deposited over the build platform. When it comes to mechanical qualities, CFR composites outperform short fibers. Due to the continuous nature of the fiber, co-extrusion printing is used in printing, or dual-head printers are used. The mechanical properties were examined for continuous-fiber nylon thermoplastic [53–55].

For improved architectures, nanofillers such as carbonaceous, nano clay, and metallic nanofiller are recycled into hydrogels, polymer matrices, thermoplastics, and resins. The sensing device, aerospace, and home sectors employ these electrically conductive nanocomposites [56]. The mechanical and thermal characteristics of ABS/montmorillonite nanocomposites were investigated; these parameters showed that FDM printed components had less strength than injection-molded ones. The PLA/clay nanocomposite, which was employed with PLA 4032D and PLA 2003D, demonstrated greater elastic modulus and thermal stability than regular PLA at various temperatures [57–59].

5.3 Approaches of FDM Technology for 3D Printed Drug Formulations

Three-dimensional (3D) printing is undergoing a remarkable evolution which is leading to its exponentially growing use. It was initially used to make molds or prototypes; however, its use expanded due to its accurate and reproducible design capabilities in a range of materials. This allowed faster fabrication of prototypes in a range of sizes, styles, materials, and colors. 3D printing is now accessible to the public and a basic fused deposition modeling (FDM) printer can be easily bought at a shopping mall. The FDM technology is remarkably cheaper than other additive manufacturing (AM) techniques due to its simplicity [60, 61].

Polymers are utilized as the raw material (filament) in fused deposition modeling (FDM), commonly referred to as material extrusion additive manufacturing technology. Typically, the filament is heated to a molten condition and then forced into the device's nozzle (3D printer). Following the G-code instructions, the nozzle head may move in three degrees of freedom (DoF) to place the extruded polymer on the build plate [62].

The use of modern additive manufacturing (AM) technology, often known as 3D printing, has increased since the 1980s. A vast variety of materials, such as polymers, metals, ceramics, food, and biomaterials, may be used due to these technologies [63]. The ability to generate items directly without requiring a whole technological infrastructure, the ability to manufacture products with complicated geometries, design equality, economical material usage, and environmental friendliness are only a few advantages of three-dimensional printing [64]. The three most important additive manufacturing (AM) processes are fused deposition modeling (FDM), selective laser sintering (SLS), and stereolithography (SLA). The first additively developed process was stereolithography, which used UV-cured resins as the building material and was based on photopolymerization [65].

This approach is well-known for its excellent accuracy in creating objects without the need for post-processing as compared to other methods. The SLS technique is a powder polymer-based printing process. This approach involves moving the laser beam in a predetermined direction, sintering the polymer powder in layers as a result of the heat created until a three-dimensional model is achieved [66]. Stratasys inventor Scot Crump created fused deposition modeling, also known as fused filament fabrication (FDM/FFF), in 1988. It was sold under the brand name FDM (US Patent No. 5 738 817). The construction material for this technique is a thermoplastic filament, which is supplied to the head at the proper melting temperature after being installed on a spool. To create a three-dimensional item with the required shape and geometry, molten material is deposited layer by layer through a nozzle of a certain diameter throughout the printing process [29, 67]. In industrial applications, the FDM technique using thermoplastic filament is the most popular choice. Of all the methods discussed, FDM is the most popular since it uses inexpensive hardware (three-dimensional printers), and a wide range of inexpensive and high-quality filaments are readily available. Technically speaking, one of the key ideas behind Industry 4.0, or the fourth industrial revolution, is 3D printing technology. Many advantages are associated with it, including the possibility to construct complicated geometries and intelligent materials, less human participation, digital data transmission, remote access, reduced waste creation, and fewer needs for final processing. Each of these traits is ideal for achieving Industry 4.0's objectives [68]. Additionally, they satisfy the ever-expanding demands of the market, which include the creation of goods for the needs of specific entities, the manufacture of goods for fast-changing client requirements, and the desire for high-quality goods at the lowest feasible production costs, particularly in low-volume production situations [69].

The initial effort to use PVA filaments and the FDM process to create fluorescence [7]. It demonstrated that the appropriate drug release pattern could be achieved by adjusting the infill density. 4-ASA and 5-ASA are utilized for colon therapy as things proceed. While 5-ASA is thermally stable and prints satisfactorily, 4-ASA's thermolabile characteristic deteriorates during printing. It demonstrates that the FDM process is appropriate for using non-thermolabile components [20].

Another area where FDM is helpful is in tablet geometry, which is not achievable with other 3D printing methods. The possibility of creating geometric forms like spheres, toruses, and pyramids has been successfully shown. It is feasible to achieve consistent geometry with diverse forms by altering the filaments' dimensions. Additionally, medication loading can be changed to meet the needs of the patient. With the right printer settings, the drug release kinetics with a specific aim may be attained. It is among the greatest methods for creating customized formulas [70, 71].

There are now three primary methods for creating 3D tablets using FDM technology: (1) Dipping-melting method: In order to create an API-containing filament for printing, the filament is dipped into a solution or dispersion (2) HME-FDM: This is the most widely used method right now for preparing 3D printed medications. The API is introduced to the conveyor together with the excipients, and the filaments containing the API are acquired by the extrusion unit. (3) Filling and shaping method: print an empty shell first, then fill in the API; printing and filling can be done in either a sequential or simultaneous fashion [6, 72–75].

Extrusion of hot melt HME is a stand-alone process for creating appropriate feedstock (filaments) for FDM 3D printing. In HME, spinning screws on a shaft pump materials through an extruder barrel at the necessary temperature. After the mixture in the barrel is run through a die, the desired product is extruded. A consistent, flexible filament whose diameter varies depending on the kind of 3D printer being used is the HME extrudate for AM [76, 77]. Crucial HME parameters: The performance of the extrusion process is greatly influenced by material, process, and equipment properties. Polymers and active pharmaceutical ingredients (APIs) are crucial for a successful HME. This process is impacted by thermal material expansion, miscibility between the polymer and API, extrudate homogeneity, and polymer and API characteristics. Temperature, pressure, torque, feed rate, die shape and diameter, screw configuration and speed, and feedstock quality are all impacted by these factors [78].

5.3.1 Coupling HME with FDM 3D Printing

In recent years, there has been a surge in fascination with 3D printing for pharmaceutical applications. In contrast to other 3D printing methods, the greatest research has been done on hot melt extrusion (HME)-based fused deposition modelling (FDM) 3D printing for patient-focused dosing. FDM 3D printing may be used with HME technology to create a continuous production process. However, in order to create HME-coupled FDM 3D printing, it is necessary to examine the critical medicinal polymers, formulation, and process parameters [78] These developments will pave the path for the creation of continuous medication delivery systems for individualized treatment. Coupling HME with FDM 3D printing process was shown in Fig. 5.1.

In order to ensure that both processes are in sync when combining HME with FDM 3D printing as a continuous production process, real-time monitoring and control are necessary. Many spectroscopic methods, including Raman, NIR, MIR,

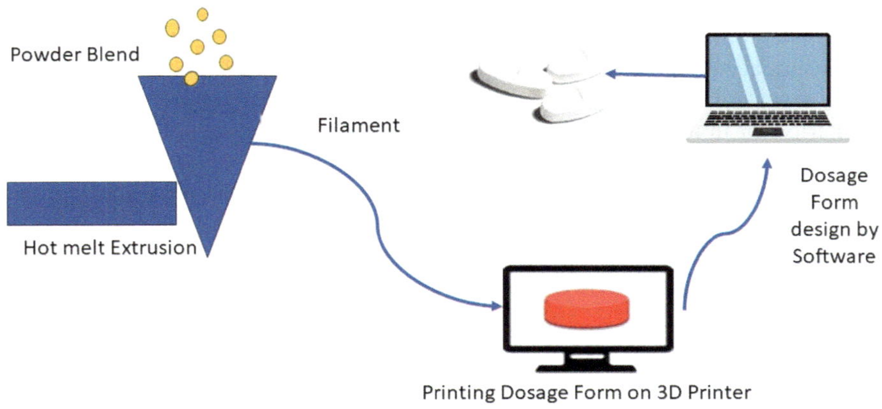

Fig. 5.1 FDM 3D printing with hot melt extrusion

FTIR, and UV/VIS, have been investigated recently as potential PAT tools for HME. However, there is not much use for these techniques in FDM 3D printing of pharmaceuticals. PAT instruments offer continuous, high-throughput material screening throughout the manufacture of medicinal products and are nondestructive [79–84].

Even though HME and FDM 3D printing are two different processes, stopping one affects the other and changes a medicine product's crucial quality characteristics. PAT instruments gather and process data quickly and efficiently. As a result, their application may improve the dependability and effectiveness of HME combined 3D printing as a CM method for producing superior, personalized pharmaceutical items. The combination of quality by design (QbD) and PAT tools will establish the CQA for pharmaceutical items. API concentration, solid state, API dispersion, filament texture diameter, melt viscosity, mechanical feedstock qualities, and 3D printing characteristics in a 3D printer are the CQA for finished drug items produced by HME-coupled 3D printing. PAT tools ought to be used in HME-coupled 3D at different stages. Zhang et al. (2017) examined the viability of combining FDM 3D printing methods with HME. The authors attempted to create paracetamol formulations with prolonged release by using several grades of HPC, HPMC polymers, Eudragit L100, Soluplus, and ethylcellulose N14. Tablets made using FDM 3D printing showed the expected prolonged release of medication compared to those made through direct compression methods [85]. Tan et al. conducted a literature study in 2018 to determine if combining HME with FDM 3D printing processes is appropriate [86]. Likewise, a number of polymers that are appropriate for HME linked FDM 3D printing techniques have been covered by Pereira GG et al. [87]. These few papers in the literature shed light on the use of polymers and PAT tools to create HME and FDM 3D printing as a continuous process, as well as how to couple both of these approaches [78].

In terms of medications, 3D printing oral dosage forms have been tried mostly for BCS class II or IV pharmaceuticals as a way to improve solubility and bioavailability (primarily accomplished by the prior HME), as well as because of the clinical limitations the drugs bring. Actually, 3D printing is seen as a benefit to help pharmaceuticals meet clinical needs. This can be achieved in one of two ways: (a) by repeatedly adjusting dosage based on body mass or age (e.g., theophylline in pediatrics) or in the case of drugs with narrow therapeutic margins (e.g., warfarin used to prevent thromboembolic events); (b) by improving organoleptic properties by taste masking and producing dosage forms appropriate for a specific age group (e.g., children), such as children; (c) using numerous medications in one unit to manage polymedication, complex therapy regimens, drug incompatibility, or the necessity for distinct release characteristics of the same medicine (e.g., metformin and glimepiride) [87].

Nonetheless, since FDM is a developing technology, it is important to recognize and tackle its drawbacks. To begin with, FDM 3D printing might not be the best option for mass production, as tablet machines tend to be quicker than printers [88]. Nonetheless, it might fill a present therapeutic need in terms of the requirement for customized therapy, acting as an adjunct or substitute to traditional industrial manufacturing [89, 90]. Second, the use of heat in drug inclusion techniques used before FDM is still a source for concern. Drug candidates are restricted to thermostable chemicals, even though HME allows high and customizable drug loading. In addition, high temperatures are needed during the printing process to melt the filament during extrusion, which might lead to problems with physical instability and deterioration. Therefore, FDM-based printing is not appropriate for pharmaceutical or biological applications involving thermosensitive medications. This indicates that FDM-specific polymers with lower melting temperatures need to be developed. Third, adding an additive to the matrix can alter the thermoplastic characteristics of the polymeric filaments, which may modify attributes like viscosity and flexibility that affect extrudability and printability. Lastly, support structures add to material waste when they are required for objects with complicated geometry or vast base areas to prevent warping by enhancing the adhesion between the specimen and the build platform. Furthermore, it is challenging to remove the inner scaffold needed to support hollow objects in methods that are scaled up [91].

When used in tandem to make pharmaceutical dosage forms and medical equipment, FDM and HME 3D printing technologies have demonstrated several benefits, simplifying the intricate procedures of traditional production techniques. The complete 3D printing process of a dosage form begins with the digital design, choosing the raw materials (polymer, drug, and excipients, if necessary), and measuring the heat of melting of the powder mixture to create filaments that, when cooled, will feed the FDM printer to create the dosage form by the computer's instructions [87].

5.3.2 FDM Technology in Pharmaceuticals

FDM technology has been widely utilized to produce a wide range of preparations due to its characteristics. For instance, this technology was used in the first study to test patient acceptability of 3D printed preparations of various sizes and shapes.

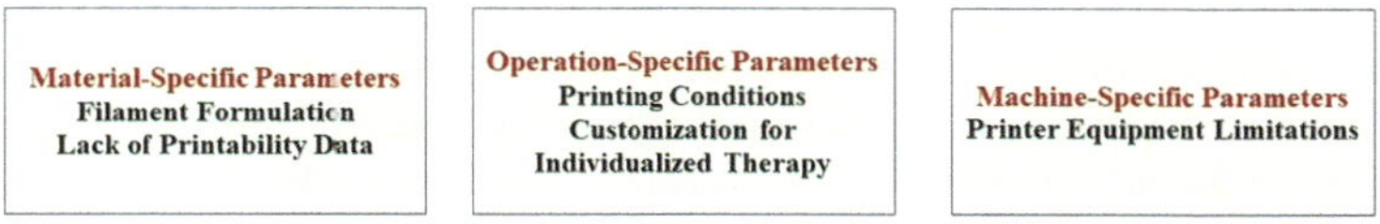

Fig. 5.2 Challenges of fused deposition modeling (FDM) 3D printing in pharmaceutical applications

Researchers also used it to prepare and test preparations of various colors, which demonstrated that smaller, circular-shaped tablets were more acceptable [92]. Furthermore, aripiprazole oral dispersion films were prepared by Jamróz et al. using FDM technology, and in vitro, research results revealed that the 3D printed films had greater dissolving rates. The creation of controlled-release formulations is another use for FDM technology. Lim et al., for instance, printed hollow scaffolds with several tiny holes for continuous medication release. The scaffold was made of a hollow base covered in a lid. The scaffolds with side holes were demonstrated to have zero-order kinetics and slow-release characteristics [93]. Multiple nozzles can be added to FDM printers to print compound preparations made up of various materials. Using paracetamol and caffeine as model drugs, Goyanes et al. used this technology in 2015 to prepare multilayer capsules and double capsules. As seen in Fig. 5.2, the double capsules are made up of one drug encapsulated in a shell made of the other drug, while the multilayer capsules are made up of one drug and one subsequent layer of another drug [94]. FDM technology has also found application in the field of transdermal drug delivery, as demonstrated by Goyanes et al. [95]. Muwaffak et al. used FDM technology in 2016 to make personalized nasal masks that helped patients cure their acne more effectively by delivering medication topically [96]. FDM technology has been used to print personalized wound dressings in the form of ears and noses [75].

5.4 Application of 3D Printing Technologies in 3D Printed Drug Formulations Modified-Release Dosage Form

5.4.1 Sustained-Release Formulations

One of the primary applications of FDM 3D printing in pharmaceuticals is the development of sustained-release formulations. These formulations are designed to release the drug at a predetermined rate, maintaining therapeutic levels over an extended period [97, 98]. A study demonstrated the use of FDM 3D printing to create gastric-floating tablets of verapamil hydrochloride in different shapes (cylinder, capsule, and hemisphere) with low infill percentages. The shapes and infill percentages significantly influenced the drug release profiles and floating behaviors, highlighting the potential of FDM for personalized sustained-release drug delivery systems. The study focused on developing sustained-release gastric-floating formulations of verapamil hydrochloride using fused deposition modeling (FDM) 3D printing technology. Results demonstrated that the drug-loaded filaments were successfully used to print gastric-floating formulations, with verapamil hydrochloride maintaining its thermal stability during the process. The different shapes and infill percentages influenced the drug release profiles and floating behaviors, with potential implications for optimizing sustained-release and gastric retention properties for improved therapeutic outcomes [99].

Chai et al. used hot hot-melt extrusion (HME) to create hydroxypropyl cellulose (HPC) filaments loaded with domperidone (DOM) for use in FDM 3D printers. These filaments were 3D printed into hollow, intragastric floating sustained-release tablets, which float due to their low density achieved by adjusting shell numbers and infill percentage. This method shows FDM 3D printers as a cost-effective way to make floating drug delivery devices [100].

Okwuosa et al. produced delayed-release, gastric-resistant tablets with a dual-extruder FDM 3D printer. They used polyvinylpyrrolidone (PVP) for the core and a methacrylic acid polymer for the enteric coating, both made using HME. This proved that FDM printers could create enteric-coated tablets in a single process. Goyanes et al. made modified-release paracetamol tablets using FDM 3D printing without needing an enteric coating. They used HME to produce paracetamol-loaded filaments mixed with different grades of hypromellose acetate succinate (HPMCAS), resulting in tablets with varying delayed-release properties based on the pH threshold of the excipients used. Li et al. combined HME and FDM to produce a novel controlled-release device for diabetes treatment. They loaded Glipizide onto PVA filaments using HME, then used a dual-extruder FDM printer to create a double-chamber table (DuoTablet) with different drug concentrations in each chamber for a sustained-release profile [101].

5.4.2 Bilayer Tablets Using FDM 3D Printing

Bilayer tablets can be designed using FDM to provide immediate and sustained drug release within a single dosage form.

Researchers developed a bilayer tablet of diclofenac sodium using FDM 3D printing, where the tablet featured a honeycomb structure for immediate release and a filled structure for sustained release. This design ensured a rapid onset of action followed by prolonged therapeutic effects, showcasing the versatility of FDM in creating complex drug delivery systems [102]. FDM 3D printing technology offers immense potential in the development of bilayer tablets, allowing for precise control over drug release profiles and the combination of multiple drugs in a single dosage form. Its ability to customize drug delivery systems, fabricate complex geometries, and improve patient compliance makes it a valuable tool in pharmaceutical research and manufacturing. As technology continues to evolve, it is expected to play a pivotal role in the future of personalized medicine and advanced drug delivery systems.

5.4.3 Extended-Release Formulations Using FDM 3D Printing

Extended-release formulations are designed to release the drug slowly over time, reducing dosing frequency and improving patient compliance. Cui et al. developed extended-release Levetiracetam tablets using FDM 3D printing with PLA as the polymer matrix. The tablets exhibited controlled drug release over extended periods, demonstrating the potential of FDM in producing effective extended-release formulations [103]. Goyanes et al. used FDM 3D printing to create modified-release Paracetamol tablets without the need for an enteric coating. They utilized HME to produce Paracetamol-loaded filaments mixed with different grades of hypromellose acetate succinate (HPMCAS), resulting in tablets with varying delayed-release properties based on the pH threshold of the excipients used [18].

Theophylline-loaded tablets were fabricated using FDM 3D printing, with different shell thicknesses to control the drug release rate. This approach demonstrated the feasibility of customizing drug release profiles through tablet design and printing parameters [18]. FDM 3D printing technology holds immense potential in the development of extended-release tablets, offering precise control over drug release profiles and the ability to fabricate complex dosage forms tailored to individual therapeutic needs. As technology continues to evolve, it is expected to play a crucial role in advancing personalized medicine and improving patient outcomes through innovative drug delivery systems [94].

The 3D printed tablets showed better extended-release rates due to smoother surfaces and tighter structures, proving that a single process can produce various formulations. Using hydroxypropyl methylcellulose (HPMC) as a matrix material, researchers printed tablets with different designs to achieve various drug release profiles, showing that 3D design effectively optimizes controlled drug release rates [94]. Goyanes et al. also made controlled-release budesonide tablets using a similar approach, combining FDM, HME, and fluid bed coating. These tablets released the drug in the small intestine and continued sustained release in the distal intestine and colon, demonstrating the feasibility of this combined method for modified-release oral dosage forms [104].

Okwuosa et al. combined FDM 3D printing and liquid dispensing to create individualized dosage forms on demand. They used polymethacrylate shells made with FDM, filled with a drug solution or suspension, to achieve controlled drug release. Adjusting the shell thickness allowed for extended-release without changing the formulation. This approach improves patient compliance by masking taste and odor and can be adapted to various liquid formulations. It also avoids the need for material compatibility with FDM's high temperatures. This work demonstrated a fully automated process using a dual-head FDM printer with a syringe-based liquid dispenser, proving FDM's capability to produce individualized dosage forms [105].

5.4.4 Rapid/Immediate-Release Dosage Forms

Creating rapid or immediate-release dosage forms using FDM 3D printing involves leveraging the technology's capability to produce intricate designs and precise drug release profiles. FDM 3D printing has been utilized to create immediate-release tablets by adjusting parameters such as infill density and layer thickness. This customization helps in achieving rapid dissolution and absorption of drugs, crucial for medications requiring quick therapeutic effects. The ability of FDM 3D printing to produce tablets with complex geometries (e.g., porous structures) enhances the surface area available for dissolution, thereby facilitating faster drug release. This approach is advantageous for drugs with high solubility and rapid absorption requirements. As FDM technology continues to advance, incorporating novel polymers and precise printing techniques will further enhance its capability to produce rapid-release dosage forms. This evolution holds promise for developing innovative pharmaceutical products that meet diverse clinical needs [86].

Although FDM 3D printing has been extensively studied for various drug delivery systems, it has not been widely adopted for producing immediate-release tablets due to their typically slower dissolution rates compared to conventionally manufactured tablets [106]. Okwuosa et al. found that FDM 3D printed Theophylline tablets made from Eudragit® E and PVP with plasticizers required 30 minutes for complete drug release. However, efforts to enhance dissolution rates have been explored, such as by using different polymeric carriers [105].

In another study, pantoprazole sodium tablets made from various polymers (PVP K12, PEG 6000, Kollidon® VA64, PEG 20000, and poloxamer 407) showed varying drug release profiles, with PVP exhibiting the fastest release completed within 10 minutes. Adjusting the infill rate during printing to increase tablet porosity further improved dissolution rates [107]. Kollamaram et al. successfully printed immediate-release formulations of Ramipril at lower temperatures using Kollidon VA64 and Kollidon 12PF as carriers, without thermal drug degradation observed on the tablets [108].

Furthermore, Solanki et al. demonstrated the feasibility of FDM 3D printing for rapid drug release formulations using haloperidol as a model drug. Tablets with 60% infill exhibited faster drug release (45 minutes) than 100% infill tablets due to their porous nature. The optimal polymer system for these formulations was a mixture of Kollidon® VA-64 and AffinisolTM 15 cP, providing flexibility and mechanical strength suitable for 3D printing [109].

These studies collectively illustrate the potential of FDM 3D printing to fabricate immediate-release dosage forms by leveraging appropriate polymers and printing parameters.

5.4.5 Drug-Loaded Implants

Kempin et al. utilized hot melt extrusion (HME) to produce quinine-loaded filaments for use in FDM 3D printers to create drug-loaded implants. They compared the drug release rates of various polymers, including Eudragit® RS, polycaprolactone (PCL), poly(L-lactide) (PLLA), and ethyl cellulose (EC). The study revealed that PCL exhibited the fastest drug release, while Eudragit and EC had the slowest. This research demonstrated the feasibility of using FDM 3D printing to manufacture drug-loaded implants, as it can produce products in almost any shape, designed to function as implants and incorporate a desired drug delivery system [107].

Genina et al. used ethylene vinyl acetate (EVA) as a drug carrier to produce drug-loaded EVA filaments via HME. The EVA filaments, loaded with indomethacin, were used in FDM 3D printers to fabricate custom-made T-shaped intrauterine systems (IUS) and subcutaneous rods (SR). The aim was to investigate the printability of different grades of EVA copolymers as new feedstock material for FDM 3D printing in drug delivery devices. The IUS and SR were successfully printed at a temperature just above the drug's melting point, proving that EVA 5 polymer has the required properties to be made into filaments for FDM 3D printing of drug delivery systems [110].

Fu et al. successfully used FDM 3D printing to produce personalized progesterone-loaded vaginal rings. Progesterone was mixed with polyethylene glycol (PEG) 4000 to form a solid dispersion, cut into pieces, and combined with a mixture of PLA and PCL (8:2) and Tween 80 in a desktop single screw extruder. The resulting filaments were used to print vaginal rings in "O," "Y," or "M" shapes. The "O" ring exhibited a higher dissolution rate due to its higher surface area/volume ratio and provided long-term sustained release of progesterone for over 7 days with diffusion-controlled release behavior. This work further confirmed that HME and FDM 3D printing are effective methods for preparing personalized and customized medications [111].

5.4.6 Dosage Forms with Multiple Medications

Fused deposition modeling (FDM) 3D printing has been explored extensively for creating dosage forms containing multiple medications, offering precise control over drug release profiles, and the ability to customize medication combinations for individual patient needs. One of the studies investigated the potential of FDM 3D printing to produce multi-layered tablets, where each layer contained a different drug. They utilized hot melt extrusion (HME) to produce drug-loaded filaments and then used FDM 3D printing to create tablets with distinct layers. This approach allowed for the controlled release of multiple drugs from a single dosage form, with each layer dissolving at a different rate [112].

Goyanes and his team explored FDM 3D printing to create polypills containing multiple active pharmaceutical ingredients (APIs). They printed tablets with compartments containing different drugs, enabling the simultaneous administration of multiple medications in one pill. This method effectively produced personalized medication regimens, improved patient adherence, and simplified treatment protocols [18]. Sadia et al. developed a dual drug release system using FDM 3D printing. They fabricated tablets with two separate compartments, each containing a different drug with a distinct release mechanism. This allowed for both medications' simultaneous yet controlled release, enhancing therapeutic efficacy and patient convenience [88].

Khaled and colleagues utilized FDM 3D printing to create multi-drug tablets with customized dissolution profiles. They incorporated various excipients and polymers to modulate drug release rates and achieve sequential release of multiple drugs. This approach highlighted the flexibility of FDM 3D printing in producing complex dosage forms tailored to specific therapeutic needs [113].

These studies collectively illustrate how FDM 3D printing can revolutionize the production of dosage forms containing multiple medications by enabling precise control over drug release profiles and the customization of medication combinations, thus enhancing the effectiveness and convenience of multi-drug therapies.

5.4.7 Complex-Shaped Medicines

Fused deposition modeling (FDM) 3D printing has opened new possibilities for producing complex-shaped medicines, enabling personalized and efficient drug delivery systems. This technology allows for the precise design and fabrication of dosage forms with intricate geometries, which can significantly enhance drug release profiles, patient adherence, and therapeutic outcomes. Goyanes and colleagues demonstrated the use of FDM 3D printing to create innovative tablet designs, such as pyramidal and cylindrical shapes, to modulate drug release rates. These complex geometries increase the surface area of the tablets, allowing for a more controlled and sustained release of the active pharmaceutical ingredient (API). The study highlighted that the shape and surface area of the tablets could be precisely controlled using 3D printing, offering new ways to optimize drug delivery [18].

Norman et al. utilized FDM 3D printing to develop gyroid lattice tablets, which possess a highly porous structure. These gyroid designs enable rapid disintegration and improved drug release rates, making them suitable for immediate-release formulations. The study showed that such complex shapes could be used to achieve desired dissolution profiles by manipulating the internal structure of the tablets [114]. Khaled and colleagues explored the potential of FDM 3D printing to produce polypills with multiple compartments, each containing a different drug. They designed and printed a complex multi-layered tablet with distinct compartments for individual APIs. This approach not only simplified the medication regimen but also allowed for the controlled release of multiple drugs from a single dosage form, enhancing patient compliance and therapeutic efficacy [113]. Trenfield et al. developed personalized, complex-shaped chewable tablets using FDM 3D printing. These tablets were designed with intricate shapes, such as animals and geometric patterns, to improve pediatric patient compliance. The study demonstrated that FDM 3D printing could be used to produce visually appealing and patient-friendly dosage forms, potentially improving adherence in specific patient populations [115].

Scoutaris et al. investigated the use of FDM 3D printing to fabricate tablets with intricate internal geometries. These designs aimed to enhance drug dissolution rates by increasing the surface area and porosity of the tablets. The study found that the internal architecture of the tablets played a crucial role in achieving the desired drug release profiles, showcasing the versatility of 3D printing in creating complex-shaped medicines [116]. In Table 5.1 some modified release formulations using FDM 3D printing are shown.

Table 5.1 List of modified release formulation using FDM 3D printing

Drug	Formulation	Shapes	Materials	Purpose	Key findings	References
Verapamil hydrochloride	Sustained-release gastric-floating	Cylinder, capsule, hemisphere	HPMC, Soluplus®	Treat hypertension and angina	Different shapes and infill percentages influenced drug release and floating behavior	[117]
Diclofenac sodium	Bilayer tablet	Tablet with honeycomb and filled structures	Polyvinyl alcohol	Quick onset and sustained release for pain relief	Bilayer design achieved fast and sustained release	[102]
Levetiracetam	Extended-release tablets	Cylinder	PLA (polylactic acid)	Antiepileptic	Provided controlled drug release over extended periods	[103]
Metformin hydrochloride	Gastro-retentive floating tablets	Capsule	PVA (polyvinyl alcohol)	Diabetes management	Impact its dissolution rate	[118]
Prednisolone	Controlled release tablet	Sphere	Polycaprolactone	Anti-inflammatory	Controlled release achieved through shell design	[2]
Domperidone	Intragastric floating delivery	Cylinder shaped tablets	Hydroxypropyl, cellulose HPC	Gastroparesis	3D printed tablets for intragastric floating delivery	[100]
Pantoprazole sodium	Immediate release tablet	Tablet	polyvinylpyrrolidone (PVP K12), polyethylene glycol 6000 (PEG 6000), Kollidon® VA64, polyethylene glycol 20,000 (PEG 20,000) and poloxamer 407		Thermosensitive drug	[107]
Progesterone	Implants	Solid dispersion	Eudragit® RS, polycaprolactone (PCL), poly(L-lactide) (PLLA), and ethyl cellulose (EC)	Vaginal rings with personalized shapes	Controlled release	[111]

5.5 Challenges and Future Needs of 3D Printed Drug Formulations Using FDM Technique

5.5.1 Challenges of 3D-FDM Technique

5.5.1.1 Material-Specific Parameters

There are two specific parameters: filament formulation and lack of printability data. The formulation of a printable filament using pharmaceutical components is crucial. The filament must possess suitable physicochemical properties, including thermal, mechanical, and rheological characteristics, as well as a consistent diameter. These properties are decisive for the feasibility of the FDM 3D printing process. Inadequate properties can render FDM printing unusable. Complex formulations often require a trial-and-error approach [11, 119]. FDM is relatively new in pharmaceutical research, and there is a lack of comprehensive studies on the printability of various polymers, posing a significant challenge.

5.5.1.2 Operation-Specific Parameters

There are two specific parameters: printing conditions and customization for individualized therapy. Parameters like printing temperature, speed, and the structure of the 3D printed object (geometry, infill pattern, and density) significantly influence the final product's quality and the dissolution behavior of the drug. These parameters must be optimized to preserve drug integrity and achieve desired mechanical properties and dimensional accuracy [11]. Adjustments in dimensions and infill density could allow personalized therapy through FDM. However, this application remains theoretical and requires more scientific knowledge and better process control to ensure reproducibility [119, 11].

5.5.1.3 Machine-Specific Parameters

Printer equipment limitation is that the currently available FDM printers are suitable for small-scale productions but are not yet efficient enough for large-scale pharmaceutical manufacturing. The production speed remains relatively slow compared to traditional manufacturing systems [11, 119].

5.5.2 Future Needs for 3D Printed Drug Formulations Using FDM

5.5.2.1 Enhanced Material Understanding

Developing a deeper understanding of the printability of various pharmaceutical polymers and creating a comprehensive database to facilitate the selection of suitable materials for specific drugs.

5.5.2.2 Optimization of Printing Parameters

Improving the optimization techniques for operation-specific parameters to ensure consistent drug release profiles and product quality.

5.5.2.3 Advanced Printer Technology

Innovating printer designs and technologies that can meet the high demands of large-scale pharmaceutical production.

5.5.2.4 Personalized Medicine

Advancing the practical application of FDM for personalized medicine by ensuring reproducibility and consistency in customized drug formulations.

5.5.2.5 Regulatory Framework

Establishing a robust regulatory framework to ensure the safety and efficacy of 3D printed drugs, including guidelines for the entire FDM printing process from filament formulation to final product testing.

By addressing these challenges and future needs, the pharmaceutical industry can better leverage the potential of FDM 3D printing for innovative drug formulations and personalized therapy solutions.

5.6 Conclusion

FDM has emerged as a prominent 3D printing technology in the pharmaceutical research domain, owing to its low cost, compact apparatus, ability to create prototypes with intricate shapes, and lack of need for organic solvents. In both personalized medicine and the creation of oral solid dosage forms with the appropriate drug release profile, the complexity of the structures generated is a significant advantage. Excellent properties are provided by fiber-reinforced polymers and nanocomposites in FDM; however, nozzle blockage may occur when the composition percentage is increased. Printing quality is influenced by variables such as infill pattern, raster angle, and layer thickness. Nanopolymer composites have drawn interest for scaffolds and tissue engineering, especially in the medical domain. However, not much study has been done on composites made of nanopolymers. Researchers are faced with a significant challenge when formulating printable filaments based on pharmaceutical components; the most limiting factors in the FDM 3D printing process are material-specific parameters; the formulation step involves developing intricate formulations to achieve desired material-specific parameters, frequently through trial and error; the main hindrance to 3D printing in pharmacological research is the paucity of data on printability of polymers; once a printable filament is produced, the next challenge is creating a high-quality product that maintains drug integrity and combines mechanical properties with desired dimensional accuracy and surface roughness; parameters like geometry, infill pattern, and density are critical for achieving desired drug. Notwithstanding advancements, issues such as inadequate resolution, low production, elevated temperature exposure, safety, and regulatory apprehensions persist, necessitating remedies to transform customized dosage forms while guaranteeing safety and effectiveness.

References

1. Khalid GM, Billa N. Solid dispersion formulations by FDM 3D printing—a review. Pharmaceutics. 2022;14(4):690.
2. Skowyra J, Pietrzak K, Alhnan MA. Fabrication of extended-release patient-tailored prednisolone tablets via fused deposition modelling (FDM) 3D printing. Eur J Pharm Sci. 2015;68:11–7.
3. Roche A, Sanchez-Ballester NM, Bataille B, Delannoy V, Soulairol I. Fused deposition modelling 3D printing and solubility improvement of BCS II and IV active ingredients–a narrative review. J Control Release. 2024;365:507–20.
4. Tahsin M. Formulation of 3D printed tablet for rapid drug release by Fused Deposition Modeling (FDM): screening polymers for drug release, drug-polymer miscibility and printability. St. John's University; 2018.
5. Mohammed A, Elshaer A, Sareh P, Elsayed M, Hassanin H. Additive manufacturing technologies for drug delivery applications. Int J Pharm. 2020;580:119245.
6. Cailleaux S, Sanchez-Ballester NM, Gueche YA, Bataille B, Soulairol I. Fused Deposition Modeling (FDM), the new asset for the production of tailored medicines. J Control Release. 2021;330:821–41.
7. Goyanes A, Buanz AB, Basit AW, Gaisford S. Fused-filament 3D printing (3DP) for fabrication of tablets. Int J Pharm. 2014;476(1–2):88–92.
8. Mazzanti V, Malagutti L, Mollica F. FDM 3D printing of polymers containing natural fillers: a review of their mechanical properties. Polymers. 2019;11(7):1094.
9. Vithani K, Goyanes A, Jannin V, Basit AW, Gaisford S, Boyd BJ. An overview of 3D printing technologies for soft materials and potential opportunities for lipid-based drug delivery systems. Pharm Res. 2019;36:1–20.
10. Prasad LK, Smyth H. 3D Printing technologies for drug delivery: a review. Drug Dev Ind Pharm. 2016;42(7):1019–31.
11. Parulski C, Jennotte O, Lechanteur A, Evrard B. Challenges of fused deposition modeling 3D printing in pharmaceutical applications: where are we now? Adv Drug Deliv Rev. 2021;175:113810.
12. Caballero-Aguilar LM, Silva SM, Moulton SE. Three-dimensional printed drug delivery systems. In: Engineering drug delivery systems. Elsevier; 2020. p. 147–62.
13. Goole J, Amighi K. 3D printing in pharmaceutics: a new tool for designing customized drug delivery systems. Int J Pharm. 2016;499(1–2):376–94.
14. Khatri P, Shah MK, Vora N. Formulation strategies for solid oral dosage form using 3D printing technology: a mini-review. J Drug Deliv Sci Technol. 2018;46:148–55.
15. Jamróz W, Szafraniec J, Kurek M, Jachowicz R. 3D printing in pharmaceutical and medical applications–recent achievements and challenges. Pharm Res. 2018;35:1–22.
16. Jennotte O, Koch N, Lechanteur A, Evrard B. Three-dimensional printing technology as a promising tool in bioavailability enhancement of poorly water-soluble molecules: a review. Int J Pharm. 2020;580:119200.
17. Ilyés K, Kovács NK, Balogh A, Borbás E, Farkas B, Casian T, et al. The applicability of pharmaceutical polymeric blends for the fused deposition modelling (FDM) 3D technique: material considerations–printability–process modulation, with consecutive effects on in vitro release, stability and degradation. Eur J Pharm Sci. 2019;129:110–23.
18. Goyanes A, Fina F, Martorana A, Sedough D, Gaisford S, Basit AW. Development of modified release 3D printed tablets (printlets) with pharmaceutical excipients using additive manufacturing. Int J Pharm. 2017;527(1–2):21–30.
19. Dizon JRC, Espera AH Jr, Chen Q, Advincula RC. Mechanical characterization of 3D-printed polymers. Addit Manuf. 2018;20:44–67.
20. Goyanes A, Buanz AB, Hatton GB, Gaisford S, Basit AW. 3D printing of modified-release aminosalicylate (4-ASA and 5-ASA) tablets. Eur J Pharm Biopharm. 2015;89:157–62.

21. Dul S, Fambri L, Pegoretti A. Fused deposition modelling with ABS–graphene nanocomposites. Compos A: Appl Sci Manuf. 2016;85:181–91.
22. Popescu D, Zapciu A, Amza C, Baciu F, Marinescu R. FDM process parameters influence over the mechanical properties of polymer specimens: a review. Polym Test. 2018;69:157–66.
23. Jiang J, Lou J, Hu G. Effect of support on printed properties in fused deposition modelling processes. Virtual Phys Prototyp. 2019;14(4):308–15.
24. Rajan K, Samykano M, Kadirgama K, Harun WSW, Rahman MM. Fused deposition modeling: process, materials, parameters, properties, and applications. Int J Adv Manuf Technol. 2022;120(3):1531–70.
25. Lalehpour A, Barari A. Post processing for fused deposition modeling parts with acetone vapour bath. IFAC-PapersOnLine. 2016;49(31):42–8.
26. Chen Y-F, Wang Y-H, Tsai J-C. Enhancement of surface reflectivity of fused deposition modeling parts by post-processing. Opt Commun. 2019;430:479–85.
27. Daminabo SC, Goel S, Grammatikos SA, Nezhad HY, Thakur VK. Fused deposition modeling-based additive manufacturing (3D printing): techniques for polymer material systems. Mater Today Chem. 2020;16:100248.
28. Bryll K, Piesowicz E, Szymański P, Ślączka W, Pijanowski M, editors. Polymer composite manufacturing by FDM 3D printing technology. MATEC Web of Conferences. EDP Sciences; 2018.
29. Shahrubudin N, Lee TC, Ramlan R. An overview on 3D printing technology: technological, materials, and applications. Procedia Manuf. 2019;35:1286–96.
30. Valino AD, Dizon JRC, Espera AH Jr, Chen Q, Messman J, Advincula RC. Advances in 3D printing of thermoplastic polymer composites and nanocomposites. Prog Polym Sci. 2019;98:101162.
31. Salem Bala A, Bin Wahab MS, Binti Ahmad M, editors. Elements and materials improve the FDM products: a review. Adv Eng Forum. 2016;16:33–51. Trans Tech Publ.
32. Singh R, Garg HK. Fused deposition modeling–a state of art review and future applications. In: Reference module in materials science and materials engineering. Elsevier Inc; 2016. p. 1–20.
33. Novakova-Marcincinova L, Novak-Marcincin J, Barna J, Torok J. Special materials used in FDM rapid prototyping technology application. In: 2012 IEEE 16th International Conference on Intelligent Engineering Systems (INES). IEEE; 2012.
34. Pakkanen J, Manfredi D, Minetola P, Iuliano L. About the use of recycled or biodegradable filaments for sustainability of 3D printing: state of the art and research opportunities. In: Sustainable design and manufacturing 2017: selected papers on Sustainable Design and Manufacturing, vol. 4; 2017. p. 776–85.
35. Haq RHA, Marwah OMF, Rahman MNA, Ho FH, Abdullah H, Ahmad S, et al. Mechanical properties of PCL/PLA/PEG composite blended with different molecular weight (MW) of PEG for Fused Deposition Modelling (FDM) filament wire. Int J Integrated Eng. 2018;10(5):187–192.
36. Menčík P, Přikryl R, Stehnová I, Melčová V, Kontárová S, Figalla S, et al. Effect of selected commercial plasticizers on mechanical, thermal, and morphological properties of poly (3-hydroxybutyrate)/poly (lactic acid)/plasticizer biodegradable blends for three-dimensional (3D) print. Materials. 2018;11(10):1893.
37. Alizadeh-Osgouei M, Li Y, Wen C. A comprehensive review of biodegradable synthetic polymer-ceramic composites and their manufacture for biomedical applications. Bioactive Mater. 2019;4:22–36.
38. Liu Z, Lei Q, Xing S. Mechanical characteristics of wood, ceramic, metal and carbon fiber-based PLA composites fabricated by FDM. J Mater Res Technol. 2019;8(5):3741–51.
39. Abdullah AM, Rahim TNAT, Mohamad D, Akil HM, Rajion ZA. Mechanical and physical properties of highly ZrO2/β-TCP filled polyamide 12 prepared via fused deposition modelling (FDM) 3D printer for potential craniofacial reconstruction application. Mater Lett. 2017;189:307–9.

40. Petroudy SD. Physical and mechanical properties of natural fibers. Advanced high strength natural fibre composites in construction. Elsevier; 2017. p. 59–83.
41. Hu R, Lim J-K. Fabrication and mechanical properties of completely biodegradable hemp fiber reinforced polylactic acid composites. J Compos Mater. 2007;41(13):1655–69.
42. Le Duigou A, Barbé A, Guillou E, Castro M. 3D printing of continuous flax fibre reinforced biocomposites for structural applications. Mater Des. 2019;180:107884.
43. Hinchcliffe SA, Hess KM, Srubar WV III. Experimental and theoretical investigation of prestressed natural fiber-reinforced polylactic acid (PLA) composite materials. Compos Part B. 2016;95:346–54.
44. Depuydt D, Balthazar M, Hendrickx K, Six W, Ferraris E, Desplentere F, et al. Production and characterization of bamboo and flax fiber reinforced polylactic acid filaments for fused deposition modelling (FDM). Polym Compos. 2018;40(5):1–13.
45. Andreeßen C, Steinbüchel A. Recent developments in non-biodegradable biopolymers: precursors, production processes, and future perspectives. Appl Microbiol Biotechnol. 2019;103(1):143–57.
46. Chen S, Lu J, Feng J. 3D-Printable ABS blends with improved scratch resistance and balanced mechanical performance. Ind Eng Chem Res. 2018;57(11):3923–31.
47. Singh S, Singh R. Mechanical characterization and comparison of additive manufactured ABS, Polyflex™ and ABS/Polyflex™ blended functional prototypes. Rapid Prototyp J. 2020;26(2):225–37.
48. Mostafa N, Syed HM, Igor S, Andrew G. A study of melt flow analysis of an ABS-Iron composite in fused deposition modelling process. Tsinghua Sci Technol. 2009;14:29–37.
49. Sa'ude N, Masood S, Nikzad M, Ibrahim M, Ibrahim M. Dynamic mechanical properties of copper-ABS composites for FDM feedstock. Int J Eng Res Appl. 2013;3(3):1257–63.
50. Zhong W, Li F, Zhang Z, Song L, Li Z. Short fiber reinforced composites for fused deposition modeling. Mater Sci Eng A. 2001;301(2):125–30.
51. Tekinalp HL, Kunc V, Velez-Garcia GM, Duty CE, Love LJ, Naskar AK, et al. Highly oriented carbon fiber–polymer composites via additive manufacturing. Compos Sci Technol. 2014;105:144–50.
52. Spoerk M, Savandaiah C, Arbeiter F, Traxler G, Cardon L, Holzer C, et al. Anisotropic properties of oriented short carbon fibre filled polypropylene parts fabricated by extrusion-based additive manufacturing. Compos A: Appl Sci Manuf. 2018;113:95–104.
53. Dickson AN, Barry JN, McDonnell KA, Dowling DP. Fabrication of continuous carbon, glass and Kevlar fibre reinforced polymer composites using additive manufacturing. Addit Manuf. 2017;16:146–52.
54. Li N, Li Y, Liu S. Rapid prototyping of continuous carbon fiber reinforced polylactic acid composites by 3D printing. J Mater Process Technol. 2016;238:218–25.
55. Dong G, Tang Y, Li D, Zhao YF. Mechanical properties of continuous kevlar fiber reinforced composites fabricated by fused deposition modeling process. Procedia Manuf. 2018;26:774–81.
56. Farahani RD, Dubé M, Therriault D. Three-dimensional printing of multifunctional nanocomposites: manufacturing techniques and applications. Adv Mater. 2016;28(28):5794–821.
57. Weng Z, Wang J, Senthil T, Wu L. Mechanical and thermal properties of ABS/montmorillonite nanocomposites for fused deposition modeling 3D printing. Mater Des. 2016;102:276–83.
58. Coppola B, Cappetti N, Di Maio L, Scarfato P, Incarnato L. 3D printing of PLA/clay nanocomposites: Influence of printing temperature on printed samples properties. Materials. 2018;11(10):1947.
59. Kim H, Fernando T, Li M, Lin Y, Tseng T-LB. Fabrication and characterization of 3D printed BaTiO3/PVDF nanocomposites. J Compos Mater. 2018;52(2):197–206.
60. Cano-Vicent A, Tambuwala MM, Hassan SS, Barh D, Aljabali AAA, Birkett M, et al. Fused deposition modelling: current status, methodology, applications and future prospects. Addit Manuf. 2021;47:102378.
61. Berman B. 3-D printing: the new industrial revolution. Bus Horiz. 2012;55(2):155–62.

62. Mwema FM, Akinlabi ET. Basics of fused deposition modelling (FDM). Springer International Publishing; 2020. p. 1–15.
63. Guo N, Leu MC. Additive manufacturing: technology, applications and research needs. Front Mech Eng. 2013;8:215–43.
64. Samykano M. Mechanical property and prediction model for FDM-3D Printed Polylactic Acid (PLA). Arab J Sci Eng. 2021;46(8):7875–92.
65. Wang J, Goyanes A, Gaisford S, Basit AW. Stereolithographic (SLA) 3D printing of oral modified-release dosage forms. Int J Pharm. 2016;503(1):207–12.
66. Peng C, Tran P. Bioinspired functionally graded gyroid sandwich panel subjected to impulsive loadings. Compos Part B. 2020;188:107773.
67. Ramya A, Vanapalli SL. 3D printing technologies in various applications. IJMET. 2016;7:396–409.
68. Tran TQ, Ng FL, Kai JTY, Feih S, Nai MLS. Tensile strength enhancement of fused filament fabrication printed parts: a review of process improvement approaches and respective impact. Addit Manuf. 2022;54:102724.
69. Przekop RE, Gabriel E, Pakuła D, Sztorch B. Liquid for Fused Deposition Modeling Technique (L-FDM)—a revolution in application chemicals to 3D printing technology: color and elements. Appl Sci. 2023;13(13):7393.
70. Goyanes A, Martinez PR, Buanz A, Basit AW, Gaisford S. Effect of geometry on drug release from 3D printed tablets. Int J Pharm. 2015;494(2):657–63.
71. Pawar R, Pawar A. 3D printing of pharmaceuticals: approach from bench scale to commercial development. Future J Pharma Sci. 2022;8(1):48.
72. Hoffmann L, Breitkreutz J, Quodbach J. Fused Deposition Modeling (FDM) 3D printing of the thermo-sensitive peptidomimetic drug enalapril maleate. Pharmaceutics. 2022;14(11):2411.
73. Quodbach J, Bogdahn M, Breitkreutz J, Chamberlain R, Eggenreich K, Elia AG, et al. Quality of FDM 3D printed medicines for pediatrics: considerations for formulation development, filament extrusion, printing process and printer design. Ther Innov Regul Sci. 2022;56(6):910–28.
74. Melocchi A, Uboldi M, Cerea M, Foppoli A, Maroni A, Moutaharrik S, et al. A graphical review on the escalation of fused deposition modeling (FDM) 3D printing in the pharmaceutical field. J Pharm Sci. 2020;109(10):2943–57.
75. Wang S, Chen X, Han X, Hong X, Li X, Zhang H, et al. A review of 3D printing technology in pharmaceutics: technology and applications, now and future. Pharmaceutics. 2023;15(2):416.
76. Repka MA, Bandari S, Kallakunta VR, Vo AQ, McFall H, Pimparade MB, et al. Melt extrusion with poorly soluble drugs—an integrated review. Int J Pharm. 2018;535(1):68–85.
77. Censi R, Gigliobianco MR, Casadidio C, Di Martino P. Hot melt extrusion: highlighting physicochemical factors to be investigated while designing and optimizing a hot melt extrusion process. Pharmaceutics. 2018;10(3):89.
78. Bandari S, Nyavanandi D, Dumpa N, Repka MA. Coupling hot melt extrusion and fused deposition modeling: critical properties for successful performance. Adv Drug Deliv Rev. 2021;172:52–63.
79. Rahman Z, Barakh Ali SF, Ozkan T, Charoo NA, Reddy IK, Khan MA. Additive manufacturing with 3D printing: progress from bench to bedside. AAPS J. 2018;20(6):101.
80. Dadou SM, Senta-Loys Z, Almajaan A, Li S, Jones DS, Healy AM, et al. The development and validation of a quality by design based process analytical tool for the inline quantification of Ramipril during hot-melt extrusion. Int J Pharm. 2020;584:119382.
81. Aho J, Bøtker JP, Genina N, Edinger M, Arnfast L, Rantanen J. Roadmap to 3D-printed oral pharmaceutical dosage forms: feedstock filament properties and characterization for fused deposition modeling. J Pharm Sci. 2019;108(1):26–35.
82. Andrews GP, Jones DS, Senta-Loys Z, Almajaan A, Li S, Chevallier O, et al. The development of an inline Raman spectroscopic analysis method as a quality control tool for hot melt extruded ramipril fixed-dose combination products. Int J Pharm. 2019;566:476–87.

83. Hitzer P, Bäuerle T, Drieschner T, Ostertag E, Paulsen K, van Lishaut H, et al. Process analytical techniques for hot-melt extrusion and their application to amorphous solid dispersions. Anal Bioanal Chem. 2017;409(18):4321–33.
84. Wesholowski J, Prill S, Berghaus A, Thommes M. Inline UV/Vis spectroscopy as PAT tool for hot-melt extrusion. Drug Deliv Transl Res. 2018;8(6):1595–603.
85. Zhang J, Feng X, Patil H, Tiwari RV, Repka MA. Coupling 3D printing with hot-melt extrusion to produce controlled-release tablets. Int J Pharm. 2017;519(1):186–97.
86. Tan DK, Maniruzzaman M, Nokhodchi A. Advanced pharmaceutical applications of hot-melt extrusion coupled with fused deposition modelling (FDM) 3D printing for personalised drug delivery. Pharmaceutics. 2018;10(4):203.
87. Pereira GG, Figueiredo S, Fernandes AI, Pinto JF. Polymer selection for hot-melt extrusion coupled to fused deposition modelling in pharmaceutics. Pharmaceutics. 2020;12(9):795.
88. Sadia M, Arafat B, Ahmed W, Forbes RT, Alhnan MA. Channelled tablets: an innovative approach to accelerating drug release from 3D printed tablets. J Control Release. 2018;269:355–63.
89. Lim SH, Kathuria H, Tan JJY, Kang L. 3D printed drug delivery and testing systems — a passing fad or the future? Adv Drug Deliv Rev. 2018;132:139–68.
90. Sandler N, Preis M. Printed drug-delivery systems for improved patient treatment. Trends Pharmacol Sci. 2016;37(12):1070–80.
91. Long J, Gholizadeh H, Lu J, Bunt C, Seyfoddin A. Application of Fused Deposition Modelling (FDM) method of 3D printing in drug delivery. Curr Pharm Des. 2017;23(3):433–9.
92. Goyanes A, Scarpa M, Kamlow M, Gaisford S, Basit AW, Orlu M. Patient acceptability of 3D printed medicines. Int J Pharm. 2017;530(1–2):71–8.
93. Basit AW, Gaisford S. 3D printing of pharmaceuticals. Springer; 2018.
94. Goyanes A, Wang J, Buanz A, Martínez-Pacheco R, Telford R, Gaisford S, et al. 3D printing of medicines: engineering novel oral devices with unique design and drug release characteristics. Mol Pharm. 2015;12(11):4077–84.
95. Goyanes A, Det-Amornrat U, Wang J, Basit AW, Gaisford S. 3D scanning and 3D printing as innovative technologies for fabricating personalized topical drug delivery systems. J Control Release. 2016;234:41–8.
96. Muwaffak Z, Goyanes A, Clark V, Basit AW, Hilton ST, Gaisford S. Patient-specific 3D scanned and 3D printed antimicrobial polycaprolactone wound dressings. Int J Pharm. 2017;527(1–2):161–70.
97. Bhattacharya S, Singh S, Shrestha S, Baghel Y, Maity D, Kumar A, et al. Recent findings and development of 3D printing technology in pharmaceutical formulation development: an extensive review. Int J Drug Dev Res. 2019;11:1–14.
98. Kristiawan RB, Imaduddin F, Ariawan D, Ubaidillah AZ. A review on the fused deposition modeling (FDM) 3D printing: filament processing, materials, and printing parameters. Open Eng. 2021;11(1):639–49.
99. Nguyen MN, Tran PH, Tran TT. A single-layer film coating for colon-targeted oral delivery. Int J Pharm. 2019;559:402–9.
100. Chai X, Chai H, Wang X, Yang J, Li J, Zhao Y, et al. Fused deposition modeling (FDM) 3D printed tablets for intragastric floating delivery of domperidone. Sci Rep. 2017;7(1):2829.
101. Ahmad M, Manzoor K, Singh S, Ikram S. Chitosan centered bionanocomposites for medical specialty and curative applications: a review. Int J Pharm. 2017;529(1–2):200–17.
102. Crişan AG, Porfire A, Iurian S, Rus LM, Lucăcel Ciceo R, Turza A, et al. Development of a bilayer tablet by fused deposition modeling as a sustained-release drug delivery system. Pharmaceuticals. 2023;16(9):1321.
103. Cui M, Pan H, Fang D, Qiao S, Wang S, Pan W. Fabrication of high drug loading levetiracetam tablets using semi-solid extrusion 3D printing. J Drug Deliv Sci Technol. 2020;57:101683.
104. Goyanes A, Chang H, Sedough D, Hatton GB, Wang J, Buanz A, et al. Fabrication of controlled-release budesonide tablets via desktop (FDM) 3D printing. Int J Pharm. 2015;496(2):414–20.

105. Okwuosa TC, Pereira BC, Arafat B, Cieszynska M, Isreb A, Alhnan MA. Fabricating a shell-core delayed release tablet using dual FDM 3D printing for patient-centred therapy. Pharm Res. 2017;34(2):427–37.
106. Kempin W, Domsta V, Grathoff G, Brecht I, Semmling B, Tillmann S, et al. Immediate release 3D-printed tablets produced via fused deposition modeling of a thermo-sensitive drug. Pharm Res. 2018;35:1–12.
107. Kempin W, Domsta V, Grathoff G, Brecht I, Semmling B, Tillmann S, et al. Immediate release 3D-printed tablets produced via fused deposition modeling of a thermo-sensitive drug. Pharm Res. 2018;35(6):124.
108. Kollamaram G, Croker DM, Walker GM, Goyanes A, Basit AW, Gaisford S. Low temperature fused deposition modeling (FDM) 3D printing of thermolabile drugs. Int J Pharm. 2018;545(1–2):144–52.
109. Solanki NG, Tahsin M, Shah AV, Serajuddin AT. Formulation of 3D printed tablet for rapid drug release by fused deposition modeling: screening polymers for drug release, drug-polymer miscibility and printability. J Pharm Sci. 2018;107(1):390–401.
110. Genina N, Holländer J, Jukarainen H, Mäkilä E, Salonen J, Sandler N. Ethylene vinyl acetate (EVA) as a new drug carrier for 3D printed medical drug delivery devices. Eur J Pharm Sci. 2016;90:53–63.
111. Fu J, Yu X, Jin Y. 3D printing of vaginal rings with personalized shapes for controlled release of progesterone. Int J Pharm. 2018;539(1–2):75–82.
112. Maroni A, Melocchi A, Parietti F, Foppoli A, Zema L, Gazzaniga A. 3D printed multi-compartment capsular devices for two-pulse oral drug delivery. J Control Release. 2017;268:10–8.
113. Khaled SA, Burley JC, Alexander MR, Yang J, Roberts CJ. 3D printing of five-in-one dose combination polypill with defined immediate and sustained release profiles. J Control Release. 2015;217:308–14.
114. Norman J, Madurawe RD, Moore CM, Khan MA, Khairuzzaman A. A new chapter in pharmaceutical manufacturing: 3D-printed drug products. Adv Drug Deliv Rev. 2017;108:39–50.
115. Trenfield SJ, Awad A, Goyanes A, Gaisford S, Basit AW. 3D printing pharmaceuticals: drug development to frontline care. Trends Pharmacol Sci. 2018;39(5):440–51.
116. Scoutaris N, Ross S, Douroumis D. Current trends on medical and pharmaceutical applications of inkjet printing technology. Pharm Res. 2016;33:1799–816.
117. Qian H, Chen D, Xu X, Li R, Yan G, Fan T. FDM 3D-printed sustained-release gastric-floating verapamil hydrochloride formulations with cylinder, capsule and hemisphere shapes, and low infill percentage. Pharmaceutics. 2022;14(2):281.
118. Ibrahim M, Barnes M, McMillin R, Cook DW, Smith S, Halquist M, et al. 3D printing of metformin HCl PVA tablets by fused deposition modeling: drug loading, tablet design, and dissolution studies. AAPS PharmSciTech. 2019;20:1–11.
119. Melocchi A, Briatico-Vangosa F, Uboldi M, Parietti F, Turchi M, von Zeppelin D, et al. Quality considerations on the pharmaceutical applications of fused deposition modeling 3D printing. Int J Pharm. 2021;592:119901.

Advances in Active Pharmaceutical Ingredient (API) Incorporation into 3D-Printed Dosage Forms

6

Koyel Kar, Sailee Chowdhury, and Priyanka Chakraborty

Abstract

With the use of active pharmaceutical components, three-dimensional printing, an emerging technology, can be used to create effective, dose-customized dosage forms. Despite its immense promise, 3DP has some drawbacks, and conventional drug production platforms are still the norm in the business. It seems widely agreed upon that 3DP technology will most certainly help personalized treatment, but it is not likely to displace traditional mass production methods. Contrarily, the 3DP approach might work well for manufacturing small batches as an adaptable manufacturing strategy that makes it possible to design adaptive clinical trials for preliminary clinical investigations. This chapter covers the latest developments in 3DP technologies for the integration of API, along with a review of the issues and concerns related to regulations.

Keywords

3D printing · Active pharmaceutical ingredients · Challenges · Regulatory consideration

K. Kar (✉) · S. Chowdhury
Department of Pharmaceutical Chemistry, BCDA College of Pharmacy & Technology, Hridaypur, West Bengal, India

P. Chakraborty
Department of Pharmacology, BCDA College of Pharmacy & Technology, Hridaypur, West Bengal, India

K. Vinchurkar, S. Mane (eds.), *Innovations in Drug Manufacturing*,
https://doi.org/10.1007/978-981-96-9075-6_6

6.1 Introduction

Rapid prototyping, sometimes referred to as additive manufacturing, is made possible by 3D printing, also known as three-dimensional printing, or 3DP technology. This method uses powdered plastics, metals, or bondable materials to create items by layer-by-layer printing. It is based on computer model files [26]. In contrast to conventional manufacturing and processing methods that eliminate materials, 3D printing technology represents a novel approach to manufacturing. The field of computer-aided design (CAD) and 3D printing technology is developing and progressing together. As a cutting-edge and practical tool, 3D printing technology has gained popularity. This essay primarily examines and compares the technologies used in traditional manufacturing vs 3D printing. By using computer-aided design software to create a model that is then cut, and transferred to a printer, and the concept of layered manufacturing, 3D printing is an "additive manufacturing" technology as opposed to traditional manufacturing techniques of "subtractive manufacturing" [9]. One after another, several new 3D printing technologies have evolved as a result of research and development. Based on their technological principles, the American Society for Testing and Materials divided 3D printing processes into seven groups: material extrusion, binder spray, powder bed fusion, vat photopolymerization, substance jetting, directed energy depositing, and sheet lamination. This is because each 3D printing technology uses different materials, deposition techniques, layering manufacturing mechanisms, and final product characteristics [33]. Global research into 3D printing technology is currently booming in the pharmaceutical industry.

In contrast to conventional preparation technologies, 3D printing allows for greater flexibility in the design of intricate three-dimensional drug structures, the modification of drug dosages and combinations, and quick manufacturing and prototyping. These benefits enable precise control of drug release to fulfill a variety of clinical needs, a high degree of creativity and flexibility in customizing pharmaceuticals, and a notable decrease in the time required for preparation development, leading to a breakthrough in drug manufacturing technology and revolutionizing the way drugs are designed, made, and used [34]. Numerous pharmaceutical items, including dispersible films, microneedles, implants, transdermal patches, controlled-release tablets, and immediate-release tablets, have been produced using three-dimensional printing technology [13].

6.2 Comparison Between 3D Printing Technologies and Traditional Manufacturing Methods

6.2.1 Production Process Comparison

There are stringent manufacturing procedures in traditional manufacturing technology. First comes conceptual design, which is followed by design for look and structure, drawing design (auxiliary design using CAD technology), processing parts using CNC machine tools following the drawings, and product production. The technology of 3D printing operates on a very basic level, utilizes CAD design on the computer first, and then sends the data to the 3D printer for basic configurations. The processed product is available for acquisition after printing.

In contrast to traditional manufacturing technologies, 3D printing technology is easy to use, doesn't require a high level of operator experience, and has a simple production process. It also produces a diverse range of products, has a flexible production technique, and provides a good working environment. It has drawn a lot of interest since it can produce a design without the need for drawings and has an eco-friendly production process [22].

6.2.2 Comprehensive Technical Comparison

Most sectors can today be satisfied by the reasonably complete state of traditional manufacturing technologies. The production mode of traditional manufacturing technology also has many manifestations in modern manufacturing technology, as shown in Fig. 6.1, including low production efficiency, high manufacturing costs, high labor intensity, numerous processing personnel, frequent processing turnover, and numerous production procedures, a poor and dangerous working environment, a high scrap rate, and more material waste. At the same time, traditional manufacturing technology is also upgrading and transforming, from the original traditional manufacturing technology to modern manufacturing technology conversion and integration.

The following traits apply to 3D printing technology: First, the CAD model can be directly driven to realize the digitalization of physical elements; sophisticated digital modeling tools can be utilized for early model design [59]; second, the material utilization rate is high. No need to process the blanks before processing; third,

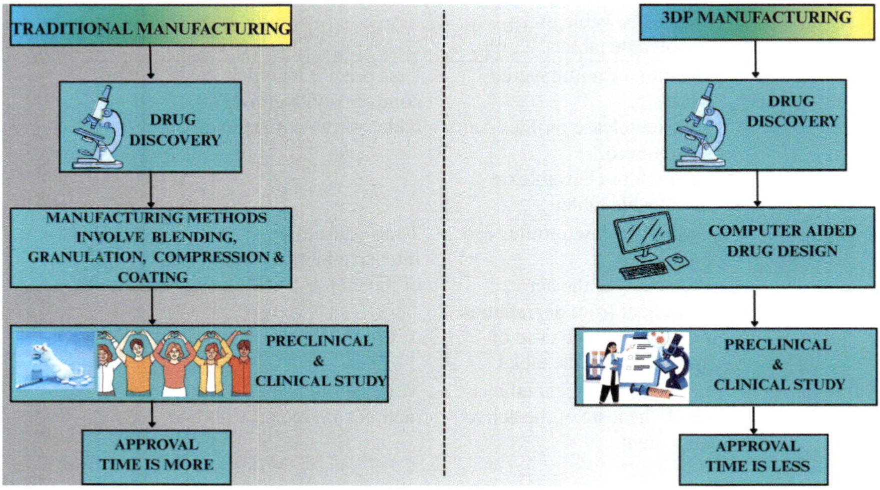

Fig. 6.1 Comparison between traditional manufacturing and 3DP manufacturing

no need for large-scale automated production lines, no fixed production workshops, reducing production costs; fourth, no need for traditional cutting tools, fixed fixtures, processing machines or molds, and can directly follow the model Data generation of physical products is simple, convenient, and flexible, which effectively shortens the product development cycle; fifth, it can easily manufacture complex parts or products that are inconvenient to manufacture using traditional methods; sixth, the processing and production environment is safe and pollution-free. The above is the analysis of its characteristics. 3D printing technology has obvious advantages compared with traditional manufacturing technology (Table 6.1).

Table 6.1 Advantages and disadvantages between 3D printing technologies and traditional manufacturing methods

Manufacturing methods	Advantages	Disadvantages	Reference
3D printing technologies	On-demand manufacturing. Dosage flexibility. Design flexibility. Dose and design flexibility. Low wastage scale-up. (scaling out instead) Can improve the taste or appearance of the tablet. Real-time-release easy to move/relocate footprint.	High cost. Limited scalability. Limited drug compatibility. Lacking regulatory approval. Low capacity. Complex formulation. Preparation step potentially needs to be limited by the properties of the ingredients. E.g., particle size and flowability.	[22]
Compression	Easy scale-up. Allows a high degree of precision in tablet weight and strength.	Limited by the properties of the ingredients (e.g., particle size and flowability).	[59]
Molding	Unique shapes. Wide range of ingredients. Create chewable or dissolvable tablets.	Less precise than the compression method.	[33]
Layering	Creation of multilayered tablets. Desired release profiles can be achieved. Creation of chewable or dissolvable tablets.	Less precise than the compression method for tablet weight and strength.	[60]
Coating	Desired release profiles can be achieved. Protection of the active ingredient from degradation. Can improve the taste or appearance of the tablet.	Time-consuming. Intensive increase in the cost of the tablet.	[11]
Sublimation	Create effervescent tablets. Mask the taste of the active ingredient.	More complex than other methods ingredients limited.	[3]

(continued)

Table 6.1 (continued)

Manufacturing methods	Advantages	Disadvantages	Reference
Direct compression	Easy process. Less time-consuming. Eliminates steps such as granulation. Reduces production costs.	Limited by properties of the ingredients (e.g., particle size and flowability).	[23]
Wet granulation	Improve flowability and compression of powders. Improve dissolution rate. Increase content uniformity.	Requires more equipment. Time-consuming.	[3]
Dry granulation	Improve flowability and compression of powders. Improve dissolution rate. Increase content uniformity.	Requires more equipment. Time-consuming.	[3]

6.3 3D Printing Technologies for the Incorporation of API in 3D-Printed Dosage Forms

Every 3D printer, which operates in a distinct mode, needs enough material to solidify before fabricating an object. Despite the variety of 3DP techniques, there are multiple steps involved in the development of a 3D-printed object:

- The process involves using computer-aided design tools to build 3D objects, optimizing their geometry to meet printer specifications, and exporting the finished product in a file format that is compatible with most printers, such as STL.
- The process of creating 3D geometry involves storing data about each vertex position, also known as OBJ, which contains additional information about coded polygonal faces or color textures.
- The file is then imported into the software, which creates layers that will be printed; the height of these layers significantly affects both the quality and speed of the printed object.
- The object is then fabricated by applying and solidifying material layers that are specific to the printing method.

The ability to quickly manufacture custom objects for use in individualized therapy or medication has made 3D printing techniques more significant in the fields of pharmaceutical and medical applications. One specific goal of the use of 3D printing in pharmaceutical technology is the creation of dose forms that are patient-centered and based on structural design. The development of a targeted-release medication is still in its infancy as a research area, delivery systems in freeform geometries. Extensive research is conducted for oral dosage forms because that route of administration remains the major and the favorite one. Some investigations are also focused on dosage forms for topical administration. The examples of 3D-printed products demonstrate the growing interest in drug design by using different 3D printing techniques.

6.3.1 Extrusion-Based Printing

Often known as additive manufacturing (AM) or additive layer manufacturing (ALM), 3D printing is a computer-aided industrial technique used to create materials into three-dimensional objects. With additive manufacturing, complex geometries can be custom-built parts with little waste. Rapid prototyping benefits from the computerized process since it allows for efficient design modifications even during the manufacturing process. Minimal material waste lowers the price of valuable items [44]. There are several AM techniques, each with unique characteristics. Binder jetting, one of the AM methods, involves moving a 3D printer head along the x, y, and z axes to deposit alternating layers of material in powder and liquid form. The binder functions as an adhesive. A concentrated energy source, such as an electron beam, plasma, or laser, is used to melt the material in the directed energy deposition process. The nozzle then drops the melted material onto a bed that is moving vertically. In material extrusion, coiled materials are either dispensed or dragged via a heated nozzle that is mounted on a moving arm. The melted material is deposited layer by layer as the platform moves vertically and the nozzle moves horizontally.

6.3.1.1 Fused Deposition Modeling

Polymers are utilized as the raw material (filament) in fused deposition modeling (FDM), commonly referred to as material extrusion additive manufacturing technology. Typically, the filament is heated to a molten condition and then forced into the device's nozzle (3D printer). Following the G-code instructions, the nozzle head can move in three degrees of freedom (DoF) to place the extruded polymer on the build plate. The machine's extruder and nozzle receive a continuous supply of filament thanks to the two rollers that rotate counter-clockwise. Layer by layer, the material is applied to the build plate until the desired product size and shape are obtained [38].

The printer nozzle moves back and forth following the original CAD model's spatial coordinates in the G-code files during the layering process, continuing until the component is created to the correct size and shape. When components of compositional gradients are needed, several extrusion nozzles can be employed in certain FDM systems (3D printers) to deposit the polymer constituents.

Since the qualities of the thermoplastic filament typically determine how well an extrusion works, different 3D printers are made to work with different types of filaments. The majority of low-cost FDM 3D printers are limited to processing a single form of thermoplastic, and the most popular kind is polylactic acid (PLA), which can be soaked in a detergent solution. Typically, the parts are stacked on the build plate (platform), which, depending on the kind of thermoplastic, can be snapped off after printing. Subsequently, the printed parts could undergo surface cleaning, sanding, painting, or milling to improve their functionality and overall look.

There are various materials used in FDM, and as stated earlier, PLA is the most adopted material by most 3D printer users at domestic and industrial levels due to the following reasons. Since polylactic acid (PLA) is bioplastic, it is safe for the environment and does not endanger the health of people or animals. Since PLA is made from entirely renewable resources such as corn, sugarcane, wheat, or any other resource that contains a lot of carbohydrates, it is considered a green substance [14]. As a result, it is advised to utilize it to make packaging containers, deli and food takeaway, and cool drink cups. Between 50 and 70 °C is the glass transition temperature of PLA, while between 180 and 220 °C is the melting point [43]. As such, it can be extruded by the most inexpensive, low-power 3D printers. Plastisol (PLA) is more resilient than acrylonitrile butadiene styrene (ABS) while having a greater friction level and being more prone to extrusion blockage.

Unlike other plastics, which have presented significant disposal issues, PLA plastics are compostable and decompose swiftly after disposal. PLA is a biopolymer that breaks down into water, biomass, inorganic salts, natural and nonpoisonous gases, and hydrolyzes or even burns when exposed to the elements. PLA has demonstrated improved tensility, flexural strengths, and a strong flexural modulus in its semicrystalline form. Most 3D printer users choose PLA since it doesn't necessarily require a hotbed for the print and platform to adhere to one another. On the other hand, graphene-doped PLA is very difficult to print on nonheated build plates and does not yield high-quality prints. A wide range of colors and textures are commercially available for purchase in PLA. Users find it appealing because of this, particularly those who manage ornamental and household 3D printers. The marketplaces for toy aficionados and CAD designers have grown due to the availability of the product in a variety of hues and textures. Toy aficionados can buy, download, and print with a variety of PLA filament colors and texture designs through the use of several databases (such as TurboSquid, CG Trader, Shapeways, Cults3D, 3DSquirrel, and Thingsverse) that the designers can use to create intriguing concepts.

Therefore, purchasers should understand the chemical makeup of the filaments they intend to employ in light of their intended uses [53]. The technique has become one of the most advanced ways to tool complicated goods quickly and produce prototypes in small- and medium-sized batches. There is a wealth of literature available on the development of a broader pool of materials for fast prototyping applications, which is the focus of current research [11]. FDM technology is being used more and more in the toy and related sectors, either as a direct manufacturing method or as a way to make injection molds for these businesses.

The possibilities for mass customization of items with FDM are immeasurable. FDM is used to create customized goods for a range of uses, including toys, car parts, interior design elements, implants, cosmetics, and so on, because of its versatility and capacity to create complex profiles [66]. FDM is also being used in the medical industry to create molds for implants, medical gadgets, and castings of implants. The most fascinating use case is the 3D printing of molds for medical implant investment casting [60]. Classic investment casting uses metallic molds and sacrificial patterns, such as wax, to generate the intricate forms of any implant.

Additional uses for FDM include the pharmaceutical sector's drug delivery components, the direct printing of conductors for the electronic industry, the manufacturing of microtrusses for biomedical scaffolding, and the direct printing of electrochemical cells for energy storage systems [15].

6.3.1.2 Semisolid Extrusion

Similar to fused deposition modeling, semisolid extrusion (SSE), also called pressure-assisted microsyringe extrusion technology or PAM, prints from a syringe that is loaded with a paste or gel rather than filaments or powder. The final product is constructed by feeding the semisolid material into a 3D printer's hot end, and it is melted and deposited there as leave-behind literature or Lbl [56, 57]. This process enables the fabrication of more complicated shapes than conventional extrusion-based 3DP technologies. The low printing temperature of semisolid extrusion makes it a viable option for thermosensitive drug administration, which is another variance [20].

This type can function at lower temperatures due to the properties of its materials. Semisolid gels and pastes naturally have lower melting points than solid filaments or powders used in classic FDM or 3D printing methods based on extrusion. Moreover, these systems are specifically designed to minimize heat exposure throughout the printing process. By carefully monitoring the temperature, it is ensured that the material doesn't get degraded or undergoes changes in quality when it is exposed to high temperatures, which is the ideal range for extrusion. The utilization of semisolid materials, like soft candy, that are ideal for making chewable tablets has been the focus of study currently. This approach has the potency to significantly increase compliance in pediatric patients [69]. These results were validated in a related study conducted by Tagami and his research group [62] who are engrossed in employing this technology to create gummy formulations for children. The group produced solutions including gelatin, syrup, water, hydroxypropyl methylcellulose (HPMC), and lamotrigine as antiepileptic. SSE's primary drawback is that, in opposition to fused deposition modeling, it prints at low resolution [6].

When compared to 3D objects created using other techniques, these may have thicker layers, coarser surface finishes, and fewer fine features. Nonetheless, technological and material advancements are ongoing; thus, the resolution issues with SSE 3D printing may be effectively resolved soon [21].

6.3.1.3 Direct Powder Extrusion

Direct powder extrusion (DPE) is enclosed in the category of extrusion-based processes. Direct powder extrusion uses a component that is obtained from hot melt extrusion (HME) and is extruded via the printer's nozzle in the form of powder or pellets rather than a filament [23].

DPE's primary benefit is its ability to get beyond drug-loading limitations that often occur with traditional HME and FDM processes. To ensure uniform medication distribution, DPE starts with a well-mixed drug–polymer mixture. To provide a constant drug content throughout printing, this combination is continually extruded. DPE makes it manageable to precisely regulate the parameters, guaranteeing precision dosage and formulation-specific flexibility. It also guarantees homogenous medication dispersion and reduces drug agglomeration. It would therefore result in the making of a single-step 3D printing manufacturing process that is faster and much affordable [54]. DPE also has the benefit of using negligible amounts of the drug and excipients, which makes it ideal for formulating mixtures for preclinical research [56, 57].

6.3.2 Powder Bed Fusion

The powder-based binding approach, which comprises the printing processes of electron beam melting (EBM), binder jetting (BJ), direct metal laser sintering (DMLS), and selective laser sintering (SLS), is another often utilized 3DP technology. These methods are applied to diverse materials and applications, and they all require distinct processes to fuse the particles and produce the finished product [61].

Binder jetting and selective laser sintering are most pertinent to pharmaceutical manufacturing. Their capacity to construct complicated designs, customization possibilities, API integration, speed, material flexibility, GMP compliance, maturity, and sustainability benefits make them exceptional. These characteristics make SLS and BJ effective and comply with regulations options for manufacturing pharmaceuticals.

6.3.2.1 Selective Laser Sintering

One of the newest and most sophisticated methods for print production is embodied by SLS. This type of printing involves spraying a thin coating of powder with a liquid binder solution in the form of droplets using an inkjet printhead; the powder particles stick together when the binder solution comes into contact with the powder bed. After that, the powder layer is selectively sintered using a CO_2 laser, and the method is continued until the necessary printlets are made [1]. When utilizing selective laser sintering (SLS), a CO_2 laser produces temperatures ranging from 1000 to 1600 °C. To precisely construct the 3D shape layer by layer, a high temperature is required to fuse or sinter the powdered material in the desired places [25].

A key component to form printlets is the liquid binder solution. Its characteristics are crucial to the accuracy and effectiveness of the printing process. Certain requirements must be met by the binder solution to guarantee optimal performance. For consistent droplet formation and distribution, surface tension, for instance, needs to fall within a certain range. In addition, meticulous control over the viscosity of the binder solution guarantees consistent droplet size and inkjet printer flow. Since the solution needs to spread readily and wet the powder surface for good adhesion, wettability and compatibility with the target powder material are important factors. The solution's spreadability, which guarantees uniform coverage of the powder bed, is equally important [7].

The viability of creating amorphous printlets using the SLS technique and the use of XRPD-chemometric models to measure the small amounts of crystalline medicine in the 3D formulations are also explored by researchers [28, 58].

SLS is not yet widely utilized in the pharmaceutical industry due to several technical and regulatory issues, not the least of which is material compatibility, which can exhibit drug degradation levels when hampered by the high localized temperatures needed to sinter powder materials [56, 57].

6.3.2.2 Binder Jetting

Based on the FDA-approved printlet, Binder Jet 3DP is a potential technology for pharmaceutical manufacturing. A liquid binder is used to selectively combine powdered material into the required layer form after it has been spread out into a layer [48]. Because binder jetting is done at room temperature, it does not require thermoplastic polymers like other printing methods. Notwithstanding its achievements, binder jetting is still relatively new, and there is plenty more to learn about its potential uses in the pharmaceutical industry.

6.3.3 Vat Photopolymerization

VAT photopolymerization is a 3DP method that uses ultraviolet (UV) light to harden a photopolymer to create 3D objects [49]. The process of solidifying or hardening the liquid photopolymer material when it is subjected to UV radiation is known as "curing" in the context of photopolymerization. This curing process determines the structure of each layer of the object. Depending on how it is cured, photopolymerization can be further divided into three categories: digital light processing (DLP), continuous liquid interface production (CLIP), and lasers (SLA) [3]. The most popular variation of VAT polymerization for the production of pharmaceuticals is SLA, which can yield completed goods of consistent quality and speed, such as microneedles and hearing aids [12].

6.3.4 Inkjet Printing

Using layer-by-layer selective ink deposition, inkjet printing (IJP) is an additive manufacturing method that allows for fine control over the structure and composition of 2D patterns or 3D objects. The demands of personalized medicine in the healthcare sector are always changing, and this technology has shown itself to be an appealing and adaptable solution.

Technologies for additive manufacturing are becoming more popular as substitutes in the medical industry. In particular, inkjet printing, or IJP, is becoming more popular for a range of pharmaceutical applications, including drug research, tissue engineering, and regenerative medicine [16]. The great level of precision in ink deposition achieved by IJP technology allows for precise control of the printed dose depending on the volume ejected from the nozzle, all while avoiding contact with the substrate [55]. Furthermore, IJP provides a significant deal of substrate versatility because designed inks can be printed on a wide range of items, such as contact lenses, films, clinical stents, microneedles (MNs), and even nails [50].

Based on the actual droplet generation method, this automated high-throughput technology is mainly divided into two parts: drop-on-demand printing (DOD) and continuous inkjet printing (CIJ) [63]. Pharmaceutical researchers' interest in DOD is expanding as a result of its low cost, high precision, and decrease in drug waste when it comes to creating different 3D dosage forms [27].

Continuous inkjet printing provides a continuous stream of ink by forcing it through a nozzle with the help of a high-pressure pump. The surface tension forces then caused this stream to break up into droplets. It is possible to modify the frequency to regulate the drop formation [36].

6.3.5 Pressure-Assisted Microsyringe

The device of pressure-assisted microsyringe employs a syringe head to incessantly expel semisolid material in layers upon layers to create three-dimensional printed objects. A mechanical, pneumatic, or solenoid piston could function as the framework for the extrusion. The semisolid mixture comprises the solvent, extra required excipients with printing-suitable attributes, and a compatible polymer mixture. The crucial role of drying after printing arises from using solvents, which could cause the finished product to shrink or deform. The printed item may also implode if the deposited layer is not strong enough to sustain the weight of the following layers. This process's primary benefit is that it doesn't use very high temperatures [8].

A pressure-assisted microsyringe was employed to create immediate-release levetiracetam tablets devoid of organic solvents. In addition to determining the influence of another polymer, polyvinyl pyrrolidone-vinyl acetate on the tablets, the polyethylene glycol-polyvinyl alcohol was used as the matrix. The dissolving and disintegration times of the formulations containing more PVP-PVAc were longer. Ginkgolide gastroretentive tablets formulated by HPMC were developed with PAM. A homogenous paste was created using cellulose and lactose to boost its formability [2].

6.3.6 Stereolithography

The course of employing ultraviolet light to photopolymerize liquid resin and harden it is the basis of stereolithography. The printer is configured top-down, with the UV source below and above the platform. The initial layer is photocured and adheres to the building platform after being tracked by the laser in the x- and y-axes, which is directed by scanning mirrors. Next, depending on how wide each layer is, the platform moves along the z-axis. Next, to continue building the three-dimensional item, the liquid resin is redistributed above the layer that has already hardened. To remove any remaining resin, the item is subsequently cleaned with alcohol. One way to reinforce is to use a UV oven for post-curing. For SLA materials to go through photo-cross-linking, they possess photo-curable properties. This printing method has the benefits of reduced heat stress and good resolution [45].

Although it offers benefits, the pharmaceutical industry uses this printing method sparingly. The dearth of suitable polymers for pharmaceutical use—none of which are classified as chemicals universally acknowledged to be safe—is one factor contributing to this. They have stability problems because of their photosensitivity and are therefore unfit for human usage. An additional constraint is the prospect of photoinitiator fragments becoming ensnared in photopolymerized structures, which may then leak out and become cytotoxic [67].

6.3.7 Digital Light Processing

It is a crucial technological advancement in additive production in 3D printing. It makes use of digital light projectors to quickly and precisely transform liquid photopolymers into solid, finely detailed things. This technology is favored for different aspects because of its excellent firmness and speed. It is a type of stereolithography technique known as "Digital Light Processing" which works by curing a photosensitive polymer with light. The fundamental concept of this technology is the way light interacts with a particular kind of polymer called a photopolymer. The polymer used for this process is known as a photopolymer that reacts to light, particularly ultraviolet light [68].

The photopolymer goes through a chemical process called photopolymerization when it is bared to UV light. The UV light is projected onto the resinous photopolymer using a digital light projector screen. Adjusting the printed structure, polymer concentration, and printer factors, such as light intensity, wavelength, and exposure duration, offers great litheness in the creation of customized drug delivery systems [37].

6.3.8 Drop-on-Demand Printer

In these printers, liquid droplets are deposited onto a substrate after being ejected from the printhead using a trigger signal only when required. The nozzle count on this kind of printer is usually high. In this type of printer, the kinetic energy of the drop is obtained from sources placed within the print-head and near the nozzle, in contrast to other inkjet printers where the expulsion of droplets is caused by atmospheric pressure. It is a low-cost, very precise technique that is reasonably straightforward. It creates tiny drips with good placement accuracy and can deposit drops of adjustable sizes. Moreover, it reduces medication waste. For printing purposes, this makes it preferred over other inkjet printing. Depending on the kind of printhead, it can be further divided into thermal and piezoelectric models. Their classification into drop-on-drop and drop-on-solid is also conferring to the substrate on which the print head deposits the droplets [10].

6.3.8.1 Thermal Inkjet Printer

Here, droplets are released through the utilization of heat energy as a trigger mechanism, and they subsequently emerge from the nozzle. The printheads contain embedded resistors that are directly exposed to the ink and generate heat when an electric current is introduced. After that, the heat causes a bubble to form in the fluid, which expands and shoots a minuscule quantity of fluid out of the nozzle in the form of a droplet. The usage of a resistor heated to 200–300 °C is the technique's primary drawback since it causes the active components in thermolabile substances to degrade [42].

6.3.8.2 Piezoelectric Inkjet Printer

In this technology, an electric voltage is used to cause a piezoelectric device, also referred to as an actuator, to alter shape. The ink is forced out of the nozzle as a result of the pressure this creates. Reloading the nozzle with fluid and preparing it for another activation occurs when the element returns to its original shape. One of the technique's main advantages is that it can work at room temperature with fluids that are less volatile and more compatible [64].

Small solenoid valves served as the basis for another fascinating printing technique dubbed "valve jet" or "electromagnetic" printing, which was applied in the pharmaceutical industry. This would assist print coarser suspensions and is favorable because of its bigger orifice widths and robustness when compared to thermal inkjet printers or piezoelectric inkjet printers [40].

For high-frequency droplet ejection, a glass inkjet device was created. Glass is inert; therefore, none of the ingredients utilized will react with it, making it a great fit for pharmaceutical implementations. By integrating UV photo-initiation with inkjet technology, more can be attained. In this sector, UV light has been engaged to quickly harden materials on demand. The ink has light-activated cross-linking functional groups, and this is sometimes aided by the accumulation of a photo-initiator [18].

6.4 Materials Used for 3D Printing

6.4.1 Polymers

6.4.1.1 Synthetic Biopolymers

6.4.1.1.1 Polyvinyl Alcohol

Because of its water solubility, dissolvability, and biodegradability, PVA is a type of polymer that is frequently used as a binder or filler in tablets that are 3D printed. Printing dosage forms can enhance their mechanical forte and medication release characteristics. Extrusion- and inkjet-based printing methods are both available for PVA. PVA filaments encumbered with either caffeine or paracetamol were utilized to create customized oral caplets by fused deposition modeling. Using PVA, researchers created tablet casing in a different study that lifted the main ingredient on gastric fluid for a minimum of 8 hours and controlled the drug's release profile, enabling zero-order release. 3D-printed PVA is also used for suppository dose forms and oral ones [30].

6.4.1.1.2 Polyvinyl Pyrrolidone

In 3D printing, PVP is often utilized. PVP has strong hydrophilicity and hydrophobicity, which improve its capability to associate with a varied range of substances. It is also nonionic. Because the amide that is linked to the apolar methylene and pyrrolidone ring methane groups, which are present along the PVP backbone and ring, allows for chemical interactions with substances that have different polarities, PVP is soluble in a varied range of polar and nonpolar liquids, including water. The carbon chain's repulsive forces also act on solvents, causing chemical interactions that give rise to polymer solubility and the inhibition of nanoparticle aggregation caused by repulsive forces. Chemical instability is therefore not caused by PVP solubility [39].

6.4.1.1.3 Polyethylene Glycol

Pharmaceutical applications can employ PEG, a polymer with various uses, in 3D printing. This water-solvable, compatible, and recyclable substance has many benefits in the pharmaceutical sector. With PEG glazes of varying molecular weights, it was applied in the drop printing process to create naproxen-PEG 3350 solid dispersions, which produced accurate doses and consistent compositional homogeneity [29].

6.4.1.1.4 Polyurethane

Because of their mechanical elasticity, water sensitivity, biocompatibility, and biodegradability, polyurethanes are used in 3D printing for the formulation of biomedical disposables. Using FDM 3D printing to produce drug-loaded tablets proved to be a highly feasible use of commercially available PU. 100 to 180 °C is the temperature range at which PU extrusion occurs [35].

6.4.1.1.5 Polylactic Acid

Three-dimensional drug-delivery devices are frequently printed using PLA, a recyclable polymer. It is regarded as safe for usage and is permitted by the US FDA. For printing purposes, fused deposition modeling can be employed since PLA possesses adequate thermoplastic characteristics. PLA filaments are made with the right evaluation when combined with the right plasticizer. To obtain the required release kinetics, PLA is mixed with an assortment of medications and ingredients. PLA is appropriate for continuous drug release, nevertheless, because of its sluggish rate of degradation [31].

6.4.1.1.6 Poly(Lactide-Co-Glycolide)

The copolymer of polyglycolic acid and polylactic acid is called polylactide-co-glycolic acid. Glycolide (GA) and lactide polymerization by ring-opening was the initial method of synthesizing this polymer in the 1970s. For the formulation of disposables for drug delivery, PLGA is a biomaterial that offers excellent biocompatibility and feasibility. High repeatability is possessed by PLGA. This polymer has higher reproductivity and purity because it is a synthetic substance and is not reliant on external environmental variables. Furthermore, PLGA is more stable than PLA and PGA, ensuring a longer drug release that may endure for several months [19].

6.4.1.1.7 Polycaprolactone

Commercial polymers like PCL are very biodegradable, biocompatible, and processable. Because ester linkage hydrolysis breaks down PCL into less hazardous chemicals like carbon dioxide and water, it causes the gradual destruction of PCL in human beings. Given that a polymeric matrix is essential for the extended proclamation of the integrated material in DDSs, these properties support the usage of PCL in the 3D printing of these materials. Furthermore, PCL's safe usage in humans was approved by the FDA [35].

6.4.1.2 Natural Biopolymers

6.4.1.2.1 Polysaccharides

In general, ether bond O-glycosidic connections bind the monosaccharide units that makeup polysaccharides' backbone. Numerous uses exist for these materials in drug delivery since they are highly stable, hydrophilic by nature, nontoxic, compatible, decomposable, and easily modifiable. In the conception of drug delivery systems via 3D printing, polysaccharides such as chitosan, hyaluronic acid, glycol chitosan, pullulan, dextrin, alginate, and cellulose are employed [52].

6.4.1.2.2 Proteins

Protein-based compounds undergo a naturally occurring, regulated breakdown. When phosphodiester links in the main polymeric chain and side chains dissolve, the polymers disintegrate through a process known as hydrolysis. This important component is being investigated for an assortment of uses. It is an animal protein that is naturally present in connective tissue. In 3D bioprinting, collagen is commonly employed [46]. There are a few problems with this strategy, though. Collagen turns liquid when this polymer is exposed to low temperatures, and as the temperature rises, it forms a fibrous structure. At roughly 37 °C, the entire gelation process of collagen may take half an hour. 3D-printed materials suffer from this moderate gelation rate [47].

6.4.2 Additives

6.4.2.1 Lactose

In pharmaceutical 3D powder bed printing, lactose can be employed as a diluent or filler. The powder mixture utilized in 3D-printed tablets can benefit from improvements in compatibility, physical firmness, and drug dispersibility. For 3D powder bed printing, lactose monohydrate binder blends are generally recommended since they can improvise mechanical characteristics. Owing to lactose's high solubility, an API that is both hydrophilic and phobic was successfully formed into a printed tablet [65].

6.4.2.2 Hydroxypropyl Methylcellulose

HPMC, a cellulose-based polymer, is widely used as a binder and diluent in 3D-printed dosage forms. HMPC is distinct from other 3D printing materials because of its low toxicity and dissolvability. HPMC is commonly printable in three dimensions through the use of an extrusion process. The hollow structure of the initial printed product could be preserved when printing HPMC, which was discovered to be readily extracted from the construction material by dissolving it in water. Researchers manufactured semisolid tablets with varying drug loading quantities at room temperature using a 3D printer based on extrusion [17].

6.5 Challenges and Regulatory Considerations of 3DP for the Integration of API

Ensuring robust quality standards and navigating complex regulatory frameworks are crucial in the pharmaceutical segment, particularly in the cutting-edge arena of 3D printing for SODF development. One important factor in overcoming these obstacles is the strategic planning that roadmaps contain. In addition to shedding light on the path toward technological advancements, roadmaps are essential resources for negotiating the complex world of regulatory compliance [24]. Roadmaps provide a methodical means of overcoming obstacles by coordinating strategic planning with regulatory control goals. Together with foreseeing regulatory roadblocks, they offer a systematic framework that outlines protocols for stringent quality requirements. By ensuring that the manufacturing progressions adhere to regulatory standards, this integration facilitates a seamless transition from conception to commercialization [41].

Although multiple SODFs with varied release profiles and geometries have been efficaciously manufactured utilizing different 3DP technologies and materials, only one of them has been certified and released onto the market. This is because 3DP technology still faces several obstacles in the drug production process, including regulatory barriers as there aren't now regulatory paths for 3DP SODFs (Fig. 6.2). To provide regulatory considerations for medical devices made utilizing 3DP technology, the FDA released a draft guidance document in 2017 titled "Technical Considerations for AM Medical Devices" [51].

It is not yet determined what the quality standards are for oral formulations that are 3D printed. It is uncertain if the existing BP testing for tablets also fully applies to 3D-printed tablets, even though the BP does outline quality requirements for tablets. The procedures used for 3DP are distinct from those used for traditional oral dose forms, although researchers adhere to the same standards of quality. The ingredients used in 3DP are a further regulatory matter. While ingredients used in 3D printing for pharmaceutical applications are either extensively utilized in polymer

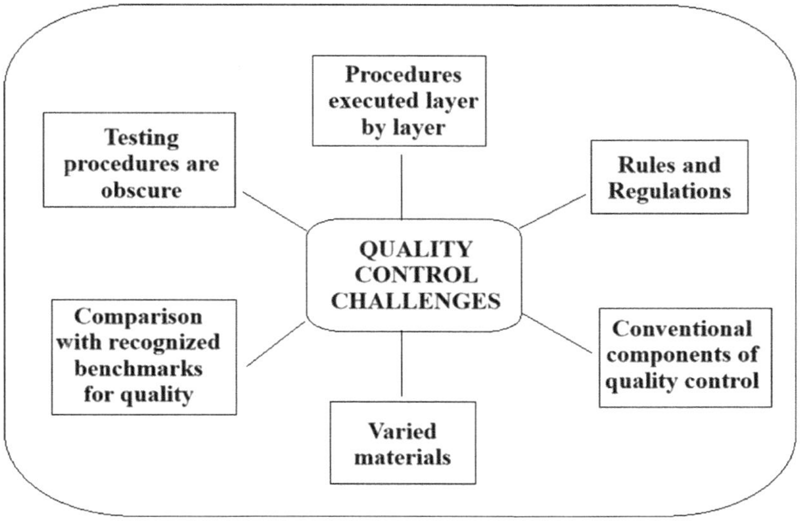

Fig. 6.2 Quality control challenges

processing or are approved for use in pharmaceutical implementations, traditional drug manufacturing processes typically use materials that are well-characterized and standardized. In contrast, 3DP involves a broader array of materials with varying properties. Regulatory bodies are attempting to assess whether materials are appropriate for use in the pharmaceutical sector, even if their position as materials varies. Quality control is a major difficulty in the manufacturing of 3D-printed SODF. The uniformity of the finished product is an issue because 3DP is an LbL process. New testing and acceptance criteria may need to be developed because standard quality control tests might not be appropriate for 3D-printed SODFs.

The process is closely watched over and managed to guarantee constant quality because variables such as material qualities, printer calibration, and printing parameters can all influence the 3D-printed SODFs' quality. Demonstrating the consistency and reproducibility of the 3DP process is a major regulatory problem. To manage the eminence of the raw materials used in the 3DP process, it is necessary to preserve the required product qualities. Manufacturers of 3D-printed SODFs can offer a more thorough production process by implementing QbD and PAT into the manufacturing process.

6.6 Conclusion and Future Outlooks of 3D Printing

With its capability to produce individualized, customized solutions that cater to the unique requirements of the patient, three-dimensional printing holds the potential to entirely transmute the pharmaceutical sector. An assortment of drug delivery devices, including pills, capsules, patches, and implants, may be produced using three-dimensional printing in pharmacies and hospitals to allow for the focused and regulated distribution of medication. Medication safety and efficiency can be enhanced, and the likelihood of adverse effects can be lessened [32]. Hospitals and pharmacies may be able to operate more efficiently and adaptably if 3D printing makes it possible to produce small quantities of goods on demand and do away with the need for extensive manufacturing and inventory management [4].

It is highly probable that shortly, 3D printing will be utilized for medication dispensing in pharmacies, hospitals, and even homes. As a result, pharmacists—who serve as the primary users—need to get ready with their knowledge and abilities for this emerging field of employment. The ability to execute these scenarios can, above all, be achieved by tackling complex practical issues that span from daily practice (as seen from the perspective of healthcare personnel) to safety-first (as seen from the standpoint of the patient). Finally, there is still no clear guidance on how to prepare or manufacture medicine using 3D printing. Therefore, major adjustments must be made while taking into account the laws as they stand now and the opinions of all relevant parties or professionals [5].

References

1. Abdulhameed O, Al-Ahmari A, Ameen W, et al. Additive manufacturing: challenges, trends, and applications. Adv Mech Eng. 2019;11
2. Aita I El, Breitkreutz J, Quodbach J. Investigation of semisolid formulations for 3D printing of drugs after prolonged storage to mimic real-life applications. Eur J Pharm Sci. 2020;146:105266.
3. Al Rashid A, Ahmed W, Khalid MY, et al. Vat photopolymerization of polymers and polymer composites: processes and applications. Addit Manuf. 2021;47:102279.
4. Algahtani MS. Assessment of pharmacist's knowledge and perception toward 3D printing technology as a dispensing method for personalized medicine and the readiness for implementation. Pharmacy. 2021;9(1):68.
5. Andreadis II, Gioumouxouzis CI, Eleftheriadis GK, et al. The advent of a new era in digital healthcare: a role for 3D printing technologies in drug manufacturing? Pharmaceutics. 2022;14(3):609.
6. Awad A, Goyanes A, Basit AW, et al. A review of state-of-the-art on enabling additive manufacturing processes for precision medicine. J Manuf Sci Eng. 2022;145
7. Awad A, Fina F, Goyanes A, et al. 3D printing: principles and pharmaceutical applications of selective laser sintering. Int J Pharm. 2020;586:119594.
8. Azad MA, Olawuni D, Kimbell G, et al. Polymers for extrusion-based 3D printing of pharmaceuticals: a holistic material–process perspective. Pharmaceutics. 2020;12:1–34.
9. Bethany CG, Jayda LE, Sarah YL, Chengpeng C, Dana MS. Evaluation of 3D Printing and Its Potential Impact on Biotechnology and the Chemical Sciences. Anal. Chem. 2014;86: 3240–3253.
10. Azizi Machekposhti S, Mohaved S, Narayan RJ, et al. Inkjet dispensing technologies: recent advances for novel drug discovery. Expert Opin Drug Discov. 2019;14(2):101–13.
11. Boparai KS, Singh R Development of rapid tooling using fused deposition modeling, in Additive Manufacturing of Emerging Materials (Springer International Publishing, Cham) 2019:251–277.
12. Bozkurt Y, Karayel E. 3D printing technology; methods, biomedical applications, future opportunities and trends. J Mater Res Technol. 2021;14:1430–50.

13. Cader HK, Rance GA, Alexander MR, et al. Water-based 3D inkjet printing of an oral pharmaceutical dosage form. Int J Pharm. 2019;564:359–68.
14. Camargo JC, Machado ÁR, Almeida EC, et al. Mechanical properties of PLA-graphene filament for FDM 3D printing. Int J Adv Manuf Technol. 2019;103(5–8):2423–43.
15. Chang P, Mei H, Zhou S. 3D printed electrochemical energy storage devices. J Mater Chem. 2019;7(9):4230–58.
16. Chowdhury H. Circular Economy Integration in Additive Manufacturing [Internet]. MDPI AG; 2023. http://dx.doi.org/10.20944/preprints202310.0087.v1.
17. Cheng Y, Qin H, Acevedo NC, et al. 3D printing of extended-release tablets of theophylline using hydroxypropyl methylcellulose (HPMC) hydrogels. Int J Pharm. 2020;591:119983.
18. Clark EA, Alexander MR, Irvine DJ, et al. 3D printing of tablets using inkjet with UV photoinitiation. Int J Pharm. 2017;529(1–2):523–30.
19. Dang Y, Guan J. Nanoparticle-based drug delivery systems for cancer therapy. Smart Mater Med. 2020;1:10–9.
20. Dumpa N, Butreddy A, Wang H, et al. 3D printing in personalized drug delivery: an overview of hot-melt extrusion-based fused deposition modeling. Int J Pharm. 2021;600:120501.
21. Funk NL, Fantaus S, Beck RCR, et al. Immediate release 3D printed oral dosage forms: how different polymers have been explored to reach suitable drug release behavior. Int J Pharm. 2022;625:122066.
22. Giangreco NP, Elias JE, Tatonetti NP. No population left behind: improving pediatric drug safety using informatics and systems biology. Br J Clin Pharmacol. 2021;88(4):1464–70.
23. Goyanes A, Allahham N, Trenfield SJ, et al. Direct powder extrusion 3D printing: fabrication of drug products using a novel single-step process. Int J Pharm. 2019;567:11847.
24. Gross BC, Erkal JL, Lockwood SY, et al. Evaluation of 3D printing and its potential impact on biotechnology and the chemical sciences. Anal Chem. 2014;86(7):3240–53.
25. Gueche YA, Sanchez-Ballester NM, Bataille B, et al. Selective laser sintering of solid oral dosage forms with copovidone and paracetamol using a CO_2 laser. Pharmaceutics. 2021;13:160.
26. Guan Yunqin. Application of 3D printing technology in 3D modeling course [J]. Quality Education in West China, 2018(6):169.
27. Gültekin HE, Tort S, Acartürk F, et al. Fabrication of three dimensional printed tablets in flexible doses: a comprehensive study from design to evaluation. J Drug Deliv Sci Technol. 2022;74:103538.
28. Hamed R, Mohamed E, Rahman Z, Khan M. 3D-printing of lopinavir printlets by selective laser sintering and quantification of crystalline fraction by XRPD-chemometric models. Int J Pharm. 2020;592
29. Hsu HY, Harris MT, Toth S, et al. Drop printing of pharmaceuticals: effect of molecular weight on PEG coated-naproxen/PEG 3350 solid dispersions. AIChE J. 2015;61(12):4502–8.
30. Huanbutta K, Sangnim T, et al. Design and development of zero-order drug release gastro retentive floating tablets fabricated by 3D printing technology. J Drug Delivery Sci Technol. 2019;52:831–7.
31. Huanbutta K, Sriamornsak P, Kittanaphon T, et al. Development of a zero-order kinetics drug release floating tablet with anti–flip-up design fabricated by 3D-printing technique. J Pharm Investig. 2021;51:213–22.
32. Huang G (2017) Research on the applications of 3D printing technology in the field of general techniques.
33. Ishita M, Gurvinder K, Amir S, Aneesah M, Cato TL. Progress in 3D Bioprinting Technology for Tissue/Organ Regenerative Engineering. Biomaterials 2020;226:119536.
34. Jacob S, Nair AB, Patel V, et al. 3D printing technologies: recent development and emerging applications in various drug delivery systems. AAPS Pharm Sci Tech. 2020;21(6)
35. Jain A, Bansal KK, Tiwari A, et al. Role of polymers in 3D printing technology for drug delivery—an overview. Curr Pharm Des. 2018;24(42):4979–90.
36. Junqueira LA, Tabriz AG, Raposo FJ, et al. Coupling of fused deposition modeling and inkjet printing to produce drug loaded 3D printed tablets. Pharmaceutics. 2022;14:159.

37. Kadry H, Wadnap S, Xu C, et al. Digital light processing (DLP) 3D-printing technology and photoreactive polymers in the fabrication of modified-release tablets. Eur J Pharm Sci. 2019;135:60–7.
38. Kamaljit SB, Singh R. Development of rapid tooling using fused deposition modeling. Springer EBooks; 2018. p. 251–77.
39. Koczkur KM, Mourdikoudis S, Polavarapu L, et al. Polyvinylpyrrolidone (PVP) in nanoparticle synthesis. Dalton Trans. 2015;44(41):17883–905.
40. Kollamaram G, Faucher A, Croker DM, et al. Valvejet technology for the production of a personalized fixed dose combination of ramipril and glimepiride: an investigative study on the stability of ramipril. Pharm Res. 2018;35(9):181.
41. Lafeber I, Tichem JM, Ouwerkerk N, et al. 3D printed furosemide and sildenafil tablets: innovative production and quality control. Int J Pharm. 2021;603:120694.
42. Lamichhane S, Bashyal S, Keum T, et al. Complex formulations, simple techniques: can 3D printing technology be the midas touch in the pharmaceutical industry? Asian J Pharm Sci. 2019;14:465–79.
43. Liao Y, Liu C, Coppola B, et al. Effect of porosity and crystallinity on 3D printed PLA properties. Polymers. 2019;11(9):1487.
44. Manideep P, Subbaratnam B, Harsha M. Design and development of pallet extruder. AIP Conference Proceedings; 2019.
45. Martinez PR, Basit AW, Gaisford S. The history, developments, and opportunities of stereolithography. In: 3D printing of pharmaceuticals. Springer; 2018.
46. Matai I, Kaur G, Seyedsalehi A, et al. Progress in 3D bioprinting technology for tissue/organ regenerative engineering. Biomaterials. 2019;226:119536.
47. Mobaraki M, Ghaffari M, Yazdanpanah A, et al. Bioinks and bioprinting: a focused review. Bioprinting. 2020;18:e00080.
48. Mostafaei A, Elliott AM, Barnes JE, et al. Binder jet 3D printing—process parameters, materials, properties, modeling, and challenges. Prog Mater Sci. 2021;119:100707.
49. Pagac M, Hajnys J, Ma QP, et al. A review of VAT photopolymerization technology: materials, applications, challenges, and future trends of 3D printing. Polymers. 2021;13:598.
50. Pollard TD, Seoane-Viaño I, Ong JJ, et al. Inkjet drug printing onto contact lenses: deposition optimization and non-invasive dose verification. Int J Pharm X. 2022;5:100150.
51. Prabhakar B, Singh RK, Yadav KS, et al. Artificial intelligence (AI) impacting diagnosis of glaucoma and understanding the regulatory aspects of AI-based software as medical device. Comput Med Imag Graph. 2021;87:101818.
52. Prajapati SK, Jain A, Jain A, et al. Biodegradable polymers and constructs: a novel approach in drug delivery. Eur Polym J. 2019;120:109191.
53. Rodríguez-Panes A, Claver J, Camacho A. The influence of manufacturing parameters on the mechanical behaviour of PLA and ABS pieces manufactured by FDM: a comparative analysis. Materials. 2018;11(8):1333.
54. Sánchez-Guirales SA, Jurado N, Kara A, et al. Understanding direct powder extrusion for fabrication of 3D printed personalized medicines: a case study for nifedipine minitablets. Pharmaceutics. 2021;13:1583.
55. Scoutaris N, Alexander MR, Gellert PR, et al. Inkjet printing as a novel medicine formulation technique. J Control Release. 2011;156(2):179–85.
56. Seoane-Viaño I, Trenfield ISJ, Basit AW, et al. Translating 3D printed pharmaceuticals: from hype to real-world clinical applications. Adv Drug Deliv Rev. 2021b;174:553–75.
57. Seoane-Viaño, Januskaite P, Alvarez-Lorenzo C, et al. Semi-solid extrusion 3D printing in drug delivery and biomedicine: personalized solutions for healthcare challenges. J Control Release. 2021a;332:367–89.
58. Sharma S, Shrestha B, Bhuyan NR, et al. Chemometric method development for the determination of naringin and verapamil. Bull Natl Res Cent. 2024;48:13.
59. Shibata Y, Itoh H, Matsuo H, et al. Differences in pharmaceutical intervention triggers for the optimization of medication by patient age: a university hospital study. Biol Pharm Bull. 2021;44(8):1060–6.

60. Singh D, Singh R, Boparai KS. Development and surface improvement of FDM pattern-based investment casting of biomedical implants: a state-of-the-art review. J Manuf Process. 2018;31:80–95.
61. Singh N, Siddiqui H, Koyalada BSR, et al. Recent advancements in additive manufacturing (AM) techniques: a forward-looking review, vol. 29. Met Mater Int; 2023. p. 2119.
62. Tagami T, Ito E, Kida R, et al. 3D printing of gummy drug formulations composed of gelatin and an HPMC-based hydrogel for pediatric use. Int J Pharm. 2021;594:120118.
63. Uddin MJ, Hassan J, Douroumis D, et al. Thermal inkjet printing: prospects and applications in the development of medicine. Technologies. 2022;10:108.
64. Vadodaria S, Mills T. Jetting-based 3D printing of edible materials. Food Hydrocoll. 2020;106:105857.
65. Van den Heuvel KA, De Wit MT, Dickhoff BH, et al. Evaluation of lactose-based 3D powder bed printed pharmaceutical drug product tablets. Powder Technol. 2021;390:97–102.
66. Whlean C, Sheahan C. Using additive manufacturing to produce injection Moulds suitable for short series production. Procedia Manufacturing. 2019;38:60–8.
67. Xu X, Robles-Martinez P, Madla CM, et al. Stereolithography (SLA) 3D printing of an anti-hypertensive polyprintlet: a case study of an unexpected photopolymer-drug reaction. Addit Manuf. 2020;33:101071.
68. Yang Y, Du T, Zhang J, et al. A 3D-engineered conformal implant releases DNA nanocomplexs for eradicating the postsurgery residual glioblastoma. Adv Sci. 2017;4(8):1600491.
69. Zuccari G, Alfei S, Marimpietri D, et al. Mini-tablets: a valid strategy to combine efficacy and safety in pediatrics. Pharmaceuticals. 2022;15:108.

Personalized Medicine: Unlocking 3D Printing's Potential in the Pharmaceutical Fields

7

Parul Gupta, Vishnu Mittal, Anjali Sharma, Devkant Sharma, and Kuldeep Vinchurkar

Abstract

Advancement in pharmacokinetics and pharmacogenomics has led to a conceptual change in the constantly evolving field of healthcare toward patient-centered care. The research of 3D printing technologies to personalize medicine to each patient's needs has been encouraged by the necessity for customized therapies in light of this advancement. The pharmaceutical industry has been cautious to adopt personalized medicine (PM) despite its revolutionary potential, which has been hindered by this technological paradigm shift. A wide variety of 3D printing methods show potential for producing dosage forms and medical equipment, such as based on nozzle extrusion, laser writing systems, and powder binder jetting. From solid and semisolid formulations to locally administered or implanted medications, these techniques have employed in a wide range of areas. Better patient compliance and efficacy are made possible by solid dosage forms, which also allow for drug combination, release profile modification, and the production of innovative medicines. Joint replacements, prostheses, and cardiovascular procedures are accessible by sustained-release implants and medical equipment. Locally applied medications, such as medicated contact lenses and wound dressings, highlight how versatile 3D printing is in the medical field. But choosing appropriate printing methods and creating pharmaceutical inks with the right physicochemical and biological characteristics are the difficult parts. The prom-

P. Gupta · V. Mittal · A. Sharma
Guru Gobind Singh College of Pharmacy, Yamunanagar, Haryana, India

D. Sharma (✉)
CH. Devi Lal College of Pharmacy, Jagadhari, Haryana, India

K. Vinchurkar
Department of Pharmaceutics, Sandip Institute of Pharmaceutical Sciences (SIPS), Affiliated To Savitribai Phule Pune University (SPPU, Pune), Nashik, Maharashtra, India

K. Vinchurkar, S. Mane (eds.), *Innovations in Drug Manufacturing*,
https://doi.org/10.1007/978-981-96-9075-6_7

ise of 3D printing in creating individualized medications for serious illnesses is encouraging, despite certain obstacles. Especially, developing a single dosage form that contains several medications has great promise for people with polypharmacy. This chapter presents an overview of 3D printing technology in customized medicine, highlighting its revolutionary role in influencing future of healthcare delivery by going over various processes, materials, and applications.

Keywords

3D printing · Personalized medicine · Medical equipment · Nozzle extrusion Laser writing systems · Powder binder jetting · Medical equipment

Abbreviations

AI	Artificial intelligence
AM	Additive manufacturing
API	Active pharmaceutical ingredients
CADD	Computer-aided design and draft
CDRH	Centre for Device and Radiological Health
CFR	Code of Federal Regulation
CJP	Continuous jet printing
CMC	Chemistry, manufacturing, and control
DLP	Digital light processing
DOD	Drop on demand
FDA	Food and Drug Administration
FDM	Fused deposition modeling
KRAS	Kirsten rat sarcoma
LOM	Laminated object manufacturing
NDDS	Novel Drug Delivery Systems
NECC	New England Compounding Centre
OSEL	The Office of Science and Engineering Laboratories
PI	Physical intelligence
PLA	Poly(lactic acid)
PM	Personalized medicine
PVA	Polyvinyl alcohol
RP	Rapid prototyping
SFF	Solid free-form technology
SLA	Stereolithography apparatus

7.1 Introduction

Drug development sector has witnessed a significant shift and expansion in treatment options, offering safer and more effective treatments. Personalized medicine (PM) has been one of the most notable developments. PM has the capacity to offer the largest safety margins and optimal responses in treatment. As a result, there are fewer adverse effects and improved patient safety [1, 2]. Drug delivery is nothing more than a technique used to precisely administer a pharmacologically active component inside the body in order to provide a safe and effective therapeutic effect. Pharmacokinetics can be balanced by controlling release profile of medicinal products, which also serves to ensure safety and efficacy [3]. Due to individual genetic differences, 'omics'-based approaches are being used to personalize drug therapy, how much they are given, and what kind of help they get. PM wants to be a part of these changes. The aims are to improve healthcare, speed up search for new medicines and discoveries, and find out how likely it is a person will get certain illnesses [4, 5]. In 1997, Phase III tests for breast cancer that included Herceptin failed because drug didn't work for everyone. But when they looked more closely, they saw response was much better in women who tested positive for raised HER2. The FDA-approved drug and diagnostic mix in 1998 after seeing it would help people who were HER2 positive (as shown by a test) [6]. European officials turned down and banned Amgen's colon cancer drug Vectibix [7] unapproved for marketing since it was determined to be inapplicable to a large number of patients. Vectibix fared better in patients whose tumours lacked a Kirsten rat sarcoma (KRAS) gene mutation, according to the company's overall analysis of the data. Permission to use the medication for those patients alone was subsequently given [8]. Therefore, a patient's gene variant profile can be used by a physician to aid in the selection of medication and therapy choices that minimize side effects and result in positive outcomes. Furthermore, PM may be used as prophylactic to avoid infections in sensitive persons since it is possible to identify an individual's sensitivity to specific diseases before they manifest. With help of PM, doctors can now offer drugs more effectively for each patient, going beyond one-size-fits-all way [1, 2, 9].

When working with dosage forms holding different active ingredients, 3D printing technology is important. This allows for making of single or multilayered pills with delayed release rates. Additive manufacturing refers to process of making 3D things using computer-controlled layers of materials in 3D printing technology. Many 3D printing methods, including stereolithography, inkjet printing, and fused deposition, are being applied in retail business these days [10]. In recent times, there has been a marked rise of use of 3D printing across drug study process. This includes research study, clinical tests, and direct medical care. Compared with normal drug types, this technology offers a wide range of benefits. Precision and accuracy can also be attained, and small doses can result in high drug-loading capacities. With the advent of 3D printing technology, healthcare practitioners now have access to an extensive range of methods for creating customized medications and medical equipment. Tablets were the first intended use for 3D printing technologies. From straightforward formulations that only included the drug in an uncommercially available dose, to intricate systems that integrated various release profiles into a single tablet and included all the required medications in a dosage customized for the patient, these systems came in a variety of forms. Three-dimensional printing (3D printing) has allowed making of steel limbs, injectable devices, and other medical goods.

The scientific community has been giving more and more attention in recent years to use of 3D printing technology in creation of medications that contain biopharmaceuticals or medications housed within nanovehicles or nanomedicines [11].

7.1.1 3D Printing

Additive manufacturing and 3D printing, which is a term for a group of methods, use a variety of technologies to build three-dimensional things layer by layer using model data. Using computer-aided design tools, 3D printing is a process of making 3D things layer by layer from digital plans [12, 13]. The earliest evidence of 3D printing's potential as a replacement for traditional tableting methods was presented in 1996 [14]. Personalized 3D-printed medications can address numerous problems for patients with poor therapeutic indices or pharmacogenetic polymorphisms [15]. Furthermore, the patient would have access to more effective medication with less risk of a negative drug reaction. Patients' chances of survival would rise even more as a result [16–18]. Therefore, several diseases designed at the time of therapy could be cured with a single dose. This improves patient compliance while having the fewest negative effects, revolutionizing the way drugs are designed and the treatments are available to patients [18, 19]. Due to the extensive features and adaptability of 3D printing technology, any dosage form with a single or many applications can be created with a preset release profile [20–24]. This methodology employs a range of healthcare providers, ranging from community pharmacies for basic and secondary care to hospital wards for tertiary care. In these locations, dispensing medications could enhance patient access, cut down on medication waste, and expedite discharge. If 3D printers were introduced into disaster zones, emergency rooms, first reaction units, and military actions, they could even be used to quickly make one-off amounts in cases where resources are limited [25]. Scientists could have more freedom with 3D printing of tiny reaction tubes for on-demand creation of active medical ingredients (API). 3D printing has ability to ease small-scale creation of different elements in comparison with normal methods. This is especially good for drugs that have low stability or high cost [26]. Assessment of a broad range of amounts is important for clinical studies [27]. The freedom of 3D printing technology allowed for creation of an ideal product with faster lead times and lower development costs by allowing a broad variety of amounts and forms to meet study criteria. Thus, without delaying care, life can be saved at the lowest possible cost. Additionally, this technology makes it possible for patients to easily achieve benefits and lessen their pain from drug side effects [28]. Advantages, disadvantages and opportunities of 3D printing are shown in Fig. 7.1.

The approach is limited, though, in that it doesn't account for printed material's heat tolerance or solvent incompatibilities. Wherever novel drug delivery systems (NDDS) may be effectively integrated with 3D printing technology, process performance must develop to address these challenges [29]. 3D printers might be used in hospital pharmacies to produce customized medications on demand, which would be advantageous both financially and logically. Therefore, 3D-printed personalized

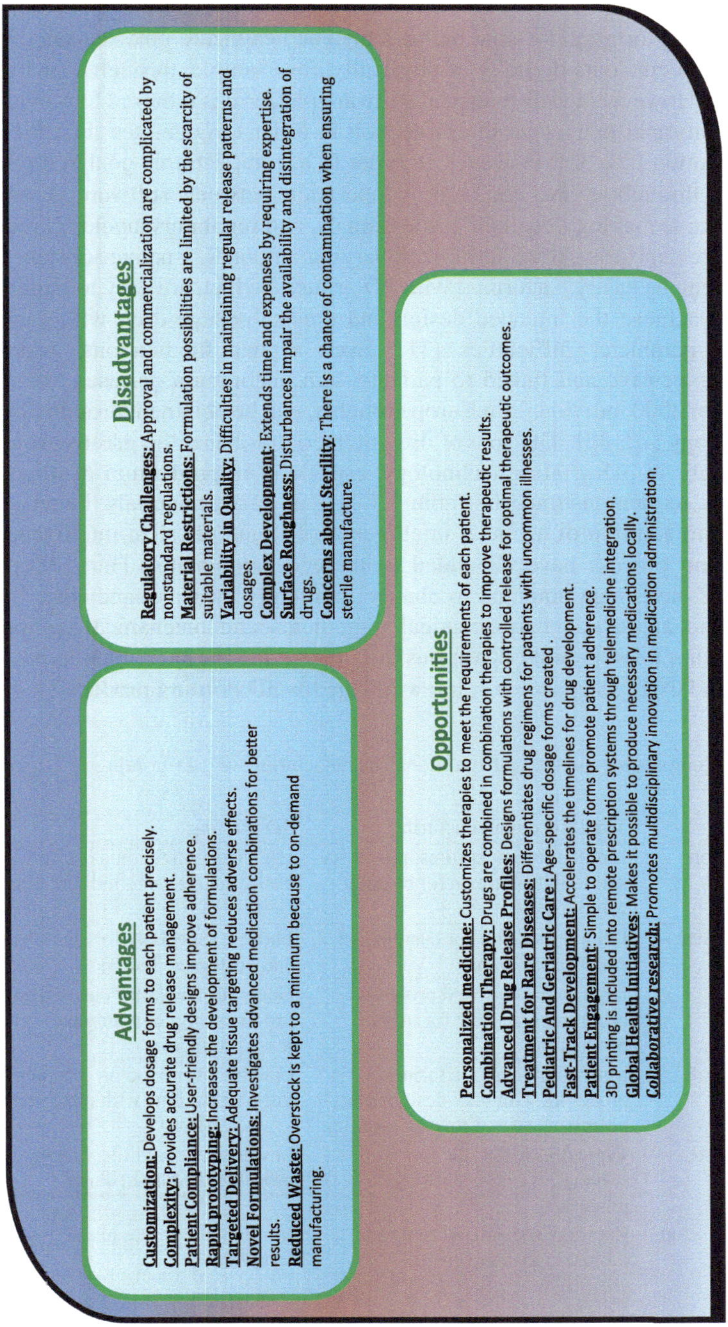

Fig. 7.1 Advantages, disadvantages, and opportunities of 3D printing

doses can take the trend on the next level of therapy by delivering affordable drugs that adequately treat the ailment, even though conventional dosages cost a lot of money and may or may not treat the patient. The healthcare provider may receive the patient-specific data digitally or physically, for example, through a smartphone application. However, a well-managed software platform is required to provide data confidentiality and patient profile protection in order to guarantee the efficacy of this intervention [20, 30]. However, in order to accomplish this goal and preserve uniformity throughout the company, cooperation between software developers, innovators in technology, medical professionals, and regulatory bodies is required. The accurate deposition of material with varying amounts of active substances and excipients can be easily performed with 3D printers, which are easy to handle. It is possible to achieve the intended design and precise dosage even with additional processing parameter difficulties [31]. Even orphan medications, which are extremely expensive and linked to patients with uncommon diseases that impact less than 1 in 2000 individuals in Europe roughly, can be obtained through 3D printing technology [22, 32]. The area of drug delivery has benefited greatly from huge breakthroughs in 3D printing technology, especially in production of micro- and nanorobots. As demonstrated in Table 7.1, use of smart materials, better control methods, and addition of artificial intelligence (AI) and physical intelligence (PI) into planning process have all added to these developments. Thus, 3D-printed microrobots have huge potential to change minimally invasive medicine. Using a low-cost and approved pharmaceutical ingredients and mechanical components while allowing for suitability of various drug molecules, and eliminating post-print finishing and drying steps are just a few of benefits 3D printing produced.

Table 7.1 Comparative analysis of traditional manufacturing vs. 3D printing in personalized medicine

Aspect	Traditional manufacturing	3D printing
Customization	Limited, often requires high costs and long lead times for custom solutions	High customization capabilities, easily adaptable to individual needs
Production time	Long, especially for custom and small-batch items	Shorter, especially for small batches and customized items
Cost	High for customized products, economies of scale for mass production	Generally lower for customized products, higher material cost for mass production
Complexity of designs	Limited by manufacturing processes, complex designs can be expensive and time-consuming	Capable of producing complex and intricate designs with relative ease
Material waste	Typically higher due to subtractive manufacturing processes	Lower due to additive manufacturing processes, minimal waste
Tooling and setup	Requires specialized tools and molds, high setup costs	Minimal tooling required, lower setup costs

(continued)

Table 7.1 (continued)

Aspect	Traditional manufacturing	3D printing
Scalability	Highly scalable for mass production, less efficient for small batches	Less scalable for mass production, more efficient for small batches and customization
Regulatory compliance	Established standards and processes, easier to ensure compliance	Emerging standards, regulatory hurdles for ensuring compliance and validation
Quality control	Well-established QC processes, consistency in large-scale production	Emerging QC processes, potential variability in small-scale production
Supply chain complexity	Complex, requires multiple suppliers and longer lead times	Simplified, potential for on-site production reducing supply chain complexity
Biocompatibility	Limited by materials that can be used in traditional manufacturing	Greater potential for biocompatible and patient-specific materials
Environmental impact	Higher due to material waste and energy consumption	Potentially lower due to reduced waste and more efficient material use
Innovation and iteration	Slower due to tooling and setup constraints	Faster, allowing rapid prototyping and iteration
Patient-specific solutions	Limited, expensive, and time-consuming	Highly suited for patient-specific solutions, more cost-effective

7.1.2 History

3D printing was proposed as a potential foundation for personal health in the 1990s. Significant advancements in the field of 3D-printed medical devices have been made possible by the FDA's Center for Device and Radiological Health (CDRH) evaluation and clearance of 3DP medical devices [33]. Thus, first 3D printing technique was used to assemble pieces. The procedure was carried out again until the last required form was obtained. Sachs et al. filed a patent on this when it was discovered for the first time at Massachusetts Institute of Technology in the early 1990s [34]. Fused deposition modeling is another 3D printing technique for which Scott Crump filed a 1989 patent application. The semiliquid heated polymer strands had to be released via a heated tube and then distributed layer by layer over a construct foundation to solidify [35]. The automobile, aerospace, medical, and tissue engineering sectors have all seen significant technological advancements, whereas 3D printing is still in its infancy in pharmaceutical sector.

7.2 Regulatory Expectations

Technical Considerations for Medical Devices Manufactured Using Additive Manufacturing was published by the US FDA in 2017. This page covers a number of standards, including design and manufacturing process aspects, tool testing, and labeling. In accordance with established protocols, it also recommends confirming the critical processes in order to provide a high degree of certainty. To meet the current requirements in the quality system rule for device approval, more paperwork has to be completed. Process validation becomes essential when further testing and inspection are not feasible to fully validate a process's outputs. Software has to be examined to make sure it is being utilized according to a set methodology and for the intended purpose [36, 37].

Regarding powder bed fusion technology, the guidelines included the following examples:

- In-process parameter monitoring, including build-space environmental factors (such as temperature, pressure, and humidity), melt pool data, and temperature at beam focus.
- Reliability of printing system's mechanical components (recoater, gantry, etc.)
- The power of energy delivery system (laser, electron beam, extruder, etc.)
- Visual inspection done by hand or automatically using predetermined acceptance criteria
- Test coupon evaluation
- Nondestructive evaluation

Any modifications made to device, the manufacturing process, or deviations from the procedure should be noted and any possible dangers should be examined. This assessment may indicate that the process needs to be revalidated as a result of the modification or deviation [36]. When thinking about making modifications to an additively manufactured device that has already been cleared or approved, manufacturers should refer to the current FDA guidance regarding their regulatory pathway. Here are a few instances of revalidation triggers unique to additive manufacturing:

- Modifications to software (such as updates or modifications to build preparation software)
- Modifications to build volume's device or component spacing or orientation
- Modifications to the software workflow
- Transfer of the machine physically
- Adjustments to postprocessing parameters or steps [38–41]

A key problem regarding rules directing 3D-printed medicine is difference between made and mixed drugs. The safety of medications has been under scrutiny due to fatal events such as the 2012 New England Compounding Center (NECC) [42] and several other hazardous safety issues at compounding enterprises [43, 44]. Similar to dosage forms, 3D-printed pharmaceutical items must be made in accordance with pharmaceutical manufacturing standards satisfy 21 CFR 200 and 300 and other relevant recommendations' criteria for current chemical, manufacturing, and control (CMC) [45, 46]. Protecting makers and buyers requires dealing crucial concerns about 3D-printed drugs, such as legal responsibility and intellectual property. Completing FDA's current controlling standards could be a big hurdle that stops them from being given to market [47]. As a result of this quickly rising technology, FDA might need to change its normal rules and provide short-term advice documents [48–50]. Despite all the legal hurdles linked to 3D printing drugs, FDA cleared Spritam® (levetiracetam), first 3D-printed pill, in August 2015 [51].

7.3 3D Printing Technologies for Personalized Drug Delivery

3D printing is a manufacturing process that uses layer after layer of material to make implants, drugs, and other equipment [52, 53]. Other names for this process are solid free-form technology (SFF), rapid prototyping (RP), and additive manufacturing (AM). Different printing methods, styles, speeds, and pictures are available for a range of printing processes nowadays [19, 54]. A top-notch computer-aided style and draft (CADD) program is now being applied to make the medicine product's style. Moreover, the design has been cut out using this program to make standard processing factors such as extruder and platform temperature, filling percentage, printing speed, etc. After finishing, the 3D printer keeps making the medical product by following directions [25, 55]. To help with the printing process, raw materials can be made into bits, threads, or binding solutions based on the learning printing method. The necessary pharmaceutical product is made by automatically adding raw components and letting them to harden layer by layer. Products may be dried, joined, and finished after printing. Unprinted material can now be collected and recovered to be used again in the printing process [25, 55, 56]. The use of 3D printing technology in healthcare business has grown within the past 15 years. This method is also used by the medicine business. 3D printing was important to patient care as well as study and development. Features of various 3D printing technologies are depicted in Table 7.2. The many 3D printing methods being studied for custom medicine distribution will be covered in the part that follows.

7.3.1 Inkjet Printing

The word "inkjet printing" refers to a broad category of devices that may provide digitally controlled liquid drop formulation and placement onto a substrate with the aid of a pattern-generating device [57]. The two primary droplet creation systems used in inkjet printing technology are drop on demand (DOD) and continuous jet (CJ) printing [58].

7.3.2 Continuous Jet

In order to make a steady stream of charged drops, CJ printing needs a packed flow. The drops in the system are pushed onto the ground by the electric plates, where they are put. Moreover, the trash formed throughout the process is retrieved and made useful again [59, 60]. Both CJ and drop on demand printing utilize a combined printer head, which can be either heat and mechanical. This gives for control over the liquid's density and drop making traits [61].

Table 7.2 Features of various 3D printing technologies

3D printing technology	Features of material	Material	Best particle size	Minimum feature size	Minimum layer thickness	Tolerance	Build speed and surface finish	Functions	Advantages	Disadvantages
Fused deposition modeling	Solid (filaments)	Polycarbonate, thermoplastics,and elastomers; polyphenyl sulfone	36 × 24 × 36 in	0.005 in.	0.0050 in.	0.0050 in.	The external finish is rough and build speed is sluggish	Tooling adjustments are made quickly, and heat is used extensively in patient and food applications, presentation models, small parts, and other settings	Plastic is used, it is less expensive; printing is also less expensive and widely available. The drug's homogeneity and friability are both high	Sanding and eliminating support that left marks are necessary; limited testing funding is anticipated for thermoplastic material warping. The process starting material may deteriorate due to high temperature
Stereolithography	Liquid (photopolymer)	Mainly photocuring polymers which arouse polypropylene, ABS, PBT, rubber; expansion of ceramic-metal alloys	59.00 × 29.50 × 19.70 in	0.004 in	0.0010 in	0.0050 in	The outside finish is modest and build rate is medium	Quick tooling patterns, intricate components, quick works, presentation models, and high heat utilization	The object's size is submicron and decimicron, and it may be printed with excellent accuracy and resolution using any other kind of 3D technology	Before printing as well as drying, equipment is expensive and time-consuming

Selective laser sintering	Powder (polymer)	Elastomers; composite; thermoplastics material such as nylon, polyamide, and polystyrene.	22.00 × 22.00 × 30.00 in	0.005 in	0.0040 in	0.0100 in	Build momentum is quick, and external finish is mediocre	Rapid tooling, less intricate parts, snap-fit parts, and increased heat usage are patterns seen	High internal microstructure and porosity, easily manageable and reproducible .	The postprinting finishing process is necessary. The interconnection's speed is limited. More energy inputs result in deterioration of beginning materials
Inkjet printing	Liquid	Natural as well as synthetic waxes, acrylic established thermopolymeric plastic, fatty esters	12.00 × 6.00 × 6.00 in	0.005 in	0.0005 in	0.0010 in	The plane's production rate and external finish are slow	Medical devices: Quick assembly pattern is extremely quick; parts are highly detailed	Excellent resolution and accuracy, material versatility, and cost-effectiveness for small batches	Limited mechanical strength, material restrictions, and difficulties with regulation and quality
Laminated object manufacturing	Paper, plastics (sheets)	Paper; composites; thermoplastics such as PVC	32.00 × 22.00 × 20.00 in	0.008 in	0.0020 in	0.0040 in	Build rate and coarse exterior finish are sobering	There are extremely few detailed parts and rapid tooling patterns	High production speed, low material waste, and material versatility	Problems with material layer bonding, postprocessing requirements, and limited detail and resolution

7.3.3 Drop on Demand

DOD printing has up to 1000 holes and is more exact and efficient in its operation. Thermal and magnetic trigger methods are the main ways of starting these printheads. Heat from the creation of electric current causes bubbles to form in the explosive material being written in the thermal printer. Due to drop creation, this causes a tiny amount of liquid to be pushed out of the tip. Heat-sensitive bioactive chemicals may degrade as a result of the high temperatures produced by thermal inkjet printing, which necessitates use of high vapor pressure solutions [59, 62]. However, when an electrical current is given, piezoelectric materials which are connected to piezoelectric printheads expand and shrink [63]. Due to the formation of a pulse that causes a fluid with a shear rate of roughly 105 s^{-1}, this shift can produce enough pressure to eject a droplet [58–65]. The main benefit of both ways is the ability to make many depositions at once using different materials and colors that are made layer by layer as needed. When using "powder bed fusion," often referred to as "solid deposition," where droplets are printed directly onto solid material, droplets arrange themselves to make different pattern layers [57, 59, 66, 67].

7.3.4 Fused Deposition Modeling

Fused deposition modeling (FDM) printers are a famous and cheap printing technology that uses an inkjet-like motor. But when the printer advances, hot plastic bits are released in place of ink, covering the sample thinly [68]. This printing technology makes use of thermoplastic polymers such as PLA, PVA, and acrylonitrile butadiene styrene [69, 70]. Molten materials (mixtures of polymers and API) are allowed to flow through the hole and are put in the form of strands in layers on a platform. These filaments solidify and then settle. Thus, fused filament fabrication is another name for the method. Feed rate, pressure drop, and nozzle diameter all affect how much material is deposited. FDM has an advantage over powder-bed printing in that it can produce multipurpose scaffolds with precise dosing systems. Additionally, by adjusting the formulation's surface area, 3D model design, or infill percentage, FDM provides good mechanical strength with varying kinetics. The adoption of FDM printing technology is restricted by limited thermoplastic material and temperature-sensitive APIs [67, 71].

7.3.5 Stereolithography

Charles Hullin created stereolithography, commonly referred to as a laser-based writing technique, in 1980 [19]. The idea is based on the process of photopolymerization, in which UV light and a photoinitiator interact to produce free radicals [57]. Certain photosensitive liquid resin surface areas in a stereolithography apparatus (SLA) are exposed to a UV laser to cause localized polymerization [72, 73]. In 1986, this technique was brought to the market [74]. When using stereolithography, ultraviolet light is permitted to reach the liquid resin's surface, changing each separate layer's exposure along the x/y-axis as the z-axis gradually changes over the build process [19]. In order to create 3D-printed models, another layer of liquid resin is applied after the previous layer sets. Up till a completed product is created, these liquid resins are layered one over the other [57]. Extra glue is taken off the component after it's finished so it may be used again. Once any remaining glue has been cleaned from the linked sections, support structures are physically removed. The kind of resin material being used will determine whether a UV flash postcuring step is necessary for photopolymer conversion. The final result often has a degree of surface roughness akin to manufactured components when bases, paints, sealants, or metallic finishes are applied [75]. While layers of hard polymer are created by stereolithography using a laser beam, circular cells (voxels) are created by digital light processing (DLP) using a high resolution projector. Given that DLP may receive the whole layer at once, it is often quicker than SLA [76]. The primary advantages of using laser-based printing as a 3D printing technique are, in fact, its time-consuming nature, smooth parts that don't need to be finished, and high-resolution objects while also requiring a high level of resolution [74, 77]. The thickness of the finished layer, which relies on the light strength that the plastic is exposed to, is an important aspect that needs to be managed in SLA printing [78].

7.3.6 Extrusion-Based Bioprinting

This method uses air or mechanical pressure to spread bioink through a tube which is intended to follow a pattern made by a computer [79]. Bioinks are objects used in 3D printing that are filled with cells and other organic ingredients. The method allows for the exact placement of tiny cell units with the least amount of process-induced cell damage. By using a screwdriver, pump, or air force on a building platform, polymer or hydrogel is generally spread from steel or plastic needles. Pneumatic methods dispense material more slowly because of compressed gas, but they work better with very thick liquid polymer. However, the hydrogel flow from the tube is generally more directly controlled by the piston-driven layers method. On the other hand, screw-based devices are useful for the dispensing of highly sticky hydrogels and offer greater spatial control [80, 81]. Scaffolds for bone [82], aortic valve [83], cartilage [84], skeletal muscle [85], brain [86], and other tissue rebuilding have been made by extrusion bioprinting. Despite all of this success, the bioprinting method's material selection and mechanical strength continue to be important problems [87].

7.3.7 Laminated Object Manufacturing

Helisys of Torrance, California, created first trade laminated object manufacturing (LOM) technology in 1991. The primary components of the system that are covered on a physical platform are the maize mechanism. A heated roller is used to bind the plate to layer below, and a laser is used to cut each section of plate layer. Layers of adhesive-coated sheet material are created by cutting, stacking, and bonding them on top of the previously stated components. Before the portion is completed, the process can be repeated [87].

7.4 Applications of 3D Printing in Personalized Medicines

7.4.1 Patient-Specific Oral Dosage Forms Fabrications

The capacity to produce oral dosage forms tailored to each patient is a key benefit of 3D printing in delivery of medicines. Oral drug manufacture is generally restricted to specified sizes and formulations by means of conventional manufacturing techniques. Pharmaceutical businesses, however, can create customized dosage forms with 3D printing that are suited to each person's unique requirements [88]. Personalized dosing is made possible by this customization, which also enhances patient adherence to prescription schedules and optimizes therapeutic results. Moreover, 3D printing makes it possible to combine medications or varied dosages into a single tablet, which simplifies treatment for patients with complicated drug regimens and allows combination therapy [89, 90].

7.4.2 Personalized Drug Delivery Implants and Devices

3D-printed implants have potential to deliver targeted and drug release sustained at site of action through combination of biocompatible materials and therapeutic ingredients. This targeted medication delivery strategy optimizes therapeutic efficacy while reducing systemic negative effects [91, 93]. To treat cardiovascular disorders, for instance, drug-eluting stents made via 3D printing have been produced. These stents can be made specifically to fit vascular anatomy of patient, and they can include medications that encourage tissue repair and stop restenosis. There are several benefits to using 3D printing for therapeutic administration, such as fast prototyping and manufacture, regulated drug release, intricate geometries, and personalization [92, 93].

7.4.3 Tissue Engineering and Regenerative Medicine

7.4.3.1 Complex Tissue Structures Biofabrications

3D printing plays a key role in area of tissue engineering and regenerative medicine by making it easier to biofabricate complex tissue forms. Researchers can now make 3D models that closely resemble real tissues thanks to the mix of plastics and live cells. This new method has huge possible benefits in organ transfers and tissue repair [89, 94]. Functional tissues including skin, cartilage, and blood arteries have been successfully made by methods. Eventually, patient-specific tissue replacements and disease models may be achieved with the help of these biofabricated tissues [95, 96].

7.4.3.2 Scaffold-Based Approaches for Tissue Regeneration

In tissue engineering, creation of scaffolds is a significant use of 3D printing. Providing a surface for cell adhesion, proliferation, and vascularization, scaffolds facilitate tissue regeneration in a temporary supporting capacity. Precise control over the structural and architectural characteristics of scaffolds made with 3D printing is made possible, enabling the adjustment of factors including mechanical robustness, porosity, and pore size [98– 100]. By adding growth hormones and bioactive components to the scaffold materials, scientists can encourage tissue regeneration, cellular differentiation, and proliferation [98, 99].

7.4.4 3D-Printed Prosthetics and Orthotics

3D printing has completely changed the prosthetics and orthotics fields by making it possible to create personalized devices with better fit, functionality, and aesthetics. To produce customized gadgets, traditional approaches frequently require labor-intensive and time-consuming operations. But quick prototyping and customization are made possible by 3D printing, which simplifies the production process [100, 101]. For those with limb loss or musculoskeletal disorders, 3D-printed prosthetics and orthotics with lightweight, durable materials such carbon fiber-reinforced plastics improve comfort, mobility, and quality of life [102, 103].

7.4.5 Surgical Instruments and Customized Implants

The production of personalized implants and surgical tools is a noteworthy use of 3D printing in delivery of healthcare. The standardized sizes and designs of traditional implants and devices may not always be able to accommodate each patient's specific anatomical needs [104]. Similarly, customized and 3D-printed surgical guides and instruments can help surgeons carry out intricate procedures more precisely and effectively [105, 106]. Through its facilitation of the development of customized medical equipment, tissue-engineered constructions, and drug delivery systems, it has accomplished this. By doing this, 3D printing has opened the door for regenerative medicines and personalized medicine.

7.4.6 For Enhanced Interactions Surface Modification of 3D-Printed Structures

Researchers can improve biocompatibility of printed materials, control immune responses, and promote cell adherence by adding nanoscale features, coatings, or biomolecules to surface of 3D-printed constructions [107]. A range of surface modification methods, including layer-by-layer assembly, electrospinning, and plasma treatment, can be utilized to customize the surface characteristics of structures produced through 3D printing. These changes minimize negative reactions, enhance tissue integration, and efficiently promote cell adhesion and proliferation [108]. Furthermore, combination of 3D printing and nanotechnology has improved interactions with biological systems and enabled precise drug delivery.

7.4.7 Wound Dressing

As a process capable to generate sophisticated architectural and functional materials that are safe and personalized, additive manufacturing opens up a new and difficult arena. The process of creating antimicrobial wound dressings tailored to each patient using polycaprolactone (PCL) and integrated silver, copper, and zinc. Hot melt extrusion was used to create metal-homogeneously loaded filaments, and 3D-printed nose and ear sculptures were produced. The wound dressings demonstrated antibacterial and extended release of several metals. It was determined that the anatomically adaptive dressings were less expensive than traditional flat dressings. In an effort to accelerate wound healing in vascular grafts and facilitate insertion of wounded vessel wounds following surgical restoration, a 3D-printed hybrid scaffold composed of homogenized pericardium matrix and poly(ethyleneglycol) (PEG) was created [109]. Aside from lowering macrophage inflammatory signal, homogenized pericardium added to PEG matrix changes scaffold's stiffness. In terms of making arterial patches and starting a new area in congenital heart defect repair, produced biomaterial was thought to be quite hopeful.

7.5 Limitations and Difficulties with Dosage Form 3D Printing

Before 3D printing is extensively employed as a production technology for customized dosage forms, there are a few obstacles that need to be addressed.

Process Challenges

- *Selection of Raw Materials:* It's important to carefully consider their printability, physical properties, heat conductivity, print fluid properties, and viscous properties in addition to their safety for human use.
- *Nozzle Mechanism:* The dose form's layers are made using tool system in 3D printing. Consistent flow of printing material is needed during ordered layer production, while printer head stops and returns. At this stage, typical problems include scraping, binder movement and bleeding, jammed printer head nozzles, and wrong powder feeding [110].
- *Powder-Based 3D Printing:* Due to critical nature of powder spillage and potential for occupational hazards, this process requires a confined or particular space to be carried out [111].

- *Finished Product Surface Imperfections*: It is caused by large-sized powder or plastic beads stacked on top of one another. Surface flaws are more likely in dosage forms created using extrusion and powder-based processes due to the drying time required. Surface flaws can also be impacted by drying speed and technique [112].
- *Mechanical Resistance:* 3D dose forms have greater friability, particularly when using a powder-based method. Good dosage form strength is dependent on production technology [113].
- Compared with traditional tablet compression procedures, the current selection of materials, colours, and surface treatments for 3D printing is somewhat restricted [113].
- When printing at high temperatures, some manufacturing processes might not be suitable for thermolabile medications [114].

7.6 Conclusion

This comprehensive study explores the meaning, workings, and kinds of 3D printing technologies that are useful for medicine distribution. 3D printing has potential to completely transform personalized medicine by providing individualized healthcare solutions that are specifically designed to match each patient's needs. Thanks to increased fit, comfort, and usefulness, this technology makes it easier to create personalized medications, medical devices, and implants that improve patient outcomes. The creation of cutting-edge medical procedures and drug delivery systems is made possible by the capacity to create intricate are not possible with conventional manufacturing techniques. Even though industry faces obstacles such changing regulatory environments, scarce material options, expensive startup costs, and the need for specialized knowledge, these problems are being quickly resolved by continuing research and developments. Particularly in areas such as bioprinting and the creation of customized medication formulations, use of 3D printing in personalized medicine has enormous promise.

References

1. Vogenberg FR, Barash CI, Pursel M. Personalized medicine Part1: evolution and development of theranostics. Pharm Ther. 2010;35:560–62, 565–567, 576.
2. Mancinelli L, Cronin M, Sadee W. Pharmacogenomics: the promise of personalized medicine. AAPS Pharm Sci. 2000;2:E4.
3. Norman J, Madurawe R, et al. A new chapter in pharmaceutical manufacturing: 3D-printed drug products. Adv Drug Deliv Rev. 2018;108:39–50.
4. Edward A. The personalized medicine coalition: goals and strategies. Am J Pharmacogenomics. 2005;5:345–55.
5. Langreth R, Waldholz M. New era of personalized medicine: targeting drugs for each unique genetic profile. Oncologist. 2005;4:426–7.
6. Cobleigh MA, Vogel CL, Tripathy D, et al. Multinational study of the efficacy and safety of humanized anti-HER2 monoclonal antibody in women who have HER2-overexpressing

metastatic breast cancer that has progressed after chemotherapy for metastatic disease. J Clin Oncol. 1999;17:2639–48.
7. Abrahams E, Silver M. The case of personalized medicine. J Diabetes Sci Tech. 2009;3:680–4.
8. Looking forward, looking back. Nat Biotechnol. 2008;26:475.
9. Jain K, Soni M, Gupta U, Jain NK. Controlled delivery of gemcitabine hydrochloride using mannosylated poly (propyleneimine) dendrimers. J Nanopart Res. 2015;17:458.
10. Diogo JH. 3D printing of pharmaceutical drug delivery systems. Arch Organic Inorganic Chem Sci. 2016;1:1.
11. Gross BC, Erkal JL, et al. Evaluation of 3D printing and its potential impact on biotechnology and the chemical sciences. Anal Chem. 2014;86:3240–53.
12. Mishra Y, Mishra V, Aljabali AAA, El-Tanani M, Naikoo GA, Charbe N, et al. 3D printed personalized colon-targeted tablets: a novel approach in ulcerative colitis management. Curr Drug Deliv. 2024;21(9):1211–25.
13. Belhabib S, Guessasma S. Compression performance of hollow structures: from topology optimisation to design 3D printing. Int J Mech Sci. 2017;133:728–39.
14. Wu B, Borland S, Giordano R, Cima MJ, Sachs EM, Cima LG. Solid free-form fabrication of drug delivery devices. J Control Release. 1996;40:77–87.
15. Bartlett S. Printing organs on demand. Lancet Respir Med. 2013;1(9):684.
16. Banks J. Adding value in additive manufacturing: researchers in the United Kingdom and Europe look to 3D printing for customization. IEEE Pulse. 2013;4(6):22–6.
17. Ursan I, Chiu L, Pierce A. Three-dimensional drug printing: a structured review. J Am Pharm Assoc. 2013;53(2):136–44.
18. Khaled SA, Burley JC, Alexander MR, Roberts CJ. Desktop 3D printing of controlled release pharmaceutical bilayer tablets. Int J Pharm. 2014;461(1–2):105–11.
19. Ventola CL. Medical applications for 3D printing: current and projected uses. Pharm. Ther. 2014;39(10):704–11.
20. Trenfield SJ, Awad A, Gaisford S, Basit AW. 3D printed medicine: a new branch of digital healthcare. Int J Pharm. 2018;548(1):586–96.
21. Trenfield SJ, Awad A, Goyanes A, Gaisford S, Basit AW. 3D printing pharmaceuticals: drug development to frontline care. Trends Pharmacol Sci. 2018;39:440–51.
22. Awad A, Trenfield SJ, Goyanes A, Gaisford S, Basit AW. Reshaping drug development using 3D printing. Drug Discov Today. 2018;23(8):1547–55.
23. Kadry H, Al-Hilal TA, Keshavarz A, et al. Multi-purposable filaments of HPMC for 3D printing of medications with tailored drug release and timed-absorption. Int J Pharm. 2018;544:285–96.
24. Tagami T, Nagata N, Hayashi N, et al. Defined drug release from 3D-printed composite tablets consisting of drug-loaded polyvinyl alcohol and a water-soluble or water-insoluble polymer filler. Int J Pharm. 2018;543:361–7.
25. Norman J, Madurawe RD, Moore CM, Khan MA, Khairuzzaman A. A new chapter in pharmaceutical manufacturing: 3D-printed drug products. Adv Drug Deliv Rev. 2017;108:39–50.
26. Hornung CH. The art of manufacturing molecules. Science. 2018;359:273–4.
27. Ku MS, Dulin W. A biopharmaceutical classification-based right-first-time formulation approach to reduce human pharmacokinetic variability and project cycle time from first-in-human to clinical proof-of-concept. Pharm Dev Technol. 2012;17:285–302.
28. Goyanes A, Robles MP, Buanz A, Basit AW, Gaisford S. Effect of geometry on drug release from 3D printed tablets. Int J Pharm. 2015;494:657–63.
29. Moulton SE, Wallace GG. 3-dimensional (3D) fabricated polymer-based drug delivery system. J Control Release. 2014;193:27–34.
30. Brooke L. Future challenges for digital healthcare. 2017. https://www.medicalnewstoday.com/articles/317022.php.
31. Chen D, Heyer S, Ibbotson S, Salonitis K, Steingrímsson JG, Thiede S. Direct digital manufacturing: definition, evolution, and sustainability implications. J Clean Prod. 2015;107:615–25.
32. Downing J. Cycle pharmaceuticals to use 3D printing to develop 'orphan drugs'. Cambridge Independent; 2018.

33. Yu DG, Zhu LM, et al. Three-dimensional printing in pharmaceutics: promises and problems. J Pharm Sci. 2008;97:3666–90.
34. Ventola CL. Medical applications for 3D printing: current and projected uses. Pharmacol Ther. 2014;39(10):704–11.
35. Vogenberg FR, Barash CI, Pursel M. Personalized medicine. Part 1: Evolution and development into theranostics. Pharm Ther. 2010;35:560–2, 565–7, 576.
36. Food and Drug Administration. Guidance for Industry: Technical Considerations for Additive Manufactured Medical Devices. Center for Devices and Radiological Health Center for Biologics Evaluation and Research, U.S. Department of Health and Human Services, 2017. Available online: https://www.fda.gov/downloads/MedicalDevices/DeviceRegulationandGuidance/GuidanceDocuments/UCM499809.pdf.
37. Food and Drug Administration. General Principles of Software Validation; Final Guidance for Industry and FDA Staff. Center for Devices and Radiological Health, Center for Biologics Evaluation and Research, U.S. Department of Health and Human Services, 2002. Available online: https://www.fda.gov/downloads/medicaldevices/.../ucm085371.pdf.
38. Deciding When to Submit a 510(k) for a Change to an Existing Device. Available online: www.fda.gov/MedicalDevices/DeviceRegulationandGuidance/GuidanceDocuments/ucm080235.htm
39. 30-Day Notices, 135-Day Premarket Approval (PMA) Supplements and 75-Day Humanitarian Device Exemption (HDE) Supplements for Manufacturing Method or Process Changes. Available online: www.fda.gov/downloads/MedicalDevices/DeviceRegulationandGuidance/GuidanceDocuments/UCM080194.pdf
40. Modifications to Devices Subject to Premarket Approval (PMA) - The PMA Supplement Decision-Making Process. Available online: https://www.fda.gov/downloads/medicaldevices/deviceregulationandguidance/guidancedocuments/ucm089360.pdf.
41. Changes or Modifications During the Conduct of a Clinical Investigation. Available online: www.fda.gov/downloads/medicaldevices/deviceregulationandguidance/guidancedocuments/ucm082158.pdf.
42. Outterson K. Regulating compounding pharmacies after NECC. N Engl J Med. 2012;367(21):1969–72.
43. Drues, M. The case of the New England Compounding Center. Healthcare Packaging, 8/11/15. Available from: http://www.healthcarepackaging.com/case-new-englandcompoundingcenter
44. Sun L. FDA finds widespread safety issues at compounding pharmacies. In Washington Post: Health & Science; 2013.
45. Food and Drug Administration. 21 CFR 200. Available online: https://www.gpo.gov/fdsys/granule/CFR-2012-title21-vol4/CFR-2012-title21-vol4-part200.
46. Food and Drug Administration. CFR 300. Available online: https://www.gpo.gov/fdsys/granule/CFR-2009-title21-vol5/CFR-2009-title21-vol5-part300.
47. Colleen D, Lisa B, Matthew J, Farah T, James B, Gail D, Celeste L, Madagan K, Maiden T, Tracy Q, John S. 3D printing of medical devices: when a novel technology meets traditional legal principles. Reedsmith. 9/12/15.
48. 3D printing of medical devices: when a novel technology meets traditional legal principles. Available online: http://www.reedsmith.com/3D-Printing-of-MedicalDevices–When-a-Novel-Technology-Meets-TraditionalLegal-Principles-09-09-2015/
49. Drues M. Printing medical devices at home is just the beginning: Part II. Healthcare Packaging. 8/12/15. Available from: http://www.healthcarepackaging.com/trends-and-issues/3d-printingadditivemanufacturing/printing-medical-devices-home-just-beginning
50. Sparrow N. FDA tackles opportunities, challenges of 3D-printed medical devices. Plastics Today: Medicine; 2014. Available online: https://www.plasticstoday.com/content/fda-tackles-opportunities-challenges-3d-printed-medicaldevices/13081585320639.
51. Pollack S, Coburn J. FDA goes 3-D. 30/11/15. Available from: http://blogs.fda.gov/fdavoice/index.php/tag/osel/.

52. Schubert C, Van Langeveld MC, Donoso LA. Innovations in 3D printing: a 3D overview from optics to organs. Br J Ophthalmol. 2014;98(2):159–61.
53. Science and society. Experts warn against bans on 3D printing. Science. 2013;342(6157):439.
54. Lipson H. New world of 3-D printing offers "completely new ways of thinking:" Q & a with author, engineer, and 3-D printing expert Hod Lipson. IEEE Pulse. 2013;4(6):12–4.
55. Khatri P, Shah MK, Vora N, Vora MS. Formulation strategies for solid oral dosage form using 3D printing technology: a minor review. J Drug Deliv Sci Technol. 2018;46:148–55.
56. United States Food and Drug Administration (USFDA). Additive Manufacturing of Medical Devices Public Workshop—Transcript for October 8th, 2014.
57. Jonathan G, Karim A. 3D printing in pharmaceutics: a new tool for designing customized drug delivery systems. Int J Pharm. 2016;499:376–94.
58. Goole J, Amighi K. 3D printing in pharmaceutics: a new tool of design customized drug delivery system. Int J Pharm. 2016;499:376–94.
59. Acosta-Vélez GF, Wu BM. 3Dpharming: direct printing of personalized pharmaceutical tablets. Pol Sci. 2016;1:2.
60. Derby B. Inkjet printing of functional and structural materials: fluid property requirements, feature stability, and resolution. Annu Rev Mater Res. 2010;40:395–414.
61. Ihalainen P, Määttänen A, Sandler N. Printing technologies for biomolecules and cell-based applications. Int J Pharm. 2015;494:585–92.
62. Alomari M, Mohamed FH, Basit AW, Gaisford S. Personalised dosing: printing a dose of one's own medicine. Int J Pharm. 2015;494:568–77.
63. Tekin E, Smith PJ, Schubert US. Inkjet printing as a deposition and patterning tool for polymers and inorganic particles. Soft Matter. 2008;4:703–13.
64. Yun YH, Kim JD, Lee BK, Cho YW. Polymer inkjet printing: construction of three-dimensional structures at micro-scale by repeated lamination. Macromol Res. 2009;17:197–202.
65. Dimitrov D, Schreve K, De Beer N. Advances in three dimensional printing. J Mew Gener Sci. 2006;4:21–9.
66. Konta AA, Pina MG, Serrano DR. Personalised 3D printed medicines: which technique and polymer is more successful? Bioengineering. 2017;4(79):1–16.
67. Fina F, Goyanes A, Gaisford S, Basit AW. Selective laser sintering (SLS) 3D printing of medicines. Int J Pharm. 2017;529(1–2):285–93.
68. Hoy MB. 3D printing: making things at the library. Med Ref Serv Q. 2013;32(1):94–9.
69. Rathees G, Venugopal JR, Chinappan A, Ezhilarasu H, Sadiq A, Ramakrishna S. 3D fabrication of polymeric scaffolds for regenerative therapy. ACS Biomater Sci Eng. 2017;3(7):1175–94.
70. Prasad LK, Smyth H. 3D printing technologies for drug delivery: a review. Drug Dev Ind Pharm. 2016;42:1019–31.
71. Wang J, Goyanes A, Gaisford S, Basit AW. Stereolithographic (SLA) 3D printing of oral modified-release dosage forms. Int J Pharm. 2016;503:207–12.
72. Carts YA. Software enables laser stereolithography. Laser Focus World. 1990;26:57.
73. Neckers DC. Stereolithography—An introduction. ChemTech. 1990;20:615–9.
74. Hull CW, inventor; UVP, Inc., assignee. Apparatus for production of three dimensional objects by stereolithography. US Patent 4575330, 1986.
75. Wong KV, Hernandez A. A review of additive manufacturing. ISRN Mech Eng. 2012;1-10:2012.
76. Economiduo SN, Lamprou DA, Douroumis D. 3D printing application for transdermal drug delivery. Int J Pharm. 2018;544(2):415–24.
77. Stansbury JW, Idacavage MJ. 3D printing with polymers: challenges among expanding options and opportunities. Dent Mater. 2016;32(1):54–64.
78. Melchels FPW, Feijen J, Grijpma DW. A review on stereolithography and its applications in biomedical engineering. Biomaterials. 2010;31:6121–30.
79. Panwar A, Tan LP. Current status of bioinks for micro-extrusion-based 3D bioprinting. Molecules. 2016;21(6):685.
80. Maher PS, Keatch RP, Donnelly K, Mackay RE, Paxton JZ. Construction of 3D biological matrices using rapid prototyping technology. Rapid Prototyp J. 2009;15(3):204–10.

81. Duarte CDF, Blaeser A, Weber M, et al. Three-dimensional printing of stem cell-laden hydrogels submerged in a hydrophobic high-density fluid. Biofabrication. 2013;5:015003.
82. Phillippi JA, Miller E, Weiss L, Huard J, Waggoner A, Campbell P. Microenvironments engineered by inkjet bioprinting spatially direct adult stem cells toward muscle and bone-like subpopulations. Stem Cells. 2008;26:127–34.
83. Duan B, Hockaday LA, Kang KH, Butcher JT. 3D bioprinting of heterogeneous aortic valve conduits with alginate/gelatin hydrogels. J Biomed Mater Res A. 2013;101:1255–64.
84. Markstedt K, Mantas A, Tournier I, Martínez ÁH, Hägg D, Gatenholm P. 3D bioprinting human chondrocytes with nanocellulose alginate bioink for cartilage tissue engineering applications. Biomacromolecules. 2015;16:1489–96.
85. Fedorovich NE, Alblas J, De WJR, Hennink WE, Verbout AJ, Dhert WA. Hydrogels as extracellular matrices for skeletal tissue engineering: state-of-the-art and novel application in organ printing. Tissue Eng. 2007;13:1905–25.
86. Hsieh FY, Lin HH, Hsu S. 3D bioprinting of neural stem cell-laden thermoresponsive biodegradable polyurethane hydrogel and potential in central nervous system repair. Biomaterials. 2015;71:48–57.
87. Suntornnond R, An J, Chua CK. Roles of support materials in 3D bioprinting. Int J Bioprint. 2017;3:83–9.
88. Karalia D, Siamidi A, Karalis V, Vlachou M. 3D-printed oral dosage forms: mechanical properties, computational approaches and applications. Pharmaceutics. 2021;13(9)
89. Jain P, Kathuria H, Dubey N. Advances in 3D bioprinting of tissues/organs for regenerative medicine and in-vitro models. Biomaterials. 2022;287:121639.
90. Dumpa N, Butreddy A, Wang H, Komanduri N, Bandari S, Repka MA. 3D printing in personalized drug delivery: An overview of hot-melt extrusion-based fused deposition modeling. Int J Pharm. 2021;600:120501.
91. Al-Litani K, Ali T, Robles Martinez P, Buanz A. 3D printed implantable drug delivery devices for women's health: formulation challenges and regulatory perspective. Adv Drug Deliv Rev. 2023;198:114859.
92. Lu J, Hu X, Yuan T, Cao J, Zhao Y, Xiong C, et al. 3D-printed poly (P-Dioxanone) stent for endovascular application: in vitro evaluations. Polymers (Basel). 2022;14(9). https://doi.org/10.3390/polym14091755.
93. Shen Y, Cui J, Yu X, Song J, Cai P, Guo W, et al. Recent advances in three-dimensional printing in cardiovascular devices: bench and bedside applications. Smart Mater Med. 2024;5(1):36–51. https://doi.org/10.1016/j.smaim.2023.07.001.
94. Ramadan Q, Zourob M. 3D bioprinting at the frontier of regenerative medicine, pharmaceutical, and food industries. Front Med Technol. 2020;2:607648. https://doi.org/10.3389/fmedt.2020.607648.
95. Di Piazza E, Pandolfi E, Cacciotti I, Del Fattore A, Tozzi AE, Secinaro A, et al. Bioprinting technology in skin, heart, pancreas and cartilage tissues: Progress and challenges in clinical practice. Int J Environ Res Public Health. 2021;18(20):10806. https://doi.org/10.3390/ijerph182010806.
96. Leberfinger AN, Dinda S, Wu Y, Koduru SV, Ozbolat V, Ravnic DJ, et al. Bioprinting functional tissues. Acta Biomater. 2019;95:32–49. https://doi.org/10.1016/j.actbio.2019.01.009.
97. Chung JJ, Im H, Kim SH, Park JW, Jung Y. Toward biomimetic scaffolds for tissue engineering: 3D printing techniques in regenerative medicine. Front Bioeng Biotechnol. 2020;8:586406. https://doi.org/10.3389/fbioe.2020.586406.
98. Han F, Wang J, Ding L, Hu Y, Li W, Yuan Z, et al. Tissue engineering and regenerative medicine: achievements, future, and sustainability in Asia. Front Bioeng Biotechnol. 2020;8:83. https://doi.org/10.3389/fbioe.2020.00083.
99. Muzzio N, Moya S, Romero G. Multifunctional scaffolds and synergistic strategies in tissue engineering and regenerative medicine. Pharmaceutics. 2021;13(6):792. https://doi.org/10.3390/pharmaceutics13060792.

100. Ligon SC, Liska R, Stampfl J, Gurr M, Mülhaupt R. Polymers for 3D printing and customized additive manufacturing. Chem Rev. 2017;117(15):10212–90. https://doi.org/10.1021/acs.chemrev.7b00074.
101. Nyberg EL, Farris AL, Hung BP, Dias M, Garcia JR, Dorafshar AH, et al. 3D-printing technologies for craniofacial rehabilitation, reconstruction, and regeneration. Ann Biomed Eng. 2017;45(1):45–57. https://doi.org/10.1007/s10439-016-1668-5.
102. Arefin AME, Khatri NR, Kulkarni N, Egan PF. Polymer 3D printing review: materials, process, and design strategies for medical applications. Polymers. 2021;13(9):1499. https://doi.org/10.3390/polym13091499.
103. Wong KC. 3D-printed patient-specific applications in orthopedics. Orthop Res Rev. 2016;8:57–66. https://doi.org/10.2147/orr.S99614.
104. Ballard DH, Trace AP, Ali S, Hodgdon T, Zygmont ME, DeBenedectis CM, et al. Clinical applications of 3D printing: primer for radiologists. Acad Radiol. 2018;25(1):52–65.
105. Betz UA, Arora L, Assal RA, Azevedo H, Baldwin J, Becker MS, et al. Game changers in science and technology-now and beyond. Technol Forecast Soc Chang. 2023;193:122588. https://doi.org/10.1016/j.techfore.2023.122588.
106. Fiani B, Newhouse A, Cathel A, Sarhadi K, Soula M. Implications of 3-dimensional printed spinal implants on the outcomes in spine surgery. J Korean Neurosurg Soc. 2021;64(4):495–504. https://doi.org/10.3340/jkns.2020.0272.
107. Tolabi H, Bakhtiary N, Sayadi S, Tamaddon M, Ghorbani F, Boccaccini AR, et al. A critical review on polydopamine surface-modified scaffolds in musculoskeletal regeneration. Front Bioeng Biotechnol. 2022;10:1008360.
108. Ilyas K, Akhtar MA, Ammar EB, Boccaccini AR. Surface modification of 3D-printed PCL/BG composite scaffolds via mussel-inspired polydopamine and effective antibacterial coatings for biomedical applications. Materials (Basel). 2022;15(23):8289.
109. Bracaglia LG, Messina MJ, Winston S, Kuo C-Y, Lerman M, Fisher JP. Printed pericardium hydrogels to promote wound healing in vascular applications. Biomacromolecules. 2017;18(11):3802–11.
110. Yu DG, Zhu L-M, Branford-White CJ, Yang XL. Three-dimensional printing in pharmaceutics: promises and problems. J Pharm Sci. 2008;97(9):3666–90.
111. Huang SH, Liu P, Mokasdar A, Hou L. Additive manufacturing and its societal impact: a literature review. Int J Adv Manuf Technol. 2013;67(5–8):1191–203.
112. Gaylo CM, Pryor TJ, Fairweather JA, Weitzel DE. Apparatus, systems and methods for use in three-dimensional printing. 2004. https://patents.google.com/patent/WO2004005014A2/en?inventor=Christopher+M+Gaylo.
113. Alhnan MA, Okwuosa TC, Muzna S, WaiWan K, Ahmed W, Arafat B. Emergence of 3D printed dosage forms: opportunities and challenges. Pharm Res. 2016;33:1817–32.
114. Goyanes A, Wang J, Buanz A, Martínez-Pacheco R, Telford R, Gaisford S, Basit AW. 3D printing of medicines: engineering novel oral devices with unique design and drug release characteristics. Pharmaceutics. 2015;12(11):4077–84.

Patent, Intellectual Property and Legal Issues in 3D Printed Pharmaceuticals

8

Hemraj Singh Rajput, Shweta Bhandari, Avinash Khadela, and Sagar Pamu

Abstract

The concept of 3D printed pharmaceuticals came with the vision of dosage individualization and thought to be one of the milestones in the advances of medical science. The technology of 3D printing has evolved tremendously in the recent years, and with this, the hope of achieving the goal of dosage individualization has evolved. This is also a reminder of responsibility for government to engage in upbringing of this new technology and frame necessary laws and regulation to improve patentability, infringements, and relevant legal issues. The major challenge can arise from the 3D printing process, materials used for printing, active pharmaceutical ingredient use, and usage in times of emergency and pandemics. Since the 3D printing technology cannot be developed by single person and is even difficult for single company to achieve any landmark in the technology, the regulations are needed to facilitate collaboration at global level for any positive outcome. The chapter sheds light on an imperative information pertaining to current scenario of patentability of 3D pharmaceutical technologies and regulations to safeguard the rights of developer at country level and global level. The scope further extends to novelty, legality, applications, need of skillsets, sales and licencing of technology, and upscaling of technology at industrial level. Nonetheless keeping in mind, the technology must be generalized to population and must not be limited to a section of the population to avoid any disparity and social stigma.

H. S. Rajput (✉) · S. Bhandari
Department of Pharmacy, Sumandeep Vidyapeeth Deemed to be University, Vadodara, Gujarat, India

A. Khadela
L M College of Pharmacy, Ahmedabad, Gujarat, India

S. Pamu
Institute of Pharmacy, Nirma University, Ahmedabad, Gujarat, India

K. Vinchurkar, S. Mane (eds.), *Innovations in Drug Manufacturing*,
https://doi.org/10.1007/978-981-96-9075-6_8

Keywords

3D printing · 3D pharmaceuticals · Intellectual property · Patents · Pharmaceutical regulations

8.1 Introduction

In the 1800s the pharmacist played a major role in preparation of medication from raw ingredients as per the doctor's prescription and patient requirement. This role was to take over with the revolution led by industrialization of medication. The role of pharmacist was shifted from compounders to pharmacy merchandising and also as educators who also provide community pharmacy services [1]. It is a challenge that mass-produced medication in patient care leading either to decreased efficacy or increased risk of adverse drug reaction. 3D printing technology can again establish the forgotten profession of pharmacist as compounders. This will probably improve patient outcome since pharmacist will have a choice to personalize the dosage, its sizes, site of release, shapes, and multidrug combinations [2].

8.2 Exploring Intellectual Property Rights in 3D Printing of Pharmaceuticals

8.2.1 Coverage of 3D Printing in Pharmaceuticals

A range of products can be 3D printed in pharmaceuticals, and majority of them are various type drug formulations, e.g., tablet, capsule, nanocapsules, polypills, microdots, microneedle, biodegradable patches, films, microparticles, caplets, implants, etc. [3].

A range of products can be covered under the 3D-printed pharmaceuticals as shown in Fig. 8.1.

When it comes to pharmaceuticals, unlike medical devices, prosthetics, and medical tools, the regulations become quite stringent to maintain the safety and efficacy of the drug. The effect of these regulation can be seen on the overall implementation of 3D technology in pharmaceutical and medical field. Majority of the 3D technology is only focused on medical devices and prosthetics while drug manufacturing through 3D printing is still in its infancy stage [4].

8.2.2 Patentability of 3D Printed Pharmaceuticals

The complexity of implementing intellectual property rights in pharmaceuticals is a major hurdle in the progress 3D printing technology in pharmaceuticals. Following are few major key points that can highlight the issue and help formulate appropriate resolution in future:

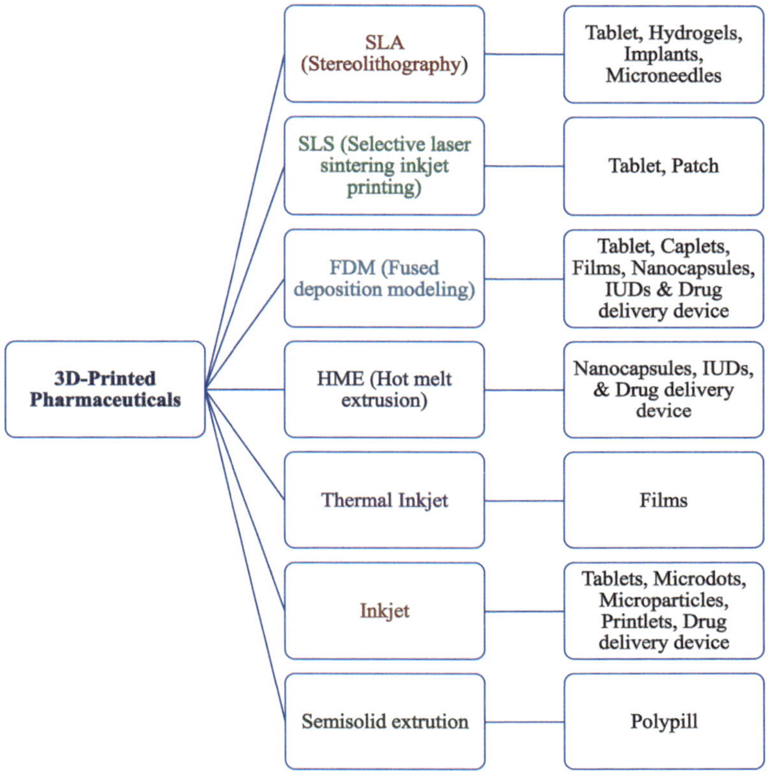

Fig. 8.1 Classification of available 3D printed pharmaceuticals

8.2.2.1 Novelty in Innovation

Existing drug formulations and related delivery mechanisms are based on the thorough research conducted by the scientific communities and pharmaceutical industries. This leads us to two obvious challenges, i.e., first, drugs which are still covered under the patent right of any institution or pharmaceutical company may not be available for the 3D printing. Secondly those drugs which are open under general license and manufacturing still fall under the government regulation that sets standards to control the safety and efficacy of the drug. Any deviation from the existing sets of standards will compromise safety and efficacy, and if no new innovation is performed, it will lead to lacking of novelty. Both situations will make it difficult to patent any 3D printed pharmaceutical product [5, 6].

8.2.2.2 Scope of Claim

The scope of patent lies within the objective of 3D printing drugs, i.e., personalization of dose, methods of adjusting doses, various processes of drug combinations, formulation as per the physiology of the patient, technology can be developed to aid patient with functional disability for easy identification, and consumption of medication. It can be said a whole new dimension of 3D technology is yet be discovered [7].

8.2.2.3 Enforcement

Though there is scope of patentability in 3D technology, it will be very difficult to implement laws and regulations to control the use of technology and tracking any infringement. The rules and regulations are political and vary from place to place [8].

8.2.3 Challenges in Implementation

Multiple major aspects from regulatory and technical perspective of 3D printing need to be addressed to overcome challenges for implementation.

8.2.3.1 Regulatory Compliance

Government bodies such as FDA and CDSCO have some considerably strict policy for the regulation and approval of drugs; this is also applicable for drugs that can be 3D printed. The majority of it is related to safety and efficacy. Several major reforms and analytical process may require to overcome this issue as it is an evolving landscape that is yet to be explored [9].

8.2.3.2 Material Compatibility

Any drug formulation comprised various additives apart from active constituent. These additives play a vital role in providing bulk, desired shape, disintegrating property, taste masking, and several other necessary characters to the drug formulation. 3D printing of drugs will require a new set of additives, which should provide similar character to the drug and also be compatible with 3D printing technology. This is one of the greatest challenges and may also require a dedicated branch in pharmaceutical science for further development of 3D printing technology [10].

8.2.3.3 Quality Control

Just like existing pharmaceutical formulation–related defects, the 3D printed drug also suffers quality issues. Though they are different from the defects observed in conventional formulation, yet they need to be controlled for an optimal dosage form. There is a stringent policy for the existing formulations, and similar policy may also need for the optimal dosage form in 3D technology [11].

8.2.3.4 Economic Viability

Like any new technology, implementation of this technology could be expensive in the beginning and gradual reduction in costing will be observed with advancement in the technology and increased demand [5].

8.3 Addressing Procurement and Enforcement of IP Rights

Like any other IP rights applicable to patents, designs, copyrights, and trademarks, IP rights are also applicable to the 3D printed pharmaceuticals. The government of bodies providing intellectual property rights considers 3D printed pharmaceuticals as any other invention and can grant patent based on the fulfilment of regulations under patent act. The challenge in 3D printing is on public disclosure of patent; it is very likely that from the provided information, any skilled person might be able to replicate the technology. It will be very difficult to both identify the accused infringing IP and prevent any future infringement [12]. Steps can be taken to enforce IP rights as follows:

1. *Standardization*: Standardized protocols need to be developed for 3D printing in pharmaceuticals; this will streamline the process of regulatory approval and will also ensure the consistency as well as quality [13].
2. *Collaborative Efforts*: There is a need of collaboration between innovator/technology provider, regulatory bodies, and pharmaceutical industries to overcome the challenges of IP infringement with appropriate IP enforcement and data protection [14].
3. *Advanced Technologies*: The help of advance blockchain technology using cryptographic hashes system for linking all steps in the 3D printing technology could be a futuristic mean of enforcing IP rights aiding both procurement and enforcement [14].

8.4 A Historical Analysis of Key Patent Applications

8.4.1 Early Innovations (1990s)

8.4.1.1 First Application

1984 was the year when first 3D printing technology invented. The scientific community recognized its application in various files so did the pharmaceutical scientist. The first known event of fabricating pharmaceuticals was recorded in the year 1993, and the technology used was based on stereolithography and selective laser sintering. This was the first event that laid foundation of 3D printing in pharmaceutical technology [15].

8.4.2 Personalization of Dosage Form (2000s)

8.4.2.1 Customization of Dosage Form

Patent applications were beginning to be filed in the early 2000s. The applications were focused on personalization of dosage form. The novelty of tailored drug release and dosage as per the individual patient need was the base of these patents.

8.4.2.2 Complex Structures

Drug delivery is very important part in drug therapy; the structure and design of drug dosage can make a significant impact on the release of the drug. 3D printing has opened gates for the possibility of infinite complex drug structure that certainly has edge over drug dosage produced using traditional methods [2].

8.4.3 Concept of Advanced Drug Delivery Systems (2010s)

8.4.3.1 Multidrug Combinations

The patent application in this time period was focused on experimenting the combination of various drugs in a single dosage form with capabilities of different release rate. The practical implication was very high for such regimen as there are so many complex disease conditions that require multidrug therapy [5].

8.4.4 First FDA Approval (2015)

8.4.4.1 Spritam (levetiracetam)

It was the first 3D printed drug that was approved by the FDA in the year 2015 for public usage. It was the milestone that has demonstrated the practical application of 3D printing in the pharmaceuticals and hence became the foundation of current ongoing research in the field of 3D printing technology. A very important part of this achievement was to meet the standards and norms assigned by the regulatory bodies [15].

8.4.5 Recent Development (2020s)

8.4.5.1 On-demand Manufacturing

Current research is focused on developing technology to allow on-site manufacturing of drug, i.e., at the site of dispensing such as hospitals and pharmacies.

8.4.5.2 Sustainable Practices

Other important aspects, i.e., eco-friendly and sustainability are the current aims of research. This will allow selection of materials that have listed impact on environment [2].

8.5 Assessing Challenges in Establishing Patent Novelty

Reproducing any technology with the help of 3D printing is quite easy nowadays. This has opened another challenge of increasing patent infringement since most of the time the design of any patent component is available online or created by any other skilled person, which can be used to print the actual component. The patent law covers the legal aspect of patent that has been printed and is physically available and not the computer-aided design. This makes it difficult for an inventor to keep the innovation to himself as with little modification similar product can be reproduced [16].

Laws in the United States and the United Kingdom allow the manufacturing the 3D parts of any component as long as the part is not patented or being used for different function and then patented for [17].

Another major aspect of the patient law included if any replicated final product is not being commercialized, it is legal to use without infringement of the US law [18].

Still to date the process of 3D printing pharmaceutical product is full of challenges. Though the technology is capable of producing a range product, the major concerns raised by researcher and regulatory bodies were related to production efficiency, drug stability, safety, efficacy, pharmacokinetics properties, and pharmacodynamic of the 3D printed drug. The consistency of final 3D printed pharmaceutical can be difficult to predict from the current 3D printing technology [19, 20]. The next challenge in 3D printing will be preparation of formulation for the pediatric population. The drug range for pediatric population is very wide and consists of preparations such as syrups and suspensions. The aim of producing such preparation is to improve the drug administration and palatability, since the success of therapy is dependent on patient medication adherence [21, 22].

For the assessment of patent novelty, a new set of guidelines is required in pharmaceutical 3D printing, and as far as it can be seen that no such guideline has been generated by regulatory bodies. Numerous patent applications have been registered for the 3D printed drug, and somehow so far only one drug has been approved for marketing; this gives an insight of challenges being faced by regulatory bodies in the approval process of 3D printed drugs [23].

8.6 Requirement of Skill Set for the Assessment of 3D Printing Technology in Pharmaceuticals [4]

There is considerable difference between the manufacturing process of conventional drug manufacturing and 3D printing technology. Similarly, the need of assessment of finished product is the priority for the successful implementation of this technology. The following points can be considered while assessing any new 3D printing pharmaceutical technology:

8.6.1 Printability Control

A sound understanding of physical and chemical properties of the materials used for 3D printing is a necessity. This includes selection of material appropriate for 3D printing such as solvents, powders, and binders.

8.6.2 Raw Materials for Binder Deposition and Binder Deposition Process

Knowledge of polymers is essential for achieving uniformity of powder layer while printing. Similarly, other associated factors such as water content, surface tension, thermal, and electrical conductivity are also important.

8.6.3 Risk Assessment

Risks such as compatibility, variability in thickness, quality, recycling, and environmental hazards must be known for the material used for 3D printing.

8.6.4 Fused Filament Fabrication

Polymer-based filaments used for 3D printing must be assessed for its viscoelastic properties, mechanical properties, and water content.

8.6.5 Fusion Printing

Laser technology is used in this process to bind particles. It is crucial to know particle size, shape, and flow property of the material during printing.

8.6.6 Other Physical and Mechanical Properties Consideration

Particle size, rheology, material behavior at different temperature, elasticity, plasticity, etc.

8.6.7 Process Analytical Technology (PAT)

The technology can be used to monitor the quality of printed layer during the process; this will ensure the quality and consistency of final product.

8.6.8 Environmental Control

Material used for the printing could be sensitive to environmental factors such as temperature, pressure, moisture, and other environmental factors.

8.6.9 Critical Process Parameters

Parameters that can affect product quality, drug release, uniformity, level of impurity, friability, hardness, crystallinity, and polymorphism are very crucial to maintain product nature.

8.6.10 Common 3D Printing Defects

Defects such as banding, leaning, warping, stringing, collapse, and residuals must be in the assessment list of pharmaceutical 3D technology.

8.7 Industrial Application of 3D Printing in Pharmaceutical Manufacturing [24]

Industrial development can happen in the key areas by focusing the following aspects of drug therapy:

8.7.1 Personalization of Drug Dosage

8.7.1.1 Individualized Treatment

Keeping in mind patient age, gender, race, and disease condition, the drug dosage administration can be adjusted.

8.7.1.2 Precision Medicine

On the basis of progression of disease condition, patient medication can be adjusted. Other factors such as patient socioeconomic status can also be considered if patient require long term therapy.

8.7.1.3 Role of 3D Printing

A precise upscaling of dosage can be achieved with the help of 3D technology.

8.7.2 Regulation of Drug Release

8.7.2.1 Custom Release Profiles

The 3D printing is capable of formulating dosage that can be immediate, sustained, delayed, or pulsating release in nature.

8.7.2.2 Unique Design

The variety of geometric formulation of the drug can be used to control quantity of drug filling and also the release of drug.

8.7.3 Personalization of Treatment for Geriatric Patient

8.7.3.1 Requirement of Personalization

Geriatric patient often suffers from multiple disease condition that needs multiple drug therapy, and it is associated with major challenge of polypharmacy, i.e., increased incidence of drug interaction and adverse drug reaction.

8.7.3.2 Polypills

The most unique advantage of 3D printing is creation of polypills. Multiple drugs can combine together in the same pill without mixing them. It is also possible to control the release of drug and hence decrease the risk of adverse drug reaction and drug interaction.

8.7.3.3 Drug Appearance

Drug can be made in various shapes, size and color, design, and encryptions. This can help patient to improve adherence by remembering the drug and its time of administration.

8.8 Personalization of Treatment for Pediatric Patients

8.8.1 Considerations

Current scenario for pediatric patient is under developmental state. Since strict regulatory norms have to be followed in pediatric dosing, very few formulations have been seen developing or under trials.

8.8.2 Possibilities of 3D Printing in Pediatric Population

Formulations that are easily chewable and appearance can help medication adherence in the pediatric population. Another aspect can be risk of overdosage in pediatric patient as drug could be seen as candy by the pediatric population.

8.9 Personalization of Treatment for Visually Impaired Patient

8.9.1 Accessibility

The biggest challenge for visually impaired patients is identification of drug, and they have to be dependent on another person for their medication. 3D printing can enable these visually impaired patients by means of Braille encryption on each medication helping them easy identification.

8.10 Exploring Infringement Issues in 3D Printed Pharmaceuticals [23]

8.10.1 Types of Infringement in Patent Law

8.10.1.1 Direct Infringement

This involves reproducing, using, and selling of patented product without appropriate approval or consent from the patent holder.

8.10.1.2 Indirect or Contributory Infringement

This involves distribution of technology outside the jurisdiction of approved patent. This could be both intentional or unintentional.

8.11 Conclusion

The pharmaceutical industry's shift toward 3D printing technology offers promising advancements, such as personalized medication and the revival of pharmacists' traditional compounding role. This technology allows for customized dosage forms, tailored drug release, and complex multidrug combinations, enhancing patient care. However, challenges remain, including stringent regulatory compliance, material compatibility, and quality control issues. The legal landscape for patenting 3D-printed pharmaceuticals is complex, with difficulties in maintaining novelty and enforcing intellectual property rights. As the technology advances, collaboration between pharmaceutical companies, regulatory bodies, and technology providers is essential. Further research and innovation are needed to address these challenges, including developing new materials and ensuring economic viability. The potential for on-demand manufacturing and sustainable practices marks a significant shift in drug distribution and manufacturing. However, issues such as patent infringement and ensuring consistent product quality highlight the need for robust regulatory frameworks and technological advancements.

8.12 Future Direction

The future of 3D printing in pharmaceuticals lies in further developing and refining the technology to address current challenges. Key areas of focus should include improving regulatory frameworks to accommodate the unique aspects of 3D printed drugs, such as ensuring safety, efficacy, and quality control. Research should continue to explore new biocompatible materials and innovative drug formulations, including personalized dosage forms for specific populations like pediatric, geriatric, and visually impaired patients.

Advancements in intellectual property protection will be crucial to safeguard innovations while fostering collaboration between pharmaceutical companies, regulatory bodies, and technology providers. The integration of advanced technologies like blockchain for secure data tracking and authentication can help address intellectual property concerns and prevent patent infringement.

Moreover, there should be a push toward developing environmentally sustainable practices in 3D printing, minimizing the environmental impact of drug manufacturing. On-demand drug manufacturing at pharmacies and hospitals could revolutionize the supply chain, making personalized medicine more accessible and cost-effective. Overall, the convergence of 3D printing technology with personalized medicine, regulatory innovations, and sustainable practices will shape the future landscape of the pharmaceutical industry.

References

1. Urick BY, Meggs EV. Towards a greater professional standing: evolution of pharmacy practice and education, 1920–202012. Pharmacy (Basel). 2019;7(3):98. https://doi.org/10.3390/pharmacy7030098.
2. Basit AW, Trenfield SJ. 3D printing of pharmaceuticals and the role of pharmacy. Pharm J. 2022;308(7959):2.
3. Gupta DK, Ali MH, Ali A, Jain P, Anwer MK, Iqbal Z, Mirza MA. 3D printing technology in healthcare: applications, regulatory understanding, IP repository and clinical trial status. J Drug Target. 2021; https://doi.org/10.1080/1061186X.2021.1935973.
4. Norman J, Madurawe RD, Moore CMV, Khan MA, Khairuzzaman A. A new chapter in pharmaceutical manufacturing: 3D-printed drug products. Adv Drug Deliv Rev. 2017;108:39–50. https://doi.org/10.1016/j.addr.2016.03.0012.
5. Wang S, Chen X, Han X, Hong X, Li X, Zhang H, et al. A review of 3D printing technology in pharmaceutics: technology and applications, now and future. Pharmaceutics. 2023;15(2):416. https://doi.org/10.3390/pharmaceutics150204163.
6. Tracy T, Wu L, Liu X, Cheng S, Li X. 3D printing: innovative solutions for patients and pharmaceutical industry. Int J Pharm. 2023;631:1224801. Available from: https://doi.org/10.1016/j.ijpharm.2022.122480.
7. Vaz VM, Kumar L. 3D printing as a promising tool in personalized medicine. AAPS PharmSciTech. 2021;22:49234. https://doi.org/10.1208/s12249-020-01905-861.
8. Basit AW, Gaisford S, editors. 3D printing of pharmaceuticals, AAPS Advances in the Pharmaceutical Sciences Series, vol. 31. Cham: Springer International Publishing; 2018. p. 237.
9. Jamróz W, Szafraniec J, Kurek M, Jachowicz R. 3D printing in pharmaceutical and medical applications—recent achievements and challenges. Pharm Res. 2018;35:176. https://doi.org/10.1007/s11095-018-2454-x.
10. Rahman Z, Ali SFB, Ozkan T, Charoo NA, Reddy IK, Khan MA. Additive manufacturing with 3D printing: progress from bench to bedside. AAPS J. 2018;20(6):1012. https://doi.org/10.1208/s12248-018-0225-63.
11. Parhi R. A review of three-dimensional printing for pharmaceutical applications: quality control, risk assessment and future perspectives. J Drug Deliv Sci Technol. 2021;64:1025712.
12. Jewell C, Stones J. 3D printing techniques in the pharmaceutical sciences—intellectual property issues. In: Basit AW, Gaisford S, editors. 3D printing of pharmaceuticals. Cham: Springer; 2018. p. 183–214.
13. Krishnan AV, Lakshman SA, Bhargav A. 3D printing and regulatory considerations. In: 3D & 4D printing methods for pharmaceutical manufacturing and personalised drug delivery: opportunities and challenges. Cham: Springer International Publishing; 2023. p. 45–68.

14. Pettersson ABV, Ballardini RM, Mimler M, Li P, Salmi M, Minssen T, et al. Core legal challenges for medical 3D printing in the EU. Healthcare. 2024;12(11):1114. https://doi.org/10.3390/healthcare1211111423.
15. Cheng S, Tracy TS, Li X. 3D printing pharmaceuticals: current status and future opportunities. Pharma Fronts. 2024;6:e192–e19412. https://doi.org/10.1055/s-0044-17825123.
16. Pearce JM. A novel approach to obviousness: an algorithm for identifying prior art concerning 3-D printing materials. World Patent Inf. 2015;42:13–8. https://doi.org/10.1016/j.wpi.2015.07.0034.
17. Wilbanks K. The challenges of 3D printing to the repair-reconstruction doctrine in patent law. George Mason Law Rev. 2013;20(4):442. Available from: https://ssrn.com/abstract=2236580 or https://doi.org/10.2139/ssrn.2236580.
18. Weinberg M. It will be awesome if they don't screw it up: 3D printing, intellectual property, and the fight over the next great disruptive technology. Public Knowledge; 2010. p. 1–121.
19. Schell KH. Compliance issues and extemporaneous preparation of medications for pediatric patients. J Pharm Technol. 1992;8(4):158–61. https://doi.org/10.1177/8755122592008004082. PMID: 101210103.
20. Gudeman J, Jozwiakowski M, Chollet J, Randell M. Potential risks of pharmacy compounding. Drugs R D. 2013;13(1):1–8. https://doi.org/10.1007/s40268-013-0005-923. PMCID: PMC3627035.
21. Gupta A, Khan MA. Challenges of pediatric formulations: a FDA science perspective. Int J Pharm. 2013;457(1):346–8. https://doi.org/10.1016/j.ijpharm.2013.08.06423.
22. Ivanovska V, Rademaker CMA, van Dijk L, Mantel-Teeuwisse AK. Pediatric drug formulations: a review of challenges and progress. Pediatrics. 2014;134(2):361–72. https://doi.org/10.1542/peds.2013-3225.23.
23. Stones JA, Jewell CM. 3D printing of pharmaceuticals: patent and regulatory challenges. Pharm Pat Anal. 2017;6(4):147–51. https://doi.org/10.4155/ppa-2017-0017.
24. Andreadis II, Gioumouxouzis CI, Eleftheriadis GK, Fatouros DG. The advent of a new era in digital healthcare: a role for 3D printing technologies in drug manufacturing? Pharmaceutics. 2022;14(3):609. https://doi.org/10.3390/pharmaceutics140306092.

Economic and Market Trends in FDM 3D Printing for Pharmaceuticals

9

Ankita Bhavsar, Shashank Dhar Tiwari, Kuldeep Vinchurkar, Rohit Doke, Koushlesh Mishra, Ankita Badoriya, and Priya Jain

Abstract

Fused deposition modeling (FDM) 3D printing has emerged as a transformative technology in pharmaceutical manufacturing, offering cost-effective and customizable drug formulations. By utilizing a layer-by-layer extrusion process, FDM enables precise control over drug composition, release kinetics, and dosage personalization, making it a promising approach for patient-centric therapies. Since the FDA's approval of the first 3D-printed drug, Spritam® (levetiracetam), in 2015, interest in this technology has surged, driving innovation in dosage form development. The economic feasibility of FDM printing in pharmaceuticals is increasingly being explored, with reductions in production costs, material waste, and supply chain complexities positioning it as a scalable alternative to conventional drug manufacturing. Market trends indicate a growing demand for personalized medicine, pushing pharmaceutical companies to invest in 3D printing solutions that can streamline drug production while ensur-

A. Bhavsar
Indukaka Ipcowala College of Pharmacy, Anand, Gujarat, India

S. D. Tiwari · K. Mishra
Shri Rama Krishna College of Pharmacy, Satna, Madhya Pradesh, India

K. Vinchurkar
Department of Pharmaceutics, Sandip Institute of Pharmaceutical Sciences (SIPS), Affiliated To Savitribai Phule Pune University (SPPU, Pune), Nashik, Maharashtra, India

R. Doke
Jaihind College of Pharmacy, Pune, Maharashtra, India

A. Badoriya (✉)
Indore Institute of Pharmacy, Indore, Madhya Pradesh, India

P. Jain
Oxford International College, Indore, India

K. Vinchurkar, S. Mane (eds.), *Innovations in Drug Manufacturing*,
https://doi.org/10.1007/978-981-96-9075-6_9

ing regulatory compliance. As advancements in printable excipients and polymer-based formulations continue, the adoption of FDM in pharmaceutical applications is expected to expand, reshaping the industry's approach to drug design and delivery.

This chapter explores the economic and market trends shaping the adoption of FDM 3D printing in the pharmaceutical sector. Key drivers include the demand for personalized medicine, regulatory advancements, and a shift toward decentralized manufacturing models. By analyzing current trends and projecting future opportunities, this study provides insights into the evolving economic landscape of FDM 3D printing in pharmaceuticals, emphasizing its potential to revolutionize the industry.

Keywords

3D printing technology · Fused deposition modeling (FDM) · Economic trends
Market trends · 3D drug product · Customized medicine · Enabling technology
Customized release profile · Local fabrication

9.1 Introduction

Three-dimensional printing (3DP) is an innovative technology that enables the fabrication of three-dimensional products through a digital design platform using a layer-by-layer approach. In recent years, 3DP has emerged as a groundbreaking advancement, significantly transforming the pharmaceutical industry by facilitating the production of novel medical products and drug delivery devices. The technology gained widespread attention following the FDA approval of the first commercial 3D-printed tablet, Spirtam® (levetiracetam), in August 2015. A key advantage of 3D printing in pharmaceuticals is its ability to develop innovative oral dosage forms with enhanced precision and customization.

Fused deposition modeling (FDM) 3D printing is rapidly evolving as a game-changing technique in pharmaceutical manufacturing, offering significant benefits such as enhanced personalization, cost-effectiveness, and streamlined production workflows. This chapter delves into the economic and market dynamics influencing the adoption of FDM 3D printing within the pharmaceutical sector. Critical factors driving this shift include the rising demand for personalized medicine, evolving regulatory frameworks, and the transition toward decentralized manufacturing models. By examining current industry trends and future prospects, this study provides a comprehensive analysis of the economic impact of FDM 3D printing in pharmaceuticals, highlighting its potential to revolutionize the field.

The origins of 3D printing technology can be traced back to the early 1990s when researchers at the Massachusetts Institute of Technology (MIT) in Cambridge, MA, United States, spearheaded by Sachs and colleagues, introduced and patented a rapid prototyping technique known as "three-dimensional printing techniques." This breakthrough innovation played a crucial role in the advancement of 3D printing, paving the way for its application in pharmaceutical research and development [1].

The adoption of 3D printing in pharmaceutical manufacturing has significantly accelerated the development of cost-effective and efficient drug production processes. This technology not only streamlines formulation design but also enhances patient adherence by enabling tailored dosage forms that improve convenience and therapeutic outcomes. Among the various 3D printing techniques applicable to pharmaceuticals, extrusion-based printing, powder-bed fusion, and inkjet-based methods have gained particular attention. These approaches offer distinct advantages in drug layering, controlled release, and complex formulation capabilities, making them integral to the evolving landscape of pharmaceutical manufacturing. This chapter provides an overview of these techniques and their impact on the industry.

This chapter also discusses different applications of 3D printing technology and highlights the impact of 3D printing as an innovative promising technology through presenting some examples as experimental studies in the fabrication of oral drug delivery systems. The study highlights the cost–benefit dynamics of using FDM, including reductions in material waste, production timelines, and distribution costs. Challenges such as regulatory compliance, scalability, and intellectual property concerns are also addressed. Furthermore, the paper examines market growth forecasts, competitive landscape, and the role of innovation in expanding applications, such as patient-specific drug formulations and on-demand production [2].

9.2 History

In the early 1990s, 3D printing has emerged as a transformative platform for personalized medicine. Notable achievements include the development of 3D-printed medical devices, with the FDA's Center for Device and Radiological Health (CDRH) revising regulations and approving several devices. The first 3D printing method applied to pharmaceuticals involved inkjet printing, where a binder solution was deposited onto a powder bed to bind particles layer by layer, forming the desired structure. This innovation originated at the Massachusetts Institute of Technology (MIT) in the early 1990s and was patented by Sachs et al.

In 1989, Scott Crump patented another ground-breaking 3D printing method, fused deposition modeling (FDM). This process involved extruding semiliquid polymer filaments through a heated nozzle and depositing them layer by layer onto a build platform to create solid structures.

Inkjet printing also played a pivotal role in producing *Spritam* (levetiracetam) tablets, the first FDA-approved 3D-printed drug for oral use, developed by Aprecia Pharmaceuticals in 2016. Today, 3D printing is a leading technology in industries such as automotive, aerospace, biomedical, and tissue engineering and is now advancing in the pharmaceutical sector. The FDA actively encourages the adoption of innovative manufacturing technologies, including 3D printing, through risk-based regulatory approaches [3, 4].

9.3 3D Technology Adoption in the Pharmaceutics

Various technical approaches exist for fabricating 3D-printed products in the pharmaceutical industry, each suited to specific applications and materials. These methods differ primarily in how layers are deposited on top of one another. Factors such as speed, precision, quality, and the properties of the materials play a critical role in determining the most appropriate 3D printing method for a given use case. Additionally, key characteristics of 3D-printed medical products, such as drug loading capacity and release profiles, can be precisely controlled by adjusting printing parameters. This can involve altering the number of printed layers in a specific area or modifying the total printing area. Fused deposition modeling (FDM) 3D printing is a rapidly evolving technology within the pharmaceutical industry. Its ability to produce personalized medicines, complex drug delivery systems, and cost-effective manufacturing solutions has positioned it as a key innovation. This review highlights the economic and market trends shaping its application in pharmaceuticals. The adoption of 3D technology in the pharmaceutical industry is a rapidly growing trend that promises to revolutionize several aspects of drug development, manufacturing, and delivery. This technology encompasses a variety of tools and methods, including 3D printing (additive manufacturing), 3D modeling, and advanced imaging techniques. 3D printing technology not only emerged as novel technique in pharmacy but it also outlooks the whole field from drug designing and development to get its approval from regulatory authorities and counsel patients regarding its benefits and advantages in personalized medicine manufacturing. The overview of how 3D technology is transforming pharmaceutical practices is described in Fig. 9.1 [5].

1. *Drug Development and Design*
   - *3D Molecular Modeling:* In the early stages of drug discovery, 3D modeling helps scientists visualize molecular structures in three dimensions, aiding in the design of more effective and targeted drug molecules. Software like molecular dynamics (MD) simulations and quantum mechanics (QM) simulations have been critical in predicting how drug molecules will interact with biological targets.
   - *Target Identification:* 3D technologies help in the design of molecules that fit perfectly into their target sites (such as receptors or enzymes) through molecular docking and simulation platforms.
2. *3D Printing for Drug Manufacturing*
   - *Additive Manufacturing in Drug Production:* 3D printing enables the production of solid dosage forms (like tablets and capsules) with complex geome-

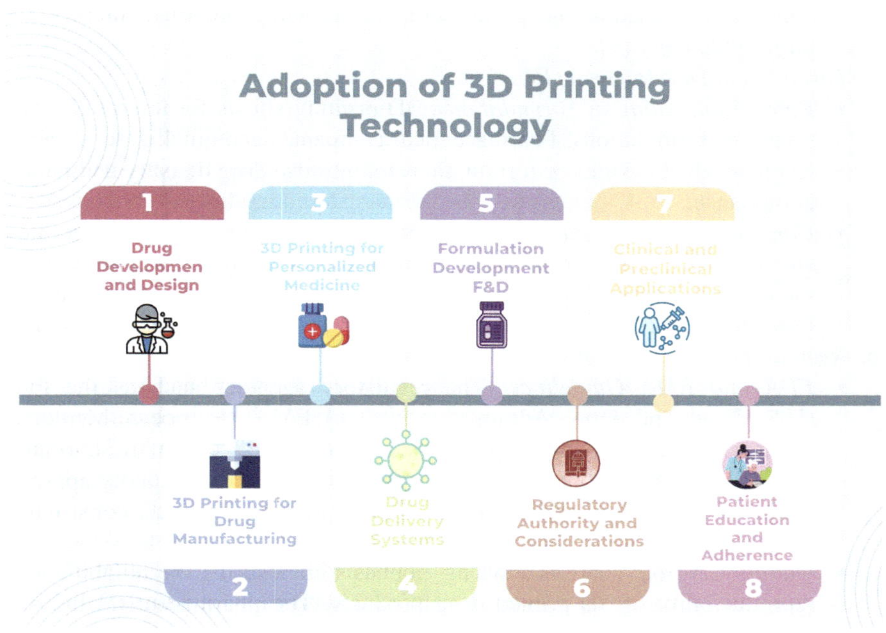

Fig. 9.1 Adoption of 3D printing technology in pharmaceutics

tries, offering precision in drug release mechanisms. This can lead to enhanced bioavailability, reduced side effects, and better patient adherence.

- *Printing Polymeric Drugs:* 3D printing is used to print complex polymeric matrices that release drugs at controlled rates, providing sustained or targeted release profiles. This is especially useful for drugs that require controlled delivery or that have a narrow therapeutic window [6, 7].

3. *3D Printing for Personalized Medicine*
   - *Customized Dosage Forms:* With 3D printing, drugs can be manufactured in personalized dosages, shapes, and release profiles tailored to an individual patient's needs. This technology can be especially useful for patients with rare conditions or those requiring a specific drug formulation.
   - *Patient-specific Tablets:* 3D printing allows for the creation of tablets that combine multiple drugs in a single dosage form. These tablets can also be designed to dissolve at different rates or at specific locations within the gastrointestinal tract, optimizing drug efficacy and minimizing side effects [8].
4. *Drug Delivery Systems*
   - *Customized Drug Release Profiles:* 3D-printed dosage forms allow for intricate designs that can control the release of drugs over time. These formulations can be designed to release drugs at specific locations in the gastrointestinal tract or at specific times, such as for chronotherapy.
   - *Microspheres and Nanocarriers:* Advances in 3D printing also support the development of drug delivery systems like nanocarriers and microspheres,

which can be used to encapsulate drugs, improving solubility, stability, and targeted delivery [9].

5. *Formulation Development (F&D)*
   - *Rapid Prototyping of Formulations:* 3D printing allows for the rapid prototyping of formulations. Pharmaceutical companies can quickly develop and test new tablet designs or formulations to optimize drug delivery and patient compliance.
   - *Complex Drug Combinations:* 3D printing can combine multiple drugs into a single device, which may enhance therapeutic outcomes, streamline treatments, and reduce the pill burden for patients, especially for chronic conditions like HIV or hypertension [10].
6. *Regulatory Considerations*
   - *FDA and EMA Guidelines:* The regulatory agencies such as the FDA (U.S. Food and Drug Administration) and EMA (European Medicines Agency) are gradually developing frameworks for the approval of 3D-printed drugs. While this technology shows significant promise, regulatory approval requires extensive validation of the printing processes, product consistency, and quality assurance.
   - *Quality Control:* There is a strong emphasis on ensuring the reliability and reproducibility of 3D-printed drug products. The pharmaceutical industry must comply with stringent regulatory guidelines to ensure patient safety, particularly as 3D printing methods can sometimes introduce variability in material properties and dosage.
7. *Clinical and Preclinical Applications*
   - *3D-printed Organs and Tissues for Testing:* Researchers are working on creating 3D-printed models of human organs and tissues for drug testing. This allows for more accurate preclinical models, enabling better predictions of drug efficacy and safety before moving to clinical trials. For instance, 3D-printed liver models are being used to test how a drug might interact with liver cells.
   - *Simulating Disease Models:* 3D technology allows for the creation of in vitro disease models that mimic human physiology more accurately than traditional 2D cell cultures. These models can be used for drug screening and toxicity testing.
8. *Patient Education and Adherence*
   - *Interactive 3D Models for Patient Education:* Pharmaceutical companies are utilizing 3D technology to create interacive models of diseases, drugs, and treatments to educate patients about their condition and the benefits of their medication. This can increase patient understanding, leading to better adherence to prescribed therapies.
   - *Innovative Packaging Solutions:* 3D printing can also be used to create patient-centric packaging designs that include easy-to-understand instructions and custom features, such as blister packs tailored to a patient's medication schedule [11, 12].

9.4 Fused Deposition Modeling

Fused deposition modeling (FDM) was developed by Stratasys in Eden Prairie, Minnesota. In this process, a plastic or wax material is extruded through a nozzle that traces the cross-sectional geometry of the part layer by layer. FDM is the second most widely used rapid prototyping technology, following stereolithography. It is one of the most common and accessible 3D printing technologies. It works by extruding a thermoplastic filament through a heated nozzle, which deposits the material layer by layer onto a build platform. The process begins with a computer-aided design (CAD) model, which is sliced into thin layers by the printer's software. The FDM printer then follows the path outlined by the software, laying down material in successive layers until the object is fully formed [13].

The 3D printers used for fused deposition modeling (FDM) feature a support base with some degree of freedom, allowing it to move vertically. Along with the base, there is an extruder that connects to the filament and is responsible for heating the filament to its melting point. The extruder then deposits the material layer by layer through a nozzle to create the desired object. The extruder is capable of moving in all three directions—x, y, and z. The process is called fused deposition modeling because the adjacent layers fuse together as they are deposited by the extruder, allowing the 3D printer to model the object. Depending on the desired surface finish, the final product may be dipped in resin, similar to the stereolithography process. The FDM is shown in Fig. 9.2. [14]

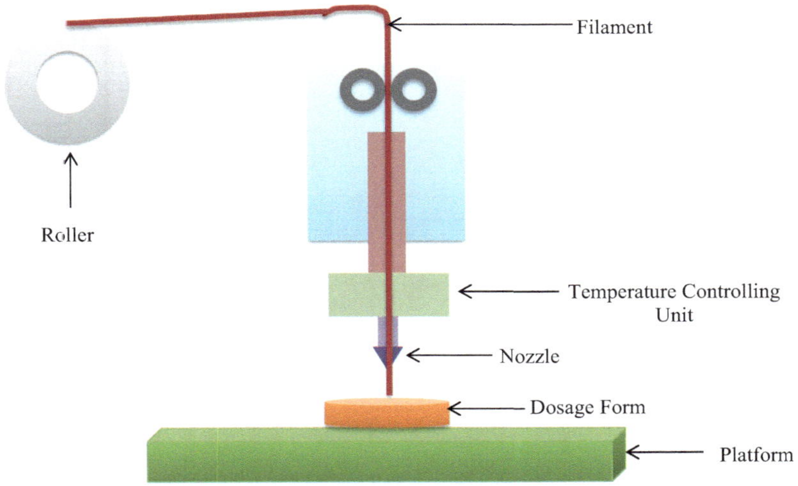

Fig. 9.2 FDM process for 3D printing

9.5 Process Parameters of FDM

Fused deposition modeling (FDM) is affected by numerous parameters, which can be broadly categorized into machine and material parameters, as illustrated in Fig. 9.3. Machine parameters are those settings configured by the 3D printer user in the slicing software during the preparation of G-code files. These include factors such as printing speed, raster angle, melt flow rate, air gap, layer thickness, in fill density, build orientation, and temperature. Conversely, material parameters pertain to the properties of the filament material, such as its thermal and mechanical characteristics, which influence both the extrusion process and the final print's performance.

The quality and performance of printed parts are heavily influenced by the selection of these parameters. Numerous studies have been conducted to evaluate the impact of various parameters on the printing process and the quality of the final prints [28]. Build orientation refers to the angle at which the longest dimension of the part is positioned relative to the build plate, typically at angles like 0°, 45°, or

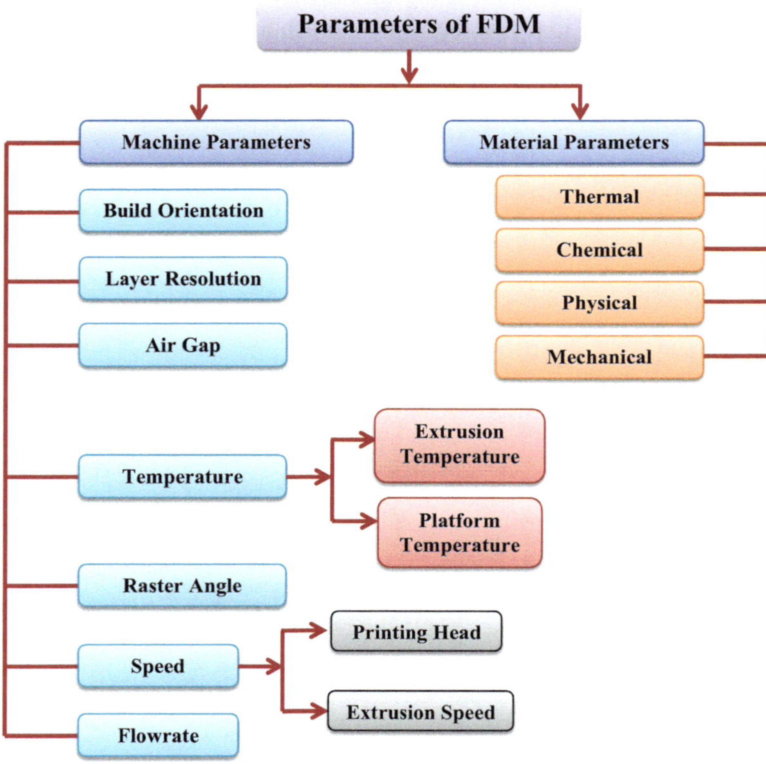

Fig. 9.3 Process parameters of FDM

90°, based on the user's preference. Layer resolution denotes the minimum thickness of each layer deposited during a single pass of the print head, ranging from a few micrometers to several millimeters, depending on the printer's precision and intended application. Extrusion temperature is the heat applied by the printer's heating elements to melt the filament for smooth extrusion. Meanwhile, platform temperature refers to the heat applied to the build plate to improve print adhesion and reduce the risk of printing failures [15, 16].

9.6 Applications of FDM

Fused deposition modeling (FDM) has become one of the most advanced methods for prototyping and rapid tooling of complex designs in small to medium production batches. Ongoing research focuses on expanding the range of materials suitable for rapid prototyping, and a substantial body of literature addresses this topic. The applications are described in Table 9.1 [17, 18].

Table 9.1 Applications of fused deposition modeling

S.No	Applications	Description
1.	Adoption for industrial practice	FDM is increasingly being utilized in industries such as toy manufacturing, either as a direct production method or for creating molds for injection molding.
2.	Mass personalization	The potential of FDM in mass customization is significant. Its flexibility and ability to create intricate profiles make it ideal for producing personalized items, including toys, automotive components, interior design pieces, implants, and beauty products
3.	Medical applications	In the medical field, FDM is used to produce molds for casting implants and medical devices. One of its notable applications is in investment casting for medical implants. Unlike traditional methods that rely on metallic molds and sacrificial patterns like wax, 3D-printed molds eliminate the need for such materials, reducing costs, time, and waste. However, challenges like poor surface quality persist, and ongoing research aims to improve the surface properties of 3D-printed molds and the resulting castings
4.	Other applications	FDM also extends to diverse fields, including the direct printing of electrochemical cells for energy storage devices, microtrusses for biomedical scaffold, drug delivery systems in pharmaceuticals, and conductors for the electronics industry.

Table 9.2 Advantages and disadvantages of FDM

S.No	Points	Advantages
1.	Affordability	FDM printers are generally more affordable than other 3D printing technologies like SLA or SLS, making them ideal for hobbyists, startups, and educational institutions. Materials (e.g., PLA, ABS) are inexpensive and widely available.
2.	Ease of use	Simple to operate with minimal training. Compatible with user-friendly software for slicing and printing.
3.	Wide range of materials	Can print with a variety of thermoplastics like PLA, ABS, PETG, and specialty materials (e.g., flexible filaments, wood-filled, or carbon-fiber composites).
4.	Accessibility	FDM printers are available in desktop sizes, making them suitable for small workspaces. Popular in schools, maker spaces, and small businesses due to their compactness and ease of integration.
5.	Customization and prototyping	Ideal for rapid prototyping with customizable designs. Produces functional prototypes with moderate mechanical strength.
6.	Low waste	Material is deposited only where needed, resulting in minimal waste compared to subtractive manufacturing.
7.	Scalability	Available in both consumer-grade and industrial-grade models for a variety of applications.

9.7 Advantages and Disadvantages of FDM

FDM is one of the most widely used 3D printing technologies due to its simplicity, cost-effectiveness, and versatility. The advantages and disadvantages of FDM are described in Table 9.2 [19, 20].

9.8 3D Printing Market Size

The global 3D printing market was valued at USD 22.39 billion in 2023 and is expected to grow from USD 27.52 billion in 2024 to USD 150.20 billion by 2032, with a compound annual growth rate (CAGR) of 23.6% during this period. The US market alone is projected to reach approximately USD 33.78 billion by 2032, driven by significant investments from both governments and major technology companies.

The rapid advancement of digitization, along with the increasing adoption of cutting-edge technologies such as smart factories, Industry 4.0, machine learning, and robotics, will drive the demand for online 3D printing in simulation applications. 3D printing technology has applications in prototyping; production, proof of concept, and others are shown in Fig. 9.4. [21]

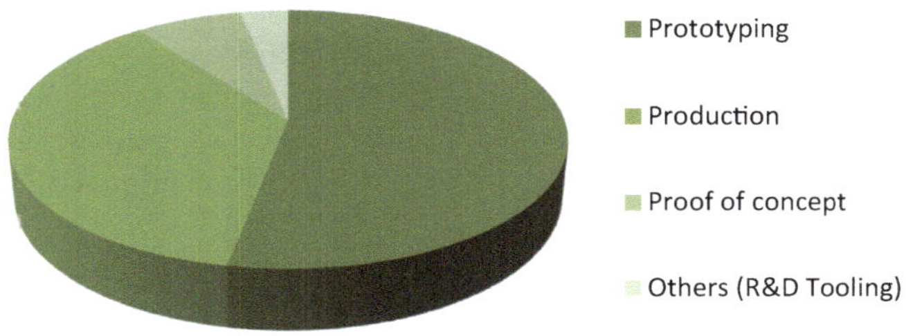

Fig. 9.4 Global 3D printing market share by applications

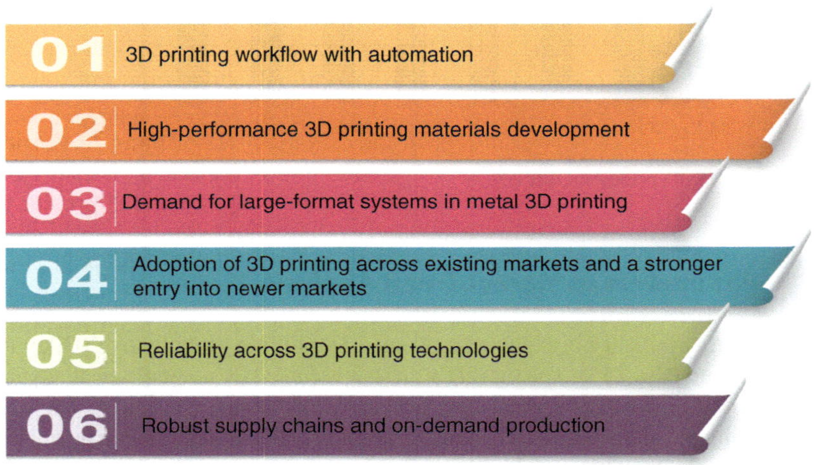

Fig. 9.5 Key market trends of 3D printing

Market trends which play an important role in 3D printing are given in Fig. 9.5.

When choosing a material for 3D printing, there are a wide range of options, and ongoing research is focused on creating new 3D-printable materials. Selecting the appropriate material is equally as crucial as choosing the right printing technology for the specific application. As 3D printing technologies evolve, new materials and increasingly advanced machines with enhanced capabilities are continually being introduced. With the current expansion of additive manufacturing, the global market for 3D-printed products and services is projected to surpass 40 billion US dollars by 2024. The industry is forecasted to grow at a compound annual rate of 29% from 2020 to 2024. The US 3D printer market size and growth is described in Fig. 9.6 [22, 23].

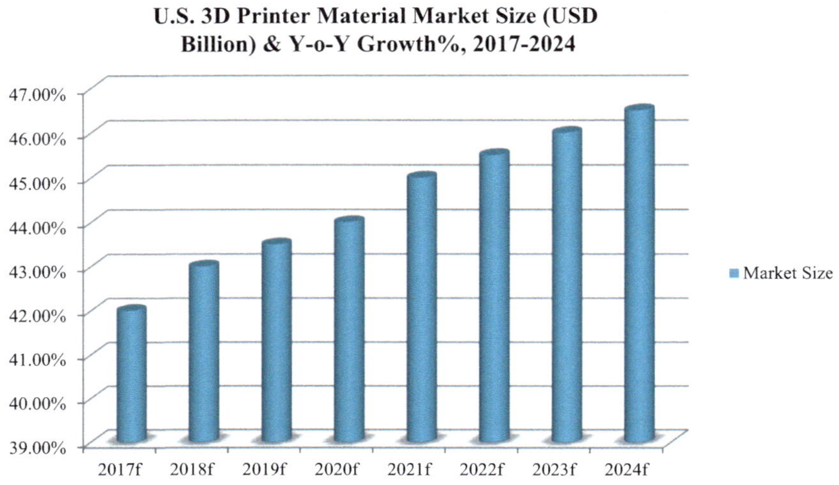

Fig. 9.6 The US 3D printer market size

9.9 Parameters of Market Trend Analysis

The 3D printing industry is expected to exceed $50 billion globally by 2030**,** with a CAGR of around 20–25%. The market's growth is fueled by technological advancements, decreasing costs, and increasing adoption across various sectors. The future of 3D printing lies in its potential to transform traditional manufacturing by enabling cost-effective, sustainable, and highly customized production. The latest generation of commercial large-format 3D printing technologies, while not as massive as BAAM, are considerably faster and more advanced, and have already seen widespread adoption across various industries. The 3D printing industry is evolving rapidly, driven by innovation, cost-efficiency, and the growing need for sustainable and customizable manufacturing solutions. The parameters are shown in Fig. 9.7 [24].

1. *Market Growth and Projections*
   - *Market size:* The global 3D printing in pharmaceuticals market is anticipated to grow at a compound annual growth rate (CAGR) exceeding 10% over the next decade.
   - *Drivers:* Increased demand for personalized medicine, the need for sustainable and efficient manufacturing, and advancements in pharmaceutical-grade materials for FDM.
   - *Regions leading adoption:*
     - North America: Early adoption due to strong R&D investments.
     - Europe: Regulatory advancements supporting personalized medicines.
     - Asia-Pacific: Emerging markets leveraging cost-effective technologies.

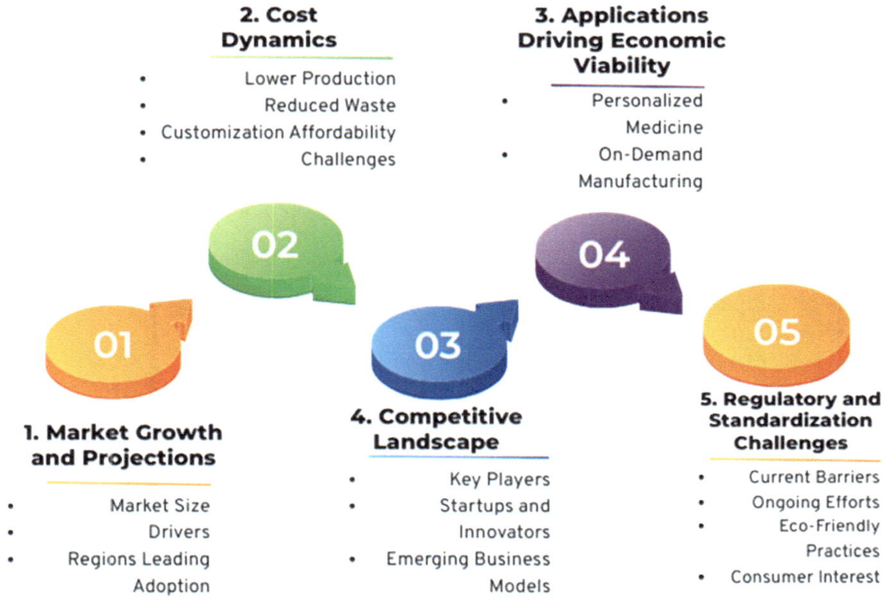

Fig. 9.7 The US 3D printer market size

2. *Cost Dynamics*

   FDM enables precise deposition of materials, significantly reducing raw material wastage compared to traditional methods.

   - *Lower Production:*
     - *Reduced waste:* Elimination of tooling and molds.
     - Ability to produce small batches economically.
     - *Customization affordability:* Costs remain stable despite individualized designs, making FDM viable for patient-specific solutions.
   - *Challenges:*
     - High initial investment for 3D printers.
     - Expensive pharmaceutical-grade filaments, though prices are declining with increased competition [25].
3. *Applications Driving Economic Viability*
   - *Personalized medicine:*
     - Tailored drug dosages based on patient needs (e.g., polypills combining multiple drugs).
     - Pediatric and geriatric formulations in unique shapes and flavors.
     - Novel drug delivery systems: Intricate designs for controlled-release systems (e.g., tablets with delayed or multi-phase release).
   - *On-demand manufacturing:*
     - Hospitals or pharmacies could produce medications on-site, reducing inventory costs and waste [26].

4. *Competitive Landscape*
   - *Key players:*
     1. Pharmaceutical giants and tech firms are collaborating to integrate FDM into drug manufacturing. Examples include partnerships between Merck and AM companies.
   - *Startups and innovators:*
     2. Small firms are focusing on material development, particularly biocompatible polymers.
     3. Academic research institutions are contributing significantly to advancing the technology.
   - *Emerging business models:*
     4. Contract manufacturing for custom drug formulations.
     5. Leasing models for FDM printers tailored for pharmaceuticals.
5. *Regulatory and standardization challenges*
   - *Current barriers:*
     6. Limited regulatory frameworks for 3D-printed drugs.
     7. FDA-approved cases like Spritam (seizure medication) serve as milestones but remain rare.
   - *Ongoing efforts:*
     8. Establishing standard protocols for testing and approving 3D-printed pharmaceuticals.
     9. Guidelines for material compatibility, dosage accuracy, and patient safety.
     10. Economic implication: Faster approvals could significantly boost market penetration and ROI for pharmaceutical companies investing in FDM.
6. *Sustainability and Market Appeal*
   - *Eco-friendly practices:*
     11. Minimal waste production aligns with global sustainability goals.
     12. Use of biodegradable and recyclable polymers under development.
   - *Consumer interest:*
     13. Growing awareness of personalized medicine increases demand for customized therapies produced via FDM.
   - *Pharmacy of the future:*
     14. The potential for localized 3D printing hubs in healthcare facilities could revolutionize how drugs are distributed and consumed [27, 28].

9.10 Insights into FDM 3D Printing in Pharmaceuticals

Here are deeper insights into specific case studies, material trends, and regulatory updates related to FDM (fused deposition modeling) in pharmaceutical 3D printing:

1. *Specific case studies*
   1.1. *Spritam (Levetiracetam)—FDA-Approved 3D-Printed Drug*
      - *Details:* Manufactured by Aprecia Pharmaceuticals using 3D printing technology (ZipDose).

- *Significance:* Spritam was the first FDA-approved 3D-printed medication, demonstrating how 3D printing can produce high-dose, fast-dissolving tablets.
- *Impact on FDM:* While the method used was not strictly FDM, it paved the way for regulatory consideration of 3D printing for pharmaceuticals, including FDM-based methods for personalized dosing.

1.2. *Personalized Polypills*
- *Project:* A collaboration between academia and pharmaceutical companies to create personalized "polypills" using FDM.
- *Details:* Polypills combine multiple drugs into a single tablet, each segment printed with a specific drug at a precise dose.
- *Outcome:* Enhanced adherence and convenience for patients with chronic conditions (e.g., cardiovascular diseases).
- *Institutions involved:* University College London, FabRx (a pioneer in pharmaceutical 3D printing).

1.3. *On-Demand Manufacturing in Hospitals*
- *Example:* Pediatric hospitals in Europe tested FDM for producing chewable tablets in customized doses and flavors.
- *Findings:* Improved palatability for children, reduced wait times for tailored dosages, and minimal waste in production.

2. *Material Trends*

2.1. *Development of Pharmaceutical-Grade Polymers*
- *Polyvinyl alcohol (PVA)*
  - Popular for FDM due to its water solubility and safety.
  - Used in controlled drug-release systems.
- *Eudragit® polymers:*
  - Enable gastroresistant tablets with controlled-release profiles.
  - Tailored for specific pH environments in the GI tract.
- *Thermoplastic polyurethanes (TPUs):*
  - Biocompatible and elastic, useful for flexible drug delivery devices (e.g., implants).

2.2. *Innovations in Filament Design*
- Drug-loaded filaments:
  - Filaments preloaded with active pharmaceutical ingredients (APIs) streamline the FDM process.
  - *Example:* FabRx's proprietary drug-loaded filaments.
- *Biodegradable materials:*
  - Growing interest in materials like polylactic acid (PLA) to meet sustainability goals.
  - PLA is biocompatible and supports immediate-release dosage forms.

2.3. *Multicomponent Printing Materials*
- *Hybrid filaments:*
  - Combining excipients for faster dissolution or extended release.
  - *Example:* Filaments containing both a binder and a disintegrant.

3. *Regulatory Updates*

3.1. *FDA Guidelines*
- *Quality control:*
  - Focus on verifying dose accuracy, mechanical integrity, and reproducibility in FDM processes.
  - Emphasis on establishing Good Manufacturing Practices (GMP) for 3D-printed pharmaceuticals.
- *Case-by-case approval:*
  - Drugs produced using 3D printing are assessed individually, with the FDA examining printing methods, materials, and drug release profiles.

3.2. *European Medicines Agency (EMA)*
- *3D printing task forces:*
  - EMA is developing specific guidelines for 3D-printed medications, including FDM-based products.
  - Areas of focus include long-term stability of drug-loaded filaments and postprint quality checks.

3.3. *Global Trends*
- *Pharmacy-level manufacturing:*
  - Regulators are exploring frameworks for in-hospital or pharmacy-based 3D printing of personalized medicines.
  - *Examples* include "point-of-care manufacturing" regulations in Canada and Australia.

4. *Challenges and Future Directions*

4.1. *Challenges*
- *API stability*
  - Ensuring the stability of heat-sensitive drugs during the FDM process.
  - Regulatory bottlenecks: Lack of harmonized global standards slows adoption.
  - Material costs: High costs of pharmaceutical-grade filaments remain a barrier.

4.2. *Future Directions*
- *Integration of AI and FDM*
  - Using AI to optimize print parameters for individual patients.
  - Expanded filament libraries: Research on biodegradable and bioabsorbable materials for temporary implants.
  - Decentralized production models: Growing interest in pharmacy-led FDM printing for remote or underserved regions [28, 29].

9.11 Conclusion

FDM 3D printing is shaping the future of pharmaceutical manufacturing by enabling economic efficiency, innovation, and patient-centric care. However, its widespread adoption depends on overcoming challenges related to cost, material availability, and regulatory acceptance. As the technology matures, its integration into mainstream pharmaceutical production could redefine the industry's economic landscape, making personalized medicine a global reality. 3D printing technology is a highly valuable and promising tool in the pharmaceutical industry, enabling a shift toward personalized medicine tailored to individual patient needs. It provides several benefits, including enhanced cost efficiency and faster manufacturing processes. By transforming traditional manufacturing methods, 3D printing improves design and production, while also reducing lead times and tooling costs for new products. This chapter highlights various fabrication techniques and notable applications of 3D printing within the healthcare sector, with a particular focus on pharmaceutical sciences. This review explores the extensive landscape of 3D printing within the manufacturing industry. Currently, 3D printing technology is emerging in various manufacturing sectors, offering significant benefits to individuals, companies, and governments. To advance the adoption of 3D printing, more information and research are needed to improve and expand its infrastructure. This paper provides an overview of different 3D printing technologies, the materials used in manufacturing, and the applications of 3D printing. Future research should focus on studying various types of 3D printing machines and identifying the most suitable materials for each machine type to further enhance the technology's effectiveness and integration.

References

1. Mwema FM. Basics of Fused Deposition Modelling (FDM), vol. 682. Springer Sciences; 2020. p. 1–15.
2. Botao H. 3D printing technology and its application in industrial manufacturing. Mater Sci Eng. 2020;782:1–6. https://doi.org/10.1088/1757-899X/782/2/022065.
3. Agashe DK. 3D printing and advance material technology. Int J Grid Distrib Comput. 2020;13(2):1899–936.
4. Fan H, et al. 3D bioprinting advances in tissue engineering: progress and challenges. Front Bioeng Biotechnol. 2022;10:1122–33. https://doi.org/10.3389/fbioe.2022.896581.
5. Jain S, et al. Artificial organ fabrication using 3D bioprinting: recent trends and applications. Biofabrication. 2023;15(2):023901. https://doi.org/10.1088/1758-5090/ab3a15.
6. Wang L, et al. Innovations in 3D-printed medical devices and tissue scaffolds. J Biomed Mater Res. 2023;111(3):312–20. https://doi.org/10.1002/jbm.b.35089.
7. Parveen S, et al. Recent advancement of 3D printing application in pharmaceutical industries. IJPR. 2020:1–10.
8. ScienceDaily. Perfecting 3D-printed blood vessels with pores. Science Daily Jan 17, 2024. https://www.sciencedaily.com/releases/2024/01/240117112935.htm.
9. Joshi S, et al. 4D printing of materials for the future: opportunities and challenges. Appl Mater. 2020;18:100490.
10. Ngo TD, et al. Additive manufacturing (3D printing): a review of materials, methods, applications and challenges. Compos B: Eng. 2018;143:172–96.
11. Jian-Yuan L, Jia A, Chee KC. Fundamentals and applications of 3D printing for novel materials. Appl Mater Today. 2017;7:120–33.
12. Van HJ. Additive manufacturing of shape memory alloy. Shape Mem Superelasticity. 2018;4(2):309–12.
13. Lili L, Yuanyuan M, Ke C, Yang Z. 3D printing complex egg white protein objects: properties and optimization. Food Bioprocess Technol. 2018;1:1–11.

14. Singh P, Raghav A. 3D food printing: a revolution in food technology. Acta Sci Nutr Health. 2018;2(2):1–2.
15. Yu-Cheng W, Toly C, Yung-Lan Y. Advanced 3D printing technologies for the aircraft industry: a fuzzy systematic approach for assessing the critical factors. Int J Adv Manuf Technol. 2018;3(3):1–10.
16. Petch M. Audi gives update on use of SLM metal 3D printing for the automotive industry. 3D Printing Industry; 2018.
17. Chuan YF, Hong NL, Mahdi MA, Wahid MH, Nay MH. Three-dimensional printed electrode and its novel applications in electronic devices. Sci Rep. 2018;1:1–11.
18. Jeongwoo L, Ho-Chan K, Jae-Won C, In HLA. A review on 3D printed smart devices for 4D printing. Int J Precis Eng Manuf-Green Technol. 2018;4(3):373–83.
19. Dankar I, et al. Impact of mechanical and microstructural properties of potato puree-food additive complexes on extrusion-based 3D printing. Food Bioprocess Technol. 2018;1:1–11.
20. Attaran M. The rise of 3-D printing: the advantages of additive manufacturing over traditional manufacturing. Bus Horiz. 2017;1:1–12.
21. Vanderploeg A, Seung-Eun L, Mamp M. The application of 3D printing technology in the fashion industry. J Int J Fash Des Technol Educ. 2017;10(2):170–9.
22. Sreehitha V. Impact of 3D printing in automotive industry. Int J Mech Prod Eng. 2017;5(2):91–4.
23. Saengchaira N, et al. A review: additive manufacturing for active electronic components. Virtual Phys Prototyp. 2016;12(1):1–16.
24. Liu Z, et al. 3D printing: printing precision and application in food sector. Trends Food Sci Technol. 2017;2(1):1–36.
25. Goulas A, Friel RJ. 3D printing with moondust. Rapid Prototyp J. 2015;22(6):864–70.
26. Joshi SC, Sheikh AA. 3D-printing in aerospace and its long-term sustainability. Virtual Phys Prototyp. 2015;10(4):175–85.
27. Yang Y, Chen Y, Wei Y, Li Y. 3D printing of shape memory polymer for functional part fabrication. Int J Adv Manuf Technol. 2015;84(9):2079–95.
28. Uriondo A, Esperon-Miguez M, Perinpanayagam S. The present and future of additive manufacturing in the aerospace sector: a review of important aspects. J Aerosp Eng. 2015;229(11):1–14.
29. Tang T, et al. Global hotspots and emerging trends in 3D bioprinting research: a bibliometric analysis. J Tissue Eng Regen Med. 2021;15(11):1129–37. https://doi.org/10.1002/term.3191.

Environmental Sustainability in 3D Printing of Pharmaceuticals

10

Shital S. Patil, Varsha N. Tambe, Snehal B. Jadhav, and Pankaj V. Dangre

Abstract

The 3D printers are used widely nowadays in pharmaceuticals. It provides eco-friendly business and reduces carbon footprints compared to other methods. 3D printers save energy and reduce the cost and wastage of material. This technology makes extensive use of biodegradable materials, which are broken down by microorganisms in a natural way, minimizing their adverse impact on the environment. The numerous applications of 3D printing in the pharmaceutical science comprise drug release, cost cutting of medicines, and drug efficacy. 3D printing reduced environmental issues such as material wastage, energy use, carbon emissions, manufacturing, and distribution. This chapter highlights 3D printing techniques utilizing a sustainable production and their environmental implications. Furthermore, the chapter investigates the case studies on utilization of 3D printing in pharmaceutical industries.

Keywords

3D printers · Pharmaceuticals · Sustainable materials · Drug release · Dosage form

10.1 Introduction

3D printing technology has advanced rapidly, having a considerable influence on both the industrial and commercial sectors [1]. Furthermore, 3D bioprinting technology has a noteworthy impression on tissue engineering and medicinal research

S. S. Patil · V. N. Tambe · S. B. Jadhav · P. V. Dangre (✉)
Department of Pharmaceutics, K K Wagh College of Pharmacy, Amrutdham, Nashik, India
e-mail: pvdangre@kkwagh.edu.in

K. Vinchurkar, S. Mane (eds.), *Innovations in Drug Manufacturing*,
https://doi.org/10.1007/978-981-96-9075-6_10

[2]. 3D printing is one of the most innovative tools in modern life. The technology also finds its promising applications in fabricating novel dosage forms on a massive scale. Demand for patient-centric medicinal product development has increased dramatically since the FDA authorized the first 3D-printed pill in 2015 [3]. Pharmaceutical businesses are always looking for new improvements in medication creation, with an emphasis on material qualities, methods, and technology. 3D-printed pharmaceuticals have resulted in breakthroughs in individualized drug doses and patient-centric products [4]. They are simple to construct and configure, and their low cost allows them to be used in small-scale production lines. Unnecessary resources and production expenses are avoided, and droplet sizes are precisely regulated enough to provide multidosing goods. Sustainable development, a crucial global imperative, requires a precise balance of social, environmental, technological, and economic considerations. The extensive literature on additive manufacturing (AM) highlights the range of research methodologies, underlining the necessity to assess emerging sustainable technologies [5]. AM's energy-efficient nature, combined with its ability to reduce material waste and inventory, presents it as a sustainable manufacturing solution.

10.1.1 3D Printing Technology in Pharmaceutical Production

The use of additive manufacturing, mainly 3D printing, in industrial settings creates a variety of potential for sustainable production in the context of industry [6]. Nonetheless, despite hopeful improvements, combining eco-friendly techniques and materials into 3D printing presents obstacles [7]. There is a significant information gap about the complete range of environmental repercussions, material limits, and overall sustainability of various 3D printing procedures. Furthermore, the translation of sustainable practices, such as the use of recyclable and biodegradable materials, from theoretical frameworks to practical applications in 3D printing still needs to be explored. Existing literature emphasizes the need for significant research into the environmental impact, material qualities, and practicality of sustainable 3D printing. This study intends to bridge the gaps described above and contribute to the long-term evolution of additive manufacturing by attaining the following objectives:

- Investigate the environmental impact of different 3D printing procedures, including energy efficiency, material efficiency, and waste generation, to better understand their sustainability profiles.
- Evaluate sustainable materials for extrusion-based 3D printing.
- Explore the impact of 3D printing on sustainable development by focusing on the utilization of recyclable resources for fabrication, environmental monitoring, and wastewater treatment.
- Identify and analyze constraints and challenges of employing sustainable materials in 3D printing, including accuracy, print quality, and structural integrity.

10.2 Environmental Impacts of Traditional Pharmaceutical Manufacturing

10.2.1 Waste Generation

The environment was affected by the notable advancements and increase in the quantity of drugs available to treat ailments and diseases. Ecosystem include terrestrial and marine environments. The environmental effects of drug manufacturing processes have a substantial influence on the value of chemistry in society [8]. Pharmaceutical waste is typically associated with hospital and pharmaceutical industry waste. However, since the 1980s, medications have been acknowledged as chemical pollutants. Three primary sources account for the majority of the complex problem of pharmaceutical residues polluting our ecosystems: the production of pharmaceuticals, the death of humans and animals, and the improper disposal of medications [9]. Large-scale production of these compounds takes place in the pharmaceutical industry, which is the primary cause of pollution in this area. Manufacturing facilities frequently discharge effluents directly into wastewater streams in spite of strict regulations. When suitable treatment protocols are either not followed or are ineffective, these effluents—which are heavy in APIs—find their way into aquatic environments. This problem is made worse in areas where pharmaceutical production is concentrated, leading to extreme localized pollution.

10.2.2 Aquatic Pollution

There are a lot of pharmaceutically active compounds (PhACs) and their by-products in lakes, rivers, and groundwater [10]. PhACs have the ability to modify microbial community composition, energy transmission, and nutrient cycling in aquatic systems. This can affect the survival and reproduction of nearly all aquatic vertebrates and invertebrates, as well as their behavior.

Chemical pollutants, including industrial and pharmaceutical chemicals and heavy metals, can alter the equilibrium of vital nutrients and oxygen levels, degrade water quality, and create environments that are hazardous or unsuitable for aquatic life [11] as represented in the Fig. 10.1. Additionally damaging to biodiversity and photosynthesis in aquatic plants, water pollution has a major negative effect on ecosystems that depend on these plants for survival [12]. Water pollution is the primary source of nutrients for both terrestrial and aquatic plants, which can then absorb it and pass it along the food chain to humans and other animals. The second prominent source of pollution is pharmaceutical residues excreted by humans and animals. Not all active pharmaceutical ingredients (APIs) are completely metabolized by the body; a sizable portion is eliminated through faces and urine, which eventually find their way into sewage systems [13]. The use of veterinary medications increases this problem as these drugs can directly enter in the environment through the use of

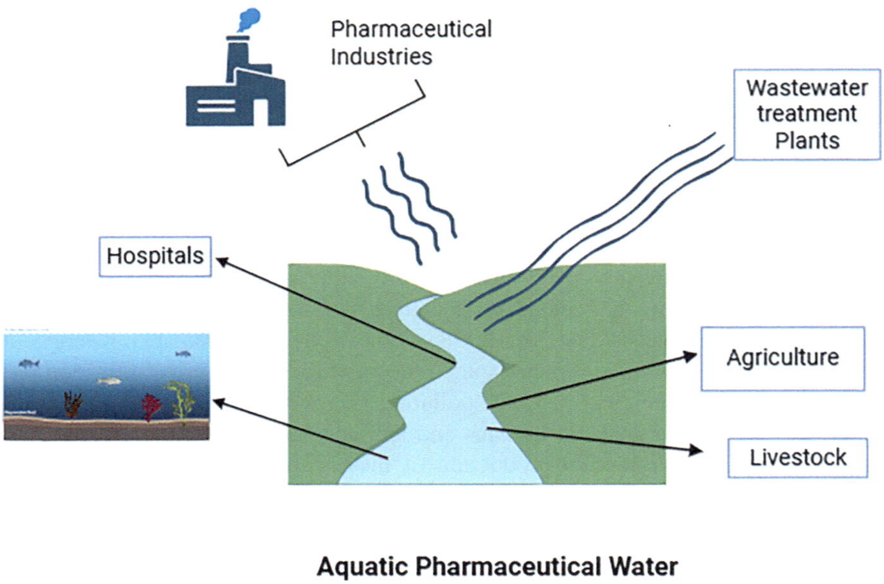

Fig. 10.1 Main pathways of pharmaceutical water system

manure in agricultural fields. Due to these factors, human and animal waste is problematic and a common cause of pharmaceutical pollution [14]. The improper disposal of obsolete or unneeded drugs can seriously affect the health of nature. Medicines that are not required need to be discarded in the trash or run through sinks and toilets. Drugs released into the environment change over time due to a variety of physical, biological, and chemical processes; they are not inert. The characteristics, actions, and possible environmental effects of the medications may alter as a result of these changes. However, it should be noted that most pharmaceuticals are developed to withstand fast disintegration in the human body while performing therapeutic activities, which contributes to their persistence in the environment.

10.2.3 Carbon Emission

In terms of trash management, CO_2 emissions, plastic consumption, pollution of air and water, and energy consumption, there is a substantial environmental effect of pharmaceutical companies [15]. Data from 2019 shows that pharmaceutical firms emit 13% more CO_2 than the automobile industry [16]. To go green, pharmaceutical businesses should prioritize investments in good manufacturing and provide standard criteria for medicine preparation along with training of employees. Since the beginning of the industrial era (about 1800), the level of carbon dioxide in the atmosphere has significantly and firstly elevated [17]. For the first time in the history of industrial era, CO_2 levels surpassed the symbolic and noteworthy 400 parts per million (ppm) threshold, according to a September 2016 report from the Scripps

Institutions of Oceanography [18]. According to research, the emission intensity of the pharmaceutical sector's carbon footprint was around 55% greater than that of the automobile industry [16]. The pharmaceutical industry produced 52 million metric tons of carbon dioxide equivalent globally in 2015, whereas 46 million metric tons of the same substance was produced by the automotive industry [19]. The healthcare business emits greenhouse gases such as anesthetic gases, nitrous oxide, carbon dioxide, hydrofluorocarbons, methane, sulfur hexafluoride, and perfluorocarbons. The creation of the above gases is linked with activities pertaining to travel, services, purchasing, and the energy needs of buildings and equipment.

10.2.4 The Effect on Human Health and Climate Change

Human health and climate change are severely affected by greenhouse gases released by the healthcare industry [20]. Extreme climate, increasing sea levels, higher temperatures, and elevated carbon dioxide levels are all results of weather change. As a result of these occurrences, people can develop respiratory allergies, asthma, cardiovascular disease, malnourishment, heat-related illnesses, and even pass away [21]. The risk of heat stroke to susceptible individuals like geriatrics and infants is increased due to elevated temperature which can lead to mortality as observed in the heatwave in Europe in 2003 which resulted in 70,000 deaths [22]. For developing effective solutions to reduce medicines, environmental impact understanding of these sources is needed. Hence, each issue needs to be addressed quickly for sustainable solutions.

10.3 Importance of Environmental Sustainability

Over the past few decades, the effect of human activities on the environment has been increasing alarmingly, and the manufacturing sector is one of the major contributors to the environment. Large amounts of natural resources are required for manufacturing activities, and they also produce waste that is large in amount and, most of the time, harmful to the environment as well. To overcome this, 3D printing technology has emerged as a potential option for these environmental issues.

10.3.1 Environmental Benefits of 3D Printing in Pharmaceuticals

10.3.1.1 Customized Dosage Form

Manufacturing dosage form by conventional methods involves a lot of chemicals and other resources usage, which differ according to the product being manufactured. It is often observed that traditional techniques result in overproduction of dosage form, eventually leading to wastage of resources. In 3D printing technology, one has definite control over the process, and designing dosage forms as per the requirement of the end-user has become possible, thus minimizing the waste amount [23].

10.3.1.2 Production as per the Demand

In traditional production techniques, dosage forms are produced in a large capacity, taking into consideration the approximate need of the product in the market, generating the requirement for maintaining a large inventory. With time, as the demand reduces, the surplus dosage form expires. 3D printing can produce the dosage form as per the requirement. This minimizes the need to maintain a large inventory and also reduces the waste associated with expired drugs.

10.3.1.3 Personalized Dosage Form

3D printing can be used to create medicine exclusively as per an individual's specific needs. This increases patient compliance and ultimately improves treatment output and reduces dose [24].

10.3.1.4 Reduction in Carbon Footprint

3D printing technology has the potential to manufacture the medicine on-site, and the intricacy and range of the pharmaceutical supply chain can be decreased. This minimizes the environmental effect generated by transportation, thereby lowering the associated carbon emission [25].

10.3.1.5 Minimized Packaging

As the medications are produced on demand and on-site in specific quantities, the need for packaging, especially secondary packaging, is reduced, and thus the waste generated by packaging material is reduced.

10.3.1.6 Use of Recyclable Material

In a few of the 3D printing technologies, recyclable materials are used. With this, it generates a circular economy. Materials like polylactic acid (PLA), polycaprolactone (PCL), cellulose materials, and polyethylene glycol (PEG) can be used and recovered using techniques like solvent recovery, mechanical grinding, and chemical recycling. The potential of 3D printing in the pharmaceutical industry to optimize production techniques, reduce waste, and improve resource efficiency in the manufacturing of medicines makes it environmentally beneficial.

10.4 Sustainable Materials Selection for 3D Printing

The selection of sustainable material for 3D printing requires considering factors like environmental friendliness, biocompatibility, and suitability for creating complex dosage forms [26]. The basic properties to be considered while selecting sustainable materials are as follows.

10.4.1 Biocompatibility

It is important to consider the safety and efficacy of the materials. It should not provoke any immune response when taken or applied to the skin. Polymers like PLA and PCL are biocompatible and do not induce any adverse reaction in the body [27].

10.4.2 Biodegradability

The material should be able to metabolize naturally after a specific time, minimizing the environmental impact. Materials like PLA are derived from corn starch, one of the popular biodegradable materials that can be used in the 3D printing of pharmaceuticals.

10.4.3 Mechanical Properties

The material should have enough mechanical strength to withstand the mechanical forces that may be applied during the printing process without deforming or breaking. The durability and elasticity of the material also need to be considered. The material should be resistant to wear and tear over a period of time, to maintain the integrity of the dosage form.

10.4.4 Chemical Stability

Material should not react with active pharmaceutical ingredients and other excipients used in the formulation. It should be compatible with other ingredients throughout its shelf-life. With this, it should be chemically inserted for body fluids as well. The properties of it should remain intact in any chemical changes in any environment.

10.4.5 Printability

Printability is a vital criterion for determining the effectiveness of an extrusion-based 3D printing process. The computational fluid dynamics (CFD) models are most commonly utilized to assess the parameters of printing such as dimensional accuracy, extrudability, and stability of 3D-printed objects. Food ink should have appropriate rheological qualities in order to print well.

10.4.6 Thermal Properties

Thermal attributes were evaluated to determine the suitability of 3D-printed phase change during the printing applications. The thermal qualities of a material determine the operating circumstances that the printed product can withstand, as well as its overall longevity and performance.

10.5 Energy Consumption and Carbon Footprint Reduction Strategies

3D printing has been used in the last few years in pharmaceuticals to customize dosage form designs to meet the patient requirement [28]. During printing, 3D printers use low energy to reduce consumption and the carbon emissions. For the carbon footprint reduction used various alternative sources as well as traditional and innovative methods are used. 3D printers use less energy, produce less waste, and permit local production, all of which lower the carbon footprint related to transportation and logistics. That being said, additive manufacturing raises certain environmental concerns. Despite not producing waste material like chips, the technique generates waste in a number of ways. Rejected prints, broken printer parts, and surplus powder or resin could all end up in a landfill. Furthermore, emissions are created both in the manufacturing process and during the use of 3D printers. Particularly, extrusion-style printers generate considerable volumes of particle pollution (PM) and volatile organic compounds (VOCs). Environmental criticism even reaches resin 3D printers. However, photopolymerization methods like stereolithography (SLA) produce less.

10.5.1 Energy Usage while in Standby

In standby mode, 3D printers need energy, just like most other machines. When measured for 1 hour, the energy consumption of all six printers ranged from 0.03 to 0.17 kWh, with DIW consuming the most. Hot melt extrusion (HME) is included in the numbers for the fused deposition modeling (FDM) printers, and a significant difference in energy consumption was found between the two: the tiny FDM printer used less energy than the large FDM printer. It was discovered that the direct powder extrusion (DPE) printer, an advancement in FDM that uses direct filament extrusion, used less energy than the large FDM printer with HME standby consumption but the same as the tiny FDM printer. Even though the selective laser sintering (SLS) printer had the highest volume, it used about the same amount of energy as the huge FDM printer and the direct ink writer (DIW) printer. There was no contribution from the standard SLA printing curing oven because it lacked a standby option.

10.5.2 The Utilization of Energy during Printing

For every one of the six printers, the energy required to produce 10 printlets was noted. The measurements take into account the energy required for printing, any subsequent cooling down processes, and the priming step (heating up, calibration, etc.). As we stated earlier, the computations also took into account the energy required for any supplementary equipment. The energy usage values ranged from 0.06 to 0.58 kWh for every printer except SLS. SLS printing requires a lot of energy due to the necessity of heating the printing chamber during the process. Its 3.08 kWh energy usage was orders of magnitude higher than comparable 3D printing processes. The carbon emission estimates ranged from 11.60 to 595.61 g CO_2 equivalent per ten printlets, even though eliminating SLS from the data limits the range to between 11.60 to 112.16 g CO_2 (eq) per ten printlets. Similar to the previously disclosed CO_2 (eq) values per tablet for a tableting machine, which vary from 2.06 to 7.71 g, the CO_2 (eq) values per printlet are 1.16 to 11.21 g [29].

10.6 Case Studies/Successes Stories

The 3D-printed drug market is still limited, though there are a growing number of startups and much innovative research being done. Here are the main pharmaceutical companies leading the push for 3D-printed medication. Table 10.1 lists application of 3D printing technology in development of different dosage forms.

Table 10.1 Application of 3D printing technology in development of different dosage forms

Method of printing	Dosage form	Drug	Polymers	Reference
Hot-melt extrusion (HME)	CR-tablet	Nifedipine	Povidone, and polyvinyl alcohol, ethylcellulose	[30]
	CR-tablet	Neomycin	Semicrystalline polyester, poly-l-lactic acid, PEG	[31]
Semi-solid extrusion (SSE)	IR-tablet	Furosemide, sildenafil	Gelucire 48/ 16, Polysorbate 80	[32]
	CR-tablet	Glipizide	HPC, polyoxyethylene, MC, lactose	[31]
	Self-nano-emulsifying drug delivery systems (SNEDDS)	Dapagliflozin propanediol monohydrate	Poloxamer 188, Capryol 90, polyethylene glycol (PEG) 6000, PEG 400, PEG 4000, and Cremophor EL	[33]
	ER-tablet	Clarithromycin	HPMC, polyvinyl pyrrolidone, ethanol	[34]

(continued)

Table 10.1 (continued)

Method of printing	Dosage form	Drug	Polymers	Reference
Fused deposition modeling (FDM)	IR-tablet	Lumefantrine	Eudragit EPO, xylitol, maltodextrin	[35]
	ER-tablet	Pramipexole	POLYOX N80, Eudragit (RSPO, RLPO, RS100, RL100)	[36]
	CR-tablet	Isoniazid, rifampicin	HPC, hypromellose acetate succinate	[37]
	SR-tablet	Propranolol HCl	D-mannitol, cellulose acetate, ethanol, acetone, dimethyl sulfoxide	[38]
		Domperidone	PVA, PLA	[39]
	FD-tablet	Captopril	PEG-6000, sodium starch glycolate, and croscarmellose sodium	[40]
	CR-tablet	Budesonide	PVA	[41]
		Acetaminophen	Soluplus, hydroxy-propyl methylcellulose (HPMC) E5	[42]
		Aripiprazole	Kollicoat® IR	[43]
Hot-melt Extrusion (HME)-coupled fused deposition modeling (FDM)-based 3D printing	SR-tablet	Naproxen	Vinyl pyrrolidone-vinyl acetate copolymer	[44]
	IR-tablet	Olanzapine	PVA/PEG graft copolymer	[45]
	SR-tablet	Ibuprofen	PVA, PEG, HPMC, Eudragit, Kollidon® vinyl acetate 64	[46]
	Gastroretentive floating tablets	Theophylline	HPC	[47]
	Ellipsoid-shaped gastric floating tablets	Propranolol hydrochloride	PVA	[34]
	IR-tablet	Itraconazole	PVP, PVA, Kollidon®CL-M	[28]
Binder jet 3D printing	Instant-dissolving tablets	Levetiracetam	MCC PH101 and Pearlitol 50C, Aerosil 200, sucralose, isopropanol	[48]

(continued)

Table 10.1 (continued)

Method of printing	Dosage form	Drug	Polymers	Reference
Powder solidification drop on solid	Implant	Isoniazide	Powder: PLLA ink: Acetone, ethanol water	[49]
	Tablets	Captopril	Powders: Maltitol maltodextrin ink: Water, polyvinyl pyrrolidone	[50]
Selective laser sintering	Orodispersible tablets	Paracetamol	HPMC, vinyl pyrrolidone—Vinyl acetate copolymer	[51]
Microneedles	Insulin	Dental SG resin, xylitol, mannitol, trehalose	Insulin skin delivery	[52]

10.6.1 Aprecia Pharmaceuticals

Aprecia Pharmaceuticals is leading the way in environmental sustainability through its innovative 3D printing technology. The company has developed a proprietary process called ZipDose Technology. ZipDose is currently the only FDA-approved product for commercial-scale pharmaceutical printing. The technology works without heat and uses a powder binder jetting technique. Rather, it uses an aqueous solution to hold several powder layers together. The result is a fast-dissolving tablet that can be filled with customized doses of up to 1000 mg. These tablets dissolve within seconds when exposed to water, making oral administration easier. Aprecia's Zip Dose technology already has a commercial application: since 2016, it has been used to produce SPRITAM, a drug used to treat seizures. The rapid-dissolve nature of the medication makes it easy to administer to children as young as 4, who may struggle to swallow more tablets. The US Food and Drugs Administration has given approval SPRITAM, the first medication manufactured via 3D printing.

10.6.2 Merck KGaA

Merck KGaA has used the powder bed fusion method and laser sintering printing techniques for widespread marketing; they report being able to produce up to 100,000 medications daily with this technique. Tablet appearance can be improved with laser sintering because it can create tablets with incredibly fine structures. Their study not only showed the value of producing clinical trials corresponding to time and money savings. Their study not only showed the value of producing clinical trials and the corresponding time and money savings but also the ability to reach production levels appropriate for large-scale manufacture on a commercial basis. The lack of solvent in the manufacturing process eliminates the need for after-processing; nonetheless, the question of what to do with excess powder that still contains API and whether to recycle it or dispose of it remains. To avoid unwanted chemical interactions between medications and resins, photocurable resins and drugs should be compatible [4].

10.6.3 FabR$_x$

FabR$_x$ is renowned biotech company in the United Kingdom that specializes in creating 3D-printed medications. The company offers two printing platforms for creating personalized printlets: The M3DIMAKER 1, designed for research and small-scale production, and the M3DIMAKER 2, which has a higher capacity for output. FabRx's innovative technology includes an interchangeable print head system that allows users to utilize various printing methods, such as semisolid extrusion, fused deposition modeling, or direct powder extrusion. Additionally, FabRx provides customers with accompanying software and pharma-ink development services.

10.6.4 GlaxoSmithKline (GSK)

A well-known pharmaceutical company improved the design and manufacturing of the Ventolin Evohaler, a widely used asthma inhaler, using 3D printing technology. Through the application of this novel strategy, GSK was able to develop a more accurate and efficient device with enhanced drug delivery and airflow. This development guaranteed precise dosage and enhanced treatment outcomes for asthma sufferers, in addition to making the inhaler simpler for patients to use.

10.6.5 MB Therapeutics

The growing organization is creating an ecosystem to design and produce customized 3D-printed medications. The MED-U Modular, a 3D printer at the core of this ecosystem, efficiently extrudes gels or pastes onto a separate build surface composed of a substance of food- or pharmaceutical-grade standard. MB Therapeutics is primarily looking to transform drug administration for children and is aiming to have its printed personalized medications available by 2026. Currently, the company is working with customers on formulation development, which involves characterizing active ingredients, developing formulations, optimizing the 3D printing process, and producing technical batches for trial.

10.6.6 Triastek

Considering emphasis on pharmaceuticals, the Chinese company succeeded in developing its own melt extrusion deposition (MED) 3D printing process. This innovative process involves using a feedstock created from API-containing powdered raw material mixed into a "movable semisolid," which is then extruded into oral tablets with customized structures for specific release profiles. Triastek recently obtained approval from the US FDA in January 2024 to move forward with the Investigational New Drug (IND) application for T22, a 3D-printed gastric retention product. With this milestone, with four 3D-printed medicine items currently undergoing the clinical development stage, Triastek has strengthened its standing as the industry leader in terms of the quantity of 3D-printed drugs under development.

10.6.7 Dutch Company

DoserThe company's DoseRx1 system is an open, GMP-qualified 3D printer capable of printing tablets with customized dosages of medication inside. The machine uses quality-controlled, refillable cartridges that contain the required formulations for printing medication. Users simply have to insert the stainless steel cartridge and select the proper dosage in the 3D printer menu. The machine, which can print 80% of all oral active pharmaceutical ingredients, can print semisolid or liquid formulations at a rate of between 100 and 1000 doses per hour and can operate at a low temperature to maintain the quality and efficacy of the active ingredients.

10.6.8 Exentis

The German company Exentis Group AG does not print pharmaceuticals itself; it has developed a unique 3D screen printing technology that can be used in cleanroom environments using a variety of materials, including bioprinting and pharmaceuticals. This technology was recently demonstrated when Exentis 3D printed his 6000 metal microfilters within 30 min and was just acquired by his CDMO pharmaceutical company in Italy. In the pharmaceutical industry, the technology is suitable for mass production of tablets with "flexibly definable release profiles" and can print up to 200 million tablets per year in a single system. The listed company says its 3D screen printing platform is already being used to develop drugs to treat diabetes, epilepsy, and Parkinson's disease, while other applications include nutritional supplements and veterinary medicine.

10.6.9 Glasgow University's

3D-printed microneedles were created by University of Glasgow researchers to deliver drugs through the skin. These microneedles that can be customized to meet

Table 10.2 Marketed formulation based on 3D printing technology [53, 54]

Dosage form	Drug name	API
Mini-tablets	Desitrend®	Levetiracetam
	Lamisil®	Terbinafine hydrochloride
	LPV/r pellets	Lopinavir and ritonavir
	Orfiril®	Sodium valproate
Chewable tablets	Isentress®	Raltegravir
Orodispersible films	Setofilm® ZUPLENZ®	Ondansetron
	EXSERVAN™	Riluzole
	SUBOXONE®	Buprenorphine and naloxone
	BELBUCA™	Buprenorphine
Sprinkle capsules	Sustiva®	Efavirenz
	Cholbam®	Cholic acid
	Nexium®	Esomeprazole magnesium
	Tasigna®	Nilotinib HCl
	Tamiflu®	Oseltamivir phosphate
	Adderall XR® or Metadate® and Ritalin®	Metilfenidato and methylphenidate hydrochloride
	AcipHex® Sprinkle™	Rabeprazole sodium
Oral powder	Reyataz®	Atazanavir sulfate
	Viread®	Tenofovir disoproxil fumarate
	Creon® Micro	Pancreatin
Oral granules	Xuriden™ and Vistogard®	Uridine triacetate
	Orkambi®	Lumacaftor + ivacaftor

the demands of the patient and particular drugs. Particularly for people who are uncomfortable with traditional injections, the 3D-printed microneedles provide a painless and minimally intrusive method of drug administration. Numerous uses for this invention, such as vaccine administration and tailored therapy, seem promising. Table 10.2 lists marketed formulations based on 3D-printed technology.

10.7 Conclusion

While the utilization of biodegradable materials in 3D printing has the potential to advance sustainability goals, inherent difficulties present significant challenges to obtaining acceptable structural quality and functional performance. Overcoming these constraints requires a multidimensional effort that includes the design of standardized printing parameters, advancements in material research, and continual innovation in 3D printing technology.

By identifying and addressing these issues, researchers and industry stakeholders may set the platform for widespread adoption of sustainable 3D printing technologies in a range of application industries. For pharmaceutical organizations, 3D printing may significantly reduce prices, waste, and environmental impact as the printer utilizes the exact of material needed for the printing.

References

1. Chan HK, Griffin J, Lim JJ, Zeng F, Chiu ASF. The impact of 3D printing technology on the supply chain: manufacturing and legal perspectives. Int J Prod Econ. 2018;205:156–62.
2. Saini G, et al. Applications of 3D bioprinting in tissue engineering and regenerative medicine. J Clin Med. 2021;10:4966.
3. Vaz VM, Kumar L. 3D printing as a promising tool in personalized medicine. AAPS PharmSciTech. 2021;22:49.
4. Tracy T, Wu L, Liu X, Cheng S, Li X. 3D printing: innovative solutions for patients and pharmaceutical industry. Int J Pharm. 2023;631:122480.
5. Kanishka K, Acherjee B. Revolutionizing manufacturing: a comprehensive overview of additive manufacturing processes, materials, developments, and challenges. J Manuf Process. 2023;107:574–619.
6. Agnusdei L, Del Prete A. Additive manufacturing for sustainability: a systematic literature review. Sustain Futur. 2022;4:100098.
7. Patel KS, Shah DB, Joshi SJ, Patel KM. Developments in 3D printing of carbon fiber reinforced polymer containing recycled plastic waste: a review. Clean Mater. 2023;9:100207.
8. Tietze LF. Domino reactions in organic synthesis. Chem Rev. 1996;96:115–36.
9. Ashiwaju BI, Uzougbo CG, Orikpete OF. Environmental impact of pharmaceuticals: a comprehensive review. Matrix Sci Pharma. 2023;7:85.
10. Ortúzar M, Esterhuizen M, Olicón-Hernández DR, González-López J, Aranda E. Pharmaceutical pollution in aquatic environments: a concise review of environmental impacts and bioremediation systems. Front Microbiol. 2022;13
11. Briffa J, Sinagra E, Blundell R. Heavy metal pollution in the environment and their toxicological effects on humans. Heliyon. 2020;6:e04691.
12. Obinna IB, Ebere Enyoh Christian. A review: water pollution by heavy metal and organic pollutants: brief review of sources, effects and progress on remediation with aquatic plants. Anal Methods Environ Chem J. 2019;2:5–38.
13. Li X, Wang B, Liu F, Yu G. Occurrence and removal of pharmaceutical contaminants in urine: a review. Water. 2023;15:1517.
14. Caban M, Stepnowski P. How to decrease pharmaceuticals in the environment? A review Environ Chem Lett. 2021;19:3115–38.
15. Moshood TD, et al. Sustainability of biodegradable plastics: new problem or solution to solve the global plastic pollution? Curr Res Green Sustain Chem. 2022;5:100273.
16. Belkhir L, Elmeligi A. Carbon footprint of the global pharmaceutical industry and relative impact of its major players. J Clean Prod. 2019;214:185–94.
17. Jones RS, West E. Environmental sustainability in veterinary anaesthesia. Vet Anaesth Analg. 2019;46:409–20.
18. Pagani M, Liu Z, LaRiviere J, Ravelo AC. High earth-system climate sensitivity determined from Pliocene carbon dioxide concentrations. Nat Geosci. 2010;3:27–30.
19. Booth A, Jager A, Faulkner SD, Winchester CC, Shaw SE. Pharmaceutical company targets and strategies to address climate change: content analysis of public reports from 20 pharmaceutical companies. Int J Environ Res Public Health. 2023;20:3206.
20. Eckelman MJ, Sherman J. Environmental impacts of the U.S. health care system and effects on public health. PLoS One. 2016;11:e0157014.
21. Redshaw CH, Stahl-Timmins WM, Fleming LE, Davidson I, Depledge MH. Potential changes in disease patterns and pharmaceutical use in response to climate change. J Toxicol Environ Health Part B. 2013;16:285–320.
22. Watts N, et al. The lancet countdown on health and climate change: from 25 years of inaction to a global transformation for public health. Lancet. 2018;391:581–630.
23. Milliken RL, Quinten T, Andersen SK, Lamprou DA. Application of 3D printing in early phase development of pharmaceutical solid dosage forms. Int J Pharm. 2024;653:123902.

24. Aimar A, Palermo A, Innocenti B. The role of 3D printing in medical applications: a state of the art. J Healthc Eng. 2019;2019:5340616.
25. Jing Q-L, Liu H-Z, Yu W-Q, He X. The impact of public transportation on carbon emissions—from the perspective of energy consumption. Sustainability. 2022;14:6248.
26. Jandyal A, Chaturvedi I, Wazir I, Raina A, Ul Haq MI. 3D printing—a review of processes, materials and applications in industry 4.0. Sustain Oper Comput. 2022;3:33–42.
27. Arif ZU, et al. Recent advances in 3D-printed polylactide and polycaprolactone-based biomaterials for tissue engineering applications. Int J Biol Macromol. 2022;218:930–68.
28. Jamróz W, Szafraniec J, Kurek M, Jachowicz R. 3D printing in pharmaceutical and medical applications—recent achievements and challenges. Pharm Res. 2018;35:176.
29. Elbadawi M, Basit AW, Gaisford S. Energy consumption and carbon footprint of 3D printing in pharmaceutical manufacture. Int J Pharm. 2023;639:122926.
30. Ayyoubi S, et al. 3D printed spherical mini-tablets: geometry versus composition effects in controlling dissolution from personalised solid dosage forms. Int J Pharm. 2021;597:120336.
31. Singh M, Jonnalagadda S. Design and characterization of 3D printed, neomycin-eluting poly-L-lactide mats for wound-healing applications. J Mater Sci Mater Med. 2021;32:44.
32. Lafeber I, et al. 3D printed furosemide and sildenafil tablets: innovative production and quality control. Int J Pharm. 2021;603:120694.
33. Algahtani MS, Mohammed AA, Ahmad J, Abdullah MM, Saleh E. 3D printing of Dapagliflozin containing self-nanoemulsifying tablets: formulation design and in vitro characterization. Pharmaceutics. 2021;13:993.
34. Chen D, et al. Preparation and in vitro evaluation of FDM 3D-printed ellipsoid-shaped gastric floating tablets with low infill percentages. AAPS PharmSciTech. 2019;21:6.
35. Fanous M, et al. Development of immediate release 3D-printed dosage forms for a poorly water-soluble drug by fused deposition modeling: study of morphology, solid state and dissolution. Int J Pharm. 2021;599:120417.
36. Gültekin HE, Tort S, Tuğcu-Demiröz F, Acartürk F. 3D printed extended release tablets for once daily use: an in vitro and in vivo evaluation study for a personalized solid dosage form. Int J Pharm. 2021;596:120222.
37. Ghanizadeh Tabriz A, et al. 3D printed bilayer tablet with dual controlled drug release for tuberculosis treatment. Int J Pharm. 2021;593:120147.
38. Algahtani MS, Mohammed AA, Ahmad J, Saleh E. Development of a 3D printed coating Shell to control the drug release of encapsulated immediate-release tablets. Polymers. 2020;12:1395.
39. Charoenying T, et al. Three-dimensional (3D)-printed devices composed of hydrophilic cap and hydrophobic body for improving buoyancy and gastric retention of domperidone tablets. Eur J Pharm Sci. 2020;155:105555.
40. Hussain A, et al. Personalised 3D printed fast-dissolving tablets for managing hypertensive crisis: in-vitro/in-vivo studies. Polymers. 2020;12:3057.
41. Deshkar, S., Rathi, M., Zambad, S. & Gandhi, K. Hot Melt Extrusion and its Application in 3D Printing of Pharmaceuticals. Curr. Drug Deliv. 18, 387–407.
42. Zhang J, et al. Hydroxypropyl methylcellulose-based controlled release dosage by melt extrusion and 3D printing: structure and drug release correlation. Carbohydr Polym. 2017;177:49–57.
43. Jamróz W, et al. 3D printing of tablets containing amorphous aripiprazole by filaments co-extrusion. Eur J Pharm Biopharm. 2018;131:44–7.
44. Kissi EO, Nilsson R, Nogueira LP, Larsson A, Tho I. Influence of drug load on the printability and solid-state properties of 3D-printed naproxen-based amorphous solid dispersion. Mol Basel Switz. 2021;26:4492.
45. Bhatt U, Malakar TK, Murty US, Banerjee S. 3D printing of immediate-release tablets containing olanzapine by filaments extrusion. Drug Dev Ind Pharm. 2021;47:1200–8.
46. Shi K, Salvage JP, Maniruzzaman M, Nokhodchi A. Role of release modifiers to modulate drug release from fused deposition modelling (FDM) 3D printed tablets. Int J Pharm. 2021;597:120315.
47. Giri BR, et al. Fabrication of Intragastric floating, controlled release 3D printed theophylline tablets using hot-melt extrusion and fused deposition modeling. Pharmaceutics. 2020;12:77.

48. Wang Z, et al. Taste masking study based on an electronic tongue: the formulation design of 3D printed Levetiracetam instant-dissolving tablets. Pharm Res. 2021;38:831–42.
49. Wu G, et al. Experimental study of PLLA/INH slow release implant fabricated by three dimensional printing technique and drug release characteristics in vitro. Biomed Eng Online. 2014;13:97.
50. Lee K-J, et al. Evaluation of critical formulation factors in the development of a rapidly dispersing captopril Oral dosage form. Drug Dev Ind Pharm. 2003;29:967–79.
51. Fina F, et al. Fabricating 3D printed orally disintegrating printlets using selective laser sintering. Int J Pharm. 2018;541:101–7.
52. Pere CPP, et al. 3D printed microneedles for insulin skin delivery. Int J Pharm. 2018;544:425–32.
53. Racaniello GF, et al. Innovative pharmaceutical techniques for Paediatric dosage forms: a systematic review on 3D printing, Prilling/vibration and microfluidic platform. J Pharm Sci. 2024;113:1726–48.
54. Strickley RG. Pediatric Oral formulations: an updated review of commercially available pediatric Oral formulations since 2007. J Pharm Sci. 2019;108:1335–65.

Challenges and Limitations of FDM 3D Printing in Pharmaceuticals

11

Gupta Ravikant, Rajoriya Vaibhav, Vengurlekar Sudha, Jain K. Sachin, and Kuldeep Vinchurkar

Abstract

This chapter explores the challenges and limitations inherent in utilizing Fused Deposition Modeling (FDM) 3D printing technology within the pharmaceutical industry. FDM 3D printing has emerged as a promising tool for the fabrication of personalized dosage forms, drug delivery systems, and medical devices, offering unique advantages such as customization, rapid prototyping, and precise control over drug release profiles. However, several hurdles impede its widespread adoption and implementation in pharmaceutical manufacturing. This chapter systematically examines these challenges, encompassing technical constraints, regulatory considerations, material selection issues, and the need for standardized processes. Moreover, it delves into the limitations associated with FDM 3D printing in terms of scalability, resolution, reproducibility, and the complexity of multi-component formulations. By shedding light on these obstacles, this chapter aims to provide a comprehensive understanding of the current state of FDM 3D printing in pharmaceuticals and pave the way for future advancements and solutions in this rapidly evolving field. With the help of case studies, the author will try to explain practical approaches. Which will provide practical insight into the facts.

G. Ravikant (✉) · V. Sudha · J. K. Sachin
Faculty of Pharmacy, Oriental University, Indore, Madhya Pradesh, India
e-mail: ravikantgupta@orientaluniversity.in

R. Vaibhav
Research Schclar, Oriental University, Indore, Madhya Pradesh, India

K. Vinchurkar
Department of Pharmaceutics, Sandip Institute of Pharmaceutical Sciences (SIPS), Affiliated To Savitribai Fhule Pune University (SPPU, Pune), Nashik, Maharashtra, India

K. Vinchurkar, S. Mane (eds.), *Innovations in Drug Manufacturing*,
https://doi.org/10.1007/978-981-96-9075-6_11

Keywords

Fused deposition modeling · 3D printing · Personalized dosage forms · Regulatory consideration · Multi-component formulations

11.1 Introduction

Fused deposition modeling (FDM) in pharmaceuticals enables personalized drug production, offering tailored medications based on individual needs and preferences [1, 2].

11.1.1 Overview of FDM 3D Printing Technology

Fused deposition modeling (FDM), also known as fused filament fabrication (FFF), is a widely used 3D printing technology developed by Scott Crump in the late 1980s [3]. FDM utilizes a thermoplastic filament to build three-dimensional objects. It involves melting the filament and depositing it layer by layer onto a print bed, gradually creating the desired object. FDM is commonly used for rapid prototyping, allowing quick production of complex parts [4].

11.1.2 Importance and Scope in Pharmaceuticals

FDM (fused deposition modeling) 3D printing is pivotal in pharmaceuticals for crafting customized medications. It enables the production of adaptable dosage forms that can contain various medicinal ingredients and offer tailored drug release rates [5]. This method is advantageous for fabricating unique product shapes and drug release profiles, which are often difficult to achieve through bulk manufacturing. In the pharmaceutical field, FDM 3D printing's potential spans a broad range of medicinal products, including quick-dissolve tablets, sustained-release drugs, and combination therapies tailored to individual needs [6]. It introduces versatility in drug formulation, dosage customization, swift production processes, and accurate control over medication release, addressing diverse therapeutic requirements [7].

FDM 3D printing in pharmaceuticals encompasses several areas:

A. *Process*: FDM 3D printing involves heating drug-loaded filaments to a molten state and extruding them layer by layer to form a three-dimensional structure. This allows for precise control over the shape, size, and composition of the dosage form [8]. In FDM 3D printing for pharmaceuticals, the process starts with the creation of a digital model of the desired drug form. Drug-loaded thermoplastic polymers are then fed into the printer, where they are heated until they reach a semi-liquid state. The printer nozzle deposits the material layer by layer onto a build platform, where it cools and solidifies to form the final product [9].

B. *Applications*: The technology is used to produce a range of pharmaceutical products, including tablets with complex structures for controlled release, multi-drug polypills tailored to individual patient needs, and devices like drug-eluting implants [10]. Controlled-release tablets are formulated by adjusting the internal structure of tablets; FDM 3D printing can control how quickly the drug is released into the body [11]. Immediate-release tablets were successfully produced using three distinct polymers – hydroxypropyl cellulose (HPC), Eudragit® EPO, and Kollidon® VA 64 – along with sodium starch glycolate as a disintegrant and drug loadings of THY up to 60%. These formulations were thoroughly characterized and optimized employing Quality by Design (QbD) principles [12]. Polypills are single pills that contain multiple drugs, which can be customized for patients who require complex medication regimens [13]. A combined polypill was also designed consisting of three cylindrical sections of 50% NFD, 33.3% SMV, and 16.6% GLZ of the total volume, with a total height of 3.2 mm [14]. Drug-eluting implants can be printed to release medication at a controlled rate directly at the target site. Al-Litani et al. [15] reported various 3D-printed implantable devices used in women's health applications and characterized by SEM, PXRD, DSC, and IR [15].

C. *Benefits*: It enables the creation of medications tailored to individual patient profiles, including dose and drug combinations. It offers the ability to design complex drug release mechanisms and geometries. It accelerates the development process from design to finished product and reduces waste by using only the necessary amount of material. It may allow for high levels of customization without the need for new tooling or molds for each new design, and medications can be printed on an as-needed basis, reducing inventory and waste on an on-demand basis. It also enables the creation of dosage forms with complex internal geometries that cannot be made with traditional manufacturing methods [16].

D. *Challenges*: Each personalized medication may require separate approval processes and regulatory approval. Ensuring consistency and quality in each print can be challenging as well, as not all pharmaceutical compounds or polymers are suitable for FDM printing. It is requiring a deep understanding of both 3D printing technology and pharmaceutical science and Initial setup costs can be high, and the cost-effectiveness for large-scale production is still being evaluated. Finding suitable pharmaceutical-grade materials that can be used in FDM printers is an ongoing area of research that makes it complex [5].

11.1.3 Objectives

An objective of the chapter aims to outline the technical obstacles like precision and scalability, address the scarcity and suitability of pharmaceutical materials for FDM printing, navigate the complex regulatory landscape for drug approval, ensure consistent quality control for safety, and assess the economic viability, including market readiness and necessary investments for adoption. Fused deposition modeling (FDM) 3D printing faces several hurdles in pharmaceutical applications, from achieving precise dosages and consistent quality to scaling up production. Material selection is critical, as they must be compatible with drugs and safe for consumption. Regulatory challenges include navigating approval processes and setting industry standards. Quality control is paramount to ensure drug safety and efficacy, requiring new testing protocols. Economically, the cost-effectiveness and market demand for personalized 3D-printed drugs are under scrutiny, alongside securing necessary investments for technological advancements. These obstacles present opportunities for innovation in drug manufacturing.

11.2 Fundamentals of FDM 3D Printing

Fused deposition modeling (FDM) is a 3D printing process that builds objects layer by layer from thermoplastic filaments. The filament is heated to its melting point and extruded through a nozzle onto a build platform, where it cools and solidifies to form a solid object [17]. This technique allows for high precision and accuracy, which is essential in pharmaceuticals for creating dosage forms with exact drug concentrations and tailored release profiles. In FDM 3D printing, objects are constructed layer by layer. The process begins with a digital model, which is sliced into thin horizontal layers by software. The printer then heats a thermoplastic filament and extrudes it through a nozzle, precisely depositing it onto the build platform to form the first layer [18]. Once a layer is complete, the build platform lowers slightly, and the nozzle adds the next layer on top. This continues until the entire object is built up from the bottom to the top, with each new layer fusing to the one below it.

Common thermoplastic materials used in FDM printing include:

A. *ABS (Acrylonitrile Butadiene Styrene)*: Known for its toughness and impact resistance.
B. *PLA (Polylactic Acid)*: Popular for its ease of use and biodegradability
C. *PETG (Polyethylene Terephthalate Glycol)*: Valued for its durability and clarity.
D. *TPU (Thermoplastic Polyurethane)*: Flexible and used for objects that require elasticity.
E. *Nylon*: Strong and durable, with good temperature resistance.

In the realm of pharmaceutical FDM 3D printing, specialized filaments are tailored to meet rigorous standards. These include ABS-based nanocomposites for enhanced properties, drug-loaded filaments produced via hot-melt extrusion that encapsulate active pharmaceutical ingredients, and eco-conscious materials for sustainable practices. Such advancements ensure that 3D-printed pharmaceuticals are safe, effective, and aligned with industry regulations [19].

11.2.1 Principles of Fused Deposition Modeling

Fused deposition modeling (FDM) operates on the principle of additive manufacturing, where objects are built by depositing melted material layer by layer. The core principles include:

1. *Material Extrusion*: A thermoplastic filament is heated and extruded through a nozzle.
2. *Layer-by-Layer Construction*: The extruded material is laid down in layers to build the 3D object.
3. *Path Planning*: The movement of the nozzle is controlled by computer-aided design (CAD) data to follow the object's geometry.
4. *Adhesion and Fusion*: Each new layer adheres to and fuses with the previous one, cooling and solidifying to form a cohesive structure.
5. *Support Structures*: Temporary structures may be printed to support overhanging features, which are removed after printing. These principles enable FDM to create complex geometries with high precision, making it a versatile tool in various industries, including pharmaceuticals [20].

Fused deposition modeling (FDM) differs from other 3D printing methods [21] in several ways, including the following:

1. *Material*: FDM uses thermoplastic filaments, while other methods like stereolithography (SLA) use liquid resin, and selective laser sintering (SLS) uses powdered material.
2. *Precision*: FDM is generally less precise than SLA or SLS due to the nature of extrusion, but it is suitable for a wide range of applications.
3. *Strength*: Objects printed with FDM are typically stronger and more durable than those printed with SLA but may be less detailed.
4. *Speed*: FDM can be slower than other methods like SLA due to the layer-by-layer extrusion process.
5. *Cost*: FDM printers are often more affordable and have lower operating costs compared to other 3D printing technologies. Each method has its advantages and is chosen based on the specific requirements of the print job, such as detail, strength, speed, and cost.

11.2.2 Components of an FDM 3D Printer

An FDM 3D printer typically consists of the following key components:

1. *Frame*: The structure that holds all parts together. Provides stability and rigidity to support the printing process.
2. *Print Bed*: The surface on which the object is printed. It can be heated to prevent warping and ensure better adhesion of the first layer.

3. *Extruder*: The part that feeds, melts, and deposits the filament. It includes a motor that pushes the filament towards the hot end to melt it.
4. *Nozzle*: The tip of the extruder where the melted filament comes out. Precision-made to allow the melted filament to extrude in a controlled manner.
5. *Filament Spool*: The roll of thermoplastic material used for printing. Holds the filament, which can be made of various materials like PLA [22], ABS, PETG, etc.
6. *Stepper Motors*: Control the movement of the print bed and extruder. Offer precise control over the movement in the *X*, *Y*, and *Z* axes.
7. *Belts and Pulleys*: Transmit movement from motors to other parts. Convert rotational motion from stepper motors into linear motion.
8. *Control Electronics*: The motherboard and processors that control the printer's operations. Include firmware that translates digital models into movements and commands for the printer.
9. *Power Supply*: Provides electricity to the printer components. Rated to handle the printer's maximum power requirements for sustained operation.

These components work together to create 3D objects through the FDM process. Each component plays a crucial role in ensuring accurate and reliable 3D printing with FDM technology.

11.2.3 Printing Process and Parameters

In fused deposition modeling (FDM) 3D printing, several key parameters influence the printing quality and the mechanical properties of the final product:

1. *Layer Height*: Determines the resolution of the print; smaller layers result in finer details. Typically ranges from 0.1 to 0.3 mm. Finer layer heights (closer to 0.1 mm) produce smoother surfaces but increase print time.
2. *Printing Speed*: Affects the print time and can impact the quality; too fast may lead to imperfections. Can vary widely, but common speeds are between 40 and 100 mm/s. Slower speeds can improve print quality, especially for intricate details.
3. *Extrusion Temperature*: Must be optimized for the specific material being used to ensure proper layer adhesion. Depends on the material. For example, PLA is usually extruded at around 180–220 °C, while ABS requires higher temperatures, around 210–250 °C.
4. *Infill Density*: Dictates the internal structure's strength and weight; higher density increases strength but also material usage and print time. Often set between 10% and 100%. Lower infill saves material and time but may compromise structural integrity. Patterns like grid, triangle, or honeycomb affect strength and print time too.
5. *Bed Temperature*: Important for bed adhesion; PLA might not need a heated bed, but ABS typically requires one at about 80–110 °C.
6. *Retraction Settings*: Help prevent stringing by pulling filament back during travel moves.

In 3D printing, an overhang is any part of a print that extends outward beyond the previous layer and lacks direct support from below. Overhangs can be challenging because gravity may cause them to sag or collapse during printing. To successfully print overhangs, one can use support structures that are built during the printing process and removed afterward. Adjust the angle of the overhang; typically, angles up to 45° can be printed without supports. Print with cooling fans to solidify the material quickly as it's deposited. Properly managing overhangs is crucial for achieving the desired geometry and surface quality in a 3D-printed object [23].

11.2.4 Material Considerations for Pharmaceutical Applications

Material considerations for pharmaceutical applications in 3D printing are crucial due to the need for:

(a) *Biocompatibility*: Materials must not cause any adverse reactions in the body. Common materials used include PLA, PCL, and biodegradable polymers that can safely dissolve in the body. The choice of material will depend on the specific application, such as whether the product is an implant, a drug delivery vehicle, or a scaffold for tissue engineering [19].
(b) *Safety*: They should be non-toxic and should not leach harmful substances.
(c) *Efficacy*: Materials must effectively deliver the drug without degrading its potency.
(d) *Regulatory Compliance*: Materials must meet standards set by bodies like the FDA or EMA.

3D printing can improve drug delivery in several ways:

(a) *Personalization*: Tailoring drug dosages and shapes to individual patient needs. 3D printing allows for the creation of medications tailored to the specific requirements of patients, such as age, weight, and medical condition. This ensures optimal therapeutic outcomes and minimizes side effects.
(b) *Complex Structures*: Creating intricate geometries that can modify drug release profiles. By manipulating the shape, size, and surface area of printed objects, it's possible to control the rate at which a drug is released into the body. For example, a porous structure can be designed to release medication slowly over time.
(c) *Multi-Drug Formulation*: Incorporating multiple drugs into a single dosage form with distinct release times. 3D printing enables the fabrication of polypills that contain several drugs with different release times, simplifying medication regimens for patients with multiple prescriptions.
(d) *Rapid Prototyping*: Allowing for quick development and testing of new drug delivery systems. The technology allows for quick design iterations and testing, accelerating the development process for new drug delivery systems and enabling rapid response to emerging health needs [24].

(e) *Cost-Effectiveness*: Reducing waste and potentially lowering manufacturing costs. It reduces material waste by using only the necessary number of raw materials to create the drug delivery device or medication. Additionally, it can potentially streamline the supply chain by enabling on-site production. By leveraging these capabilities, 3D printing has the potential to revolutionize the field of drug delivery, making it more efficient and personalized.

11.3 Challenges in FDM 3D Printing for Pharmaceuticals

FDM 3D printing for pharmaceuticals presents several challenges:

1. *Drug Stability*: High temperatures used in FDM can degrade sensitive pharmaceutical compounds. The extrusion process in FDM involves high temperatures that can cause thermal degradation of drugs, leading to reduced efficacy or altered drug properties [25]. Ensuring that the active pharmaceutical ingredients (APIs) remain stable throughout the process is crucial.
2. *Precise Dosing*: Achieving accurate drug concentration within printed objects is critical and challenging. It's vital to control the amount of drug incorporated into the printed object accurately. This requires precise calibration of the printer and careful formulation of the printing material to ensure consistent drug release.
3. *Material Limitations*: Finding suitable filaments that are biocompatible and can be used to deliver drugs effectively. The range of materials suitable for FDM that are also biocompatible and approved for drug contact is limited. Researchers must develop new filaments that can reliably deliver drugs and meet safety standards [26]. Figure 11.1 represents the challenges and limitations inherent in utilizing fused deposition modeling (FDM) 3D printing technology.
4. *Regulatory Compliance*: Meeting stringent health regulations for medical-grade products can be complex. Pharmaceutical products produced via FDM must comply with regulations regarding quality, safety, and efficacy. This includes validation of the printing process and ensuring that the final product meets all necessary guidelines.
5. *Scalability*: Adapting FDM for mass production while maintaining quality and consistency is difficult. Addressing these challenges is essential for the successful application of FDM in pharmaceutical manufacturing. While FDM is excellent for prototyping and small-scale production, scaling up to industrial manufacturing levels while maintaining product quality is a significant hurdle. This involves optimizing the printing process for high-volume production without compromising on precision or quality.

Overcoming these challenges requires ongoing research and development, as well as collaboration between regulatory bodies, manufacturers, and healthcare professionals.

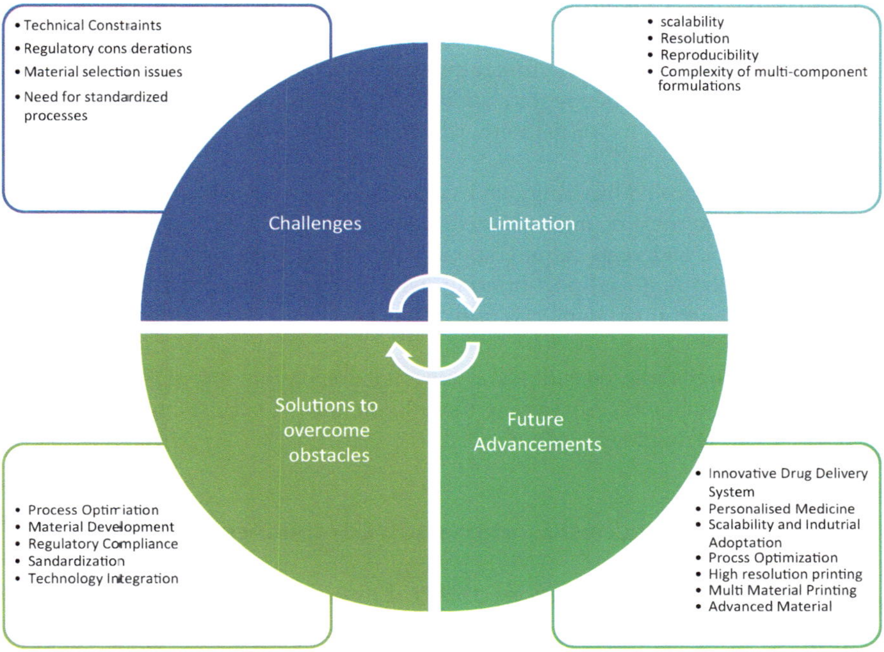

Fig. 11.1 Challenges and limitations inherent in utilizing fused deposition modeling (FDM) 3D printing technology

11.3.1 Technical Constraints and Limitations

1. *Resolution and Surface Finish*: FDM typically has lower resolution compared to other 3D printing technologies, which can result in rougher surface finishes that may require post-processing. The layer-by-layer deposition method inherent in FDM results in visible layer lines, which can affect the aesthetic and functional aspects of the printed part. Achieving high-resolution details is limited by the size of the extrusion nozzle, with smaller nozzles providing finer details but increasing print time.
2. *Material Restrictions*: The range of materials that can be used in FDM is limited by the need for them to be thermoplastic and able to withstand the extrusion process. FDM printers can only use materials that are available in filament form and that melt at a temperature their extruder can handle. This limits the use of materials with higher melting points or those that degrade at high temperatures.
3. *Mechanical Property Limitations*: Parts produced by FDM can have anisotropic properties, meaning they may be weaker in one direction due to the layer-by-layer construction. The strength of FDM-printed parts is often less in the z-axis (vertical) direction due to the nature of layer adhesion. This can affect the part's overall structural integrity and is a critical consideration in design and application.

4. *Post-Processing*: Often necessary to improve the appearance and function of FDM-printed parts, which can include sanding, painting, or chemical smoothing. To achieve a smooth surface or to meet certain dimensional tolerances, FDM-printed parts often require additional finishing steps such as sanding, acetone vapor smoothing, or painting, which adds time and cost to the manufacturing process.
5. *Support Removal*: Overhangs and complex geometries often require support structures that must be manually removed after printing. Complex designs with overhangs or undercuts require support structures during printing. These supports must be removed post-printing, which can be time-consuming and may damage the part if not done carefully.

Understanding these constraints is essential for optimizing FDM 3D printing processes and outcomes. Addressing these limitations is part of ongoing advancements in FDM technology [26].

11.3.2 Regulatory Considerations and Compliance Hurdles

1. *Good Manufacturing Practices (GMP)*: Ensuring the printing process meets GMP standards to guarantee product quality and safety. FDM 3D printing facilities must adhere to GMP to ensure products are consistently produced and controlled according to quality standards. For example, the printer's environment must be controlled to prevent contamination.
2. *Material Safety*: Verifying that materials used are safe for human use, often requiring biocompatibility testing. All materials used must be tested for biocompatibility and toxicity. For instance, a filament used in an implantable device must undergo extensive testing to ensure it does not elicit an immune response.
3. *Product Testing*: Conducting rigorous testing to ensure the printed product performs as intended and is safe for patients. Printed pharmaceuticals must undergo stability testing, dissolution testing, and other pharmacokinetic evaluations. An example would be testing a printed tablet to ensure it releases the drug at the intended rate.
4. *Documentation*: Maintaining detailed records of the manufacturing process, materials used, and quality control measures. Comprehensive documentation is required throughout the development and production process. This includes records of raw material sourcing, batch records, and quality control results.
5. *Approval Process*: Navigating the complex approval process with regulatory bodies like the FDA or EMA, which can be time-consuming and resource-intensive. Gaining regulatory approval can be challenging due to the novelty of 3D printing in pharmaceuticals. An example is the FDA's approval of SPRITAM®, the first 3D-printed drug, which required demonstration of the product's safety and efficacy through clinical trials.

Meeting these regulatory requirements is essential for the successful adoption of FDM 3D printing in the pharmaceutical industry. Navigating these regulatory pathways is crucial for bringing 3D-printed pharmaceutical products to market.

11.3.3 Material Selection Challenges

1. *Thermal Stability*: Finding materials that can withstand the high temperatures of the FDM process without degrading. Materials must not decompose or lose their properties at the high temperatures required for FDM printing. For example, PEEK (polyether ether ketone) is a material with high thermal stability that is used in FDM for high-performance parts [27].
2. *Biocompatibility*: Ensuring materials are safe for medical use and do not cause adverse reactions in patients. Materials used for medical applications must be non-toxic and compatible with the human body. PLA (polylactic acid) is commonly used for medical implants and drug delivery systems due to its biocompatibility and biodegradability.
3. *Mechanical Properties*: Selecting materials that have the necessary strength, flexibility, and durability for the intended application. The material must possess the necessary strength, elasticity, and durability. ABS (acrylonitrile butadiene styrene) is often chosen for its good mechanical properties and is used in consumer products and automotive components [28].
4. *Chemical Resistance*: Materials must resist degradation from drugs or bodily fluids. Materials should resist chemicals they may come into contact with, including drugs and bodily fluids. PETG (polyethylene terephthalate glycol) is known for its chemical resistance and is used in food containers and medical devices.
5. *Regulatory Approval*: Materials must meet regulatory standards for safety and efficacy. Materials must comply with regulations such as those set by the FDA for medical devices. Titanium is an example of a material that is often used in medical devices due to its strength, biocompatibility, and acceptance by regulatory bodies.

Selecting the right material for FDM 3D printing requires balancing these factors to meet the specific needs of the application. Addressing these challenges is crucial for the successful application of FDM in various industries, especially healthcare.

11.3.4 Standardization Issues in Printing Processes

1. *Material Properties*: Lack of standardized criteria for evaluating the performance of 3D printing materials. There's no standard for how to measure the tensile strength of a 3D-printed part, which can vary based on print orientation. For example, a part printed vertically may have different strength characteristics than one printed horizontally.

2. *Print Quality*: No universal standards for resolution, accuracy, and surface finish of printed parts. The lack of standards for print quality means that two printers may produce parts with different tolerances or surface roughness, affecting the part's functionality. For instance, a gear printed on one machine may not mesh smoothly with a gear printed on another due to slight differences in dimensions.
3. *Post-Processing*: Variability in methods and results of post-processing techniques. Without standardized post-processing methods, two identical parts can have different mechanical properties or aesthetics after treatment. For example, one company's method of vapor smoothing might result in a glossier finish compared to another.
4. *Machine Calibration*: Differences in calibration procedures across different printers. Printers from different manufacturers may require unique calibration steps, leading to inconsistencies in print quality. A printer from one brand might interpret a file differently than another, resulting in variations in the final product.
5. *Quality Assurance*: Challenges in establishing consistent quality assurance practices for 3D-printed products. The absence of standardized quality assurance protocols can lead to variability in the final product's performance. For example, a medical implant might have different porosity levels depending on the manufacturer's internal quality control measures. Standardization is key to ensuring consistency and reliability across the 3D printing industry. Addressing these standardization issues is essential for the broader adoption and reliability of 3D printing technologies [29].

11.4 Material Development for FDM Printing in Pharmaceuticals

1. *Biocompatibility*: Ensuring materials are safe for ingestion or implantation and do not cause adverse reactions. Materials must be developed to be non-toxic and suitable for human use. For example, medical-grade PLA is used for drug delivery devices due to its biodegradability and compatibility with the human body [30].
2. *Drug Compatibility*: Developing materials that are compatible with a wide range of pharmaceuticals without affecting their efficacy. Materials should not react with the drugs they carry. PVA (polyvinyl alcohol) is often used as a filament for drug-loaded prints because it dissolves in water, allowing for drug release.
3. *Controlled Release*: Engineering materials that can facilitate controlled drug release profiles. Developing materials that can provide specific release rates for drugs. For instance, composite filaments with a blend of biodegradable polymers can be engineered to dissolve at different rates, controlling the release of the drug.
4. *Printability*: Creating materials that can be easily printed with FDM technology while maintaining consistent quality. Materials must flow consistently through the printer nozzle and solidify correctly. ABS is commonly used due to its good flow properties and strength post-printing [31].

5. *Regulatory Compliance*: Ensuring all new materials meet stringent regulatory standards for safety and effectiveness. New materials must comply with regulations such as those set by the FDA. An example is the development of bioresorbable filaments that have been approved for use in surgical implants. Advancements in these areas are crucial for the expansion of FDM printing in the pharmaceutical industry. These developments are key to leveraging FDM printing for personalized medicine and other pharmaceutical applications.

11.4.1 Pharmaceutical-Grade Materials for FDM Printing

1. *PLA (Polylactic Acid)*: Biodegradable and biocompatible, making it suitable for temporary implants and drug delivery systems.
2. *PVA (Polyvinyl Alcohol)*: Water-soluble, often used for creating temporary structures or as a drug release mechanism.
3. *PETG (Polyethylene Terephthalate Glycol)*: Chemical resistant and safe for contact with the human body, used in medical device manufacturing.
4. *ABS (Acrylonitrile Butadiene Styrene)*: Strong and durable, suitable for non-implantable medical devices and equipment.
5. *PEEK (Polyether Ether Ketone)*: High thermal stability and biocompatibility, used for high-performance medical implants.
6. *TPU (Thermoplastic Polyurethane)*: Flexible and biocompatible, ideal for items like flexible tubing or cushioning in medical devices.
7. *PC (Polycarbonate)*: Durable with high impact strength, used in applications requiring transparency and toughness, such as protective equipment.

Each of these materials is selected based on the specific requirements of the pharmaceutical application, such as biodegradability, compatibility with drugs, and mechanical properties. These materials are chosen for their properties that align with pharmaceutical applications, such as biocompatibility and controlled dissolution rates [32].

11.4.2 Properties and Characteristics of Suitable Polymers

Polymers that are ideal for FDM 3D printing exhibit a range of essential properties, including the ability to endure the elevated temperatures of the FDM process without breaking down, robust mechanical strength to maintain shape and structure post-printing, and sufficient flexibility for certain applications. They also possess appropriate flow properties when melted, ensuring seamless extrusion and strong layer bonding. Among the most commonly utilized polymers for FDM are ABS, which is valued for its toughness, pliability, and resistance to heat; PLA, favored for its user-friendliness and solid mechanical attributes; and PET-G, which strikes an excellent balance between sturdiness and ductility. The selection of these materials is typically influenced by the specific needs of the printed item, such as its required durability, elasticity, or heat tolerance. Some examples are:

1. *Soluplus®*: This graft copolymer serves as a matrix to enhance the dissolution of drugs that are not easily soluble. It is particularly useful in processes involving hot-melt extrusion [33].
2. *Kollicoat® IR*: As a graft copolymer of polyvinyl alcohol and polyethylene glycol, it is applied to coat tablets that are designed to dissolve quickly. Its properties allow for the creation of flexible and soluble films [34].
3. *Kollidon® SR*: This polymer blend, consisting of polyvinyl acetate and povidone, is utilized to fabricate solid dosages that release the drug slowly over time, providing a controlled release mechanism [35].
4. *Ethyl Cellulose*: Recognized for its ability to form films that modulate drug release, this polymer also adjusts the flow properties of printing inks to ensure proper adhesion during the printing process.

These materials are chosen for their stability under heat, structural integrity, compatibility with drugs, and their capacity to produce specific drug release patterns in printed medicinal forms.

11.4.3 Advancements in Material Science and Formulation Strategies

1. *Enhanced Durability*: Progress has been made in improving the interlayer adhesion and overall strength of 3D-printed pharmaceutical items, with a particular emphasis on materials such as PLA. The focus on materials like PLA has led to significant improvements in the physical properties of 3D-printed objects. Researchers are finding ways to enhance the interlayer bonding, which results in increased mechanical strength and stability of the printed pharmaceutical forms. This is crucial for ensuring that the printed drugs can withstand handling and storage without losing their integrity.
2. *Personalized Medication*: There's a surge in the development of bespoke medical devices and implants that release drugs, which are designed to meet specific dosage, shape, size, and release profile requirements for individual patients. The ability to customize medication is a game-changer in pharmaceuticals. With 3D printing, it's now possible to create medical devices and implants that can deliver drugs in a controlled manner, tailored to the patient's specific needs [36]. This means that doses can be adjusted, and the rate at which the drug is released can be fine-tuned, providing a more effective treatment regimen.
3. *Diverse Medical Uses*: The application of 3D and 4D printing is expanding into areas like tissue engineering, drug delivery mechanisms, surgical instruments, diagnostic tools, and prosthetic devices, aiming to offer more targeted and efficient patient treatments. The scope of 3D printing in medicine is broadening. For

instance, tissue engineering can benefit from 3D-printed scaffolds that support cell growth and tissue formation. In drug delivery, 3D-printed devices can provide novel ways to administer medications, such as through dissolvable films or slow-release implants. Surgical tools and diagnostic devices are also being 3D printed for enhanced precision and customization [37].

4. *Innovative Materials and Processes*: New materials and printing processes are being introduced to overcome the drawbacks of traditional 3D printing methods. These innovations are enhancing print speeds, supporting cellular growth for bioprinting applications, and enabling the creation of intricate shapes for use in medicine. The development of new materials that are biocompatible and have the desired mechanical properties is ongoing. Additionally, advancements in printing techniques are allowing for faster production times while maintaining high-quality outputs. Bioprinting, which involves printing with cells, is seeing improvements that could lead to breakthroughs in creating living tissues or organs. This shift is leading towards a personalized approach in medicine production, moving away from bulk manufacturing to creating medication that is customized for each patient's unique needs. These advancements represent a significant shift towards personalized healthcare, where treatments are tailored to the individual rather than a one-size-fits-all approach.

11.5 Process Optimization in FDM Printing

1. *Energy Consumption*: Optimizing energy consumption involves adjusting printer settings to use the least amount of energy necessary to create a part. This can be achieved by modifying temperature settings, print speed, and layer height to find a balance that reduces energy use without affecting print quality.
2. *Processing Time*: To optimize processing time, the focus is on reducing the overall print duration while maintaining part quality. This can involve increasing print speeds, adjusting layer heights for faster build times, and streamlining the printing path to minimize movements that do not contribute to part formation.
3. *Dimensional Accuracy*: Achieving high dimensional accuracy requires precise calibration of the printer and careful selection of print parameters like layer thickness, nozzle temperature, and print speed. The goal is to ensure that the final part dimensions are as close as possible to the design specifications.
4. *Material Usage*: Minimizing material usage can be done by optimizing infill patterns and densities, which dictate how much material is used inside the part. Choosing the right infill can maintain part strength while using less material, leading to cost savings and reduced waste.
5. *Mechanical Strength*: Enhancing mechanical strength involves selecting appropriate materials and optimizing print parameters that affect the interlayer bonding and structural integrity of the part. Parameters such as extrusion temperature, print speed, and layer height can be adjusted to improve the mechanical properties of the printed object.

By systematically adjusting these parameters, it's possible to produce high-quality FDM prints more efficiently and cost-effectively. Researchers often use design of experiments (DOE) and other statistical methods to identify optimal parameter settings that achieve the desired outcomes.

11.5.1 Parameters Influencing Print Quality and Reproducibility

In the realm of FDM (fused deposition modeling) 3D printing, a variety of factors play a pivotal role in determining the fidelity and consistency of printed objects:

1. *Speed of Printing*: This parameter governs how quickly each layer is deposited, impacting not only the print's duration but also its structural integrity, surface texture, and overall aesthetic. The rate at which the printer deposits material can significantly affect the print's structural integrity. A faster speed might lead to quicker prints but can compromise detail and strength, while a slower speed improves detail and strength but increases print time.
2. *Thermal Conditions*: The temperatures at which the filament is extruded and the print bed is maintained are critical for ensuring proper layer adhesion, structural solidity, and the quality of the final print. The extrusion temperature must be high enough to ensure good flow and adhesion of the material but not so high as to cause warping or stringing. Similarly, the heated bed temperature must be optimized to prevent warping and ensure the first layer sticks well.
3. *Layer Resolution*: The height of each printed layer defines the print's detail level; finer layers yield higher detail at the expense of increased printing time. A lower layer height (higher resolution) can produce smoother surfaces and more detailed prints, but it also means more layers are needed, increasing print time. Conversely, a higher layer height (lower resolution) results in faster prints but with rougher surfaces [38].
4. *Infill Strategy*: The pattern used to fill the interior of the print affects its weight, strength, and material consumption. The pattern and density of the infill can be adjusted to balance strength and material usage. Sparse infills use less material and print faster but offer less strength, while dense infills increase strength and weight but use more material and take longer to print.
5. *Print Orientation*: The angle at which a part is printed can alter its surface quality and mechanical characteristics. The orientation of the part on the build platform affects the direction of layer lines, which can impact the part's appearance and mechanical properties. Some orientations may require support structures, which can affect surface finish where they are removed.
6. *Placement on the Printing Surface*: Where a part sits on the printing platform can influence its adherence to the platform and stability throughout the printing process. Proper placement on the build platform is crucial for good adhesion. Parts should be evenly distributed to avoid warping and to ensure consistent heating across all parts.

7. *Extrusion Path Width*: The thickness of each extrusion path plays into the density and robustness of the final product. The width of the extrusion paths affects how closely the lines of filament are packed together, influencing the part's density and strength. A wider path can increase strength but may lead to a rougher surface finish.

Optimal adjustment of these factors is essential for producing high-quality prints and ensuring that such quality can be reliably replicated. Analytical methods like the Taguchi approach and ANOVA are commonly employed to evaluate these factor impacts and refine them for enhanced print outcomes [39]. By understanding and controlling these factors, one can significantly improve the quality of FDM prints and achieve high reproducibility. It often involves a series of tests and adjustments to find the optimal settings for a given printer, material, and part design.

11.5.2 Optimization Techniques for Printing Parameters

1. *Printer Calibration*: It is essential to fine-tune your printer, which includes making sure the print bed is level, the nozzle is at the correct height, and the right amount of filament is being extruded. This foundational step involves adjusting your printer to ensure it operates correctly. Bed leveling is crucial to prevent prints from warping or not adhering to the bed. Nozzle height adjustment is necessary to avoid scraping the bed or leaving too much space, which can affect adhesion. The extrusion multiplier controls the amount of filament extruded, ensuring that the printer lays down the correct amount of material.
2. *Experimental Design Approaches*: Methods like Taguchi's orthogonal arrays and full and fractional factorial designs help in understanding how different printing parameters affect each other and the final print. These are structured methods for conducting experiments to systematically study the effects of various parameters. The Taguchi method uses orthogonal arrays to study parameter variations with a reduced number of experiments. Full factorial designs test all possible combinations of parameters [40], while fractional factorial designs test a subset, saving time and resources.
3. *Statistical Modeling*: Response surface methodology (RSM) uses a series of designed experiments to create a statistical model that can guide you towards optimal print settings. RSM is used to model and analyze problems in which several variables influence the response variable, and the goal is to optimize this response. It involves designing experiments to obtain data, fitting a response surface model, and finding optimal conditions.
4. *Bio-Inspired Algorithms (Genetic Algorithms-GA)*: Optimization techniques such as genetic algorithms mimic natural evolutionary processes to determine the best parameter settings for your prints. GAs simulate the process of natural selection by creating a population of solutions, evaluating their fitness, and then combining and mutating them to produce new generations of solutions. Over

time, the algorithm converges on an optimal or near-optimal set of parameters [41].
5. *Machine Learning Predictions*: Artificial neural networks (ANNs) can learn from past print data to predict which parameters will yield high-quality prints. ANNs can predict optimal printing parameters by learning from data. They are trained using data from previous prints, learning the relationship between parameters and print quality, and can then predict settings for new prints.
6. *Approximate Reasoning*: Fuzzy logic provides a way to make decisions with imprecise information, which can be useful in adjusting complex printing parameters. Fuzzy logic is used for decision-making with imprecise information. It's particularly useful in controlling complex systems where binary logic is insufficient. In FDM printing, it can help adjust parameters that don't have a clear right or wrong setting but rather a range of acceptable values.

These strategies are employed to refine settings like layer resolution, infill percentage, printing speed, and thermal management to achieve a balance between print quality, time, and material usage. Each technique offers a different approach to optimizing print quality and can be chosen based on the specific needs and constraints of your printing process.

11.5.3 Quality Control and Assurance in FDM Printing Processes

1. *Initial Quality Assessments*: Before any printing starts, it's crucial to ensure that the design files are error-free and optimized for printing. For example, using software to check for thin walls or unsupported overhangs can prevent print failures. Additionally, checking that the filament is dry and free from defects will help avoid issues like poor layer adhesion or nozzle clogs.
2. *In-Process Monitoring*: Modern FDM printers often come equipped with sensors that can detect issues in real-time. For instance, a printer might have a filament sensor that pauses the print if it runs out of material or detects a jam. Some printers also use cameras to monitor the print layer-by-layer, allowing for immediate intervention if a problem arises. Modern FDM printers often come equipped with sensors that can detect issues in real time.
3. *Post-Printing Inspection*: After the object is printed, it undergoes various checks to ensure it meets the desired standards. Dimensional accuracy might be verified using digital calipers to measure the dimensions against the CAD model [42]. Surface finish could be examined under a microscope to check for any unexpected textures or defects. Mechanical properties such as strength and flexibility might be tested using machines that apply force until the part breaks, ensuring it can withstand its intended use. After the object is printed, it undergoes various checks to ensure it meets the desired standards.
4. *Feedback-Based Error Compensation*: This approach involves using data collected during the printing process to adjust future prints. For example, if a part consistently comes out slightly smaller than intended, the printer's software can

be adjusted to compensate for this shrinkage on subsequent prints. This approach involves using data collected during the printing process to adjust future prints.

5. *Quality Management Systems*: Implementing a system that standardizes quality checks can greatly improve consistency. This might involve creating a checklist that operators follow for each print, ensuring that every step from design to post-processing is completed correctly. Regular training sessions can keep operators up-to-date on best practices, and periodic audits of the process can help identify areas for improvement. Implementing a system that standardizes quality checks can greatly improve consistency. By employing these methods, manufacturers can ensure that their FDM 3D-printed parts are consistently high-quality and fit for their intended applications.

11.6 Regulatory Framework for FDM Printing in Pharmaceuticals

1. *Regulatory Oversight*: Various regulatory bodies, including the FDA's CDRH in the USA, are tasked with overseeing the approval process for pharmaceutical products created using 3D printing technology [43].
2. *Framework Development*: The MHRA introduced a proposed framework in March 2021 to facilitate the development and supply of personalized medicines, which encompasses 3D printing methods at the point of care.
3. *Standardization and Engagement*: The establishment of uniform procedures and active involvement with regulatory authorities are crucial to harness the full potential of 3D printing in drug innovation while maintaining high standards of quality and compliance. This emphasizes the ongoing development and importance of regulatory collaboration to ensure the responsible integration of FDM 3D printing within the pharmaceutical sector.

11.6.1 Overview of Regulatory Requirements and Guidelines

1. *Compliance with Safety Protocols*: FDM 3D printing operations must align with established safety protocols to ensure both operator and product safety. This encompasses guidelines for equipment usage and material handling. For instance, an FDM 3D printer must have proper enclosures to prevent accidental contact with heated components. Additionally, materials like ABS filament should be handled in well-ventilated areas to mitigate the risk of inhaling fumes.
2. *Medical Device Regulations*: The FDA outlines specific directives for the design, production, and testing of 3D-printed medical devices. These directives are part of a broader quality system that guarantees the device's safety and efficacy. As an example, a 3D-printed prosthetic limb must undergo rigorous testing to meet FDA standards. This includes verifying biocompatibility, mechanical strength, and durability to ensure patient safety [44].

3. *Adherence to Quality Systems*: Producers are required to follow stringent quality systems that govern the entire manufacturing process. This is to certify that products are consistently manufactured to meet quality specifications. A company producing dental implants via FDM technology would need to document each step of their manufacturing process, from design to sterilization, ensuring traceability and consistency in line with quality system regulations.
4. *Food Safety in 3D Printing*: For 3D-printed items intended for food contact, materials must be non-toxic and safe for consumption. The FDA provides methods and considerations for ensuring that products meet these food safety standards. If a company wants to produce 3D-printed cookie cutters, they must use food-safe PLA filament and ensure that the end product can be cleaned effectively to prevent foodborne illnesses [45].
5. *Premarket Approval Process*: Devices are subjected to a premarket approval process based on their classification, which reflects the level of risk they pose. This process can vary in complexity from one device to another. A high-risk medical device like a 3D-printed heart valve would require a more extensive premarket approval process compared to a low-risk device such as a surgical instrument handle.

These examples illustrate how regulations and guidelines are applied in practice to ensure safety and quality in FDM 3D printing. It is important for manufacturers to stay informed about the specific requirements relevant to their products and operations.

11.6.2 Challenges in Regulatory Approval for FDM-Printed Pharmaceutical Products

1. *Guidance Clarity*: The industry is in need of explicit guidelines for the adoption of FDM 3D printing in creating personalized medications, particularly for use directly at healthcare facilities. The pharmaceutical industry is still awaiting comprehensive regulatory frameworks that specifically address the nuances of FDM 3D printing. For example, there's uncertainty about how to implement Good Manufacturing Practices (GMP) for drugs that are printed on demand at pharmacies or clinics.
2. *Ensuring Formulation Integrity*: A key hurdle is the establishment of reliable quality and safety protocols for medications produced via FDM 3D printing to maintain high standards. The integrity of 3D-printed drugs must be assured, which involves validating the consistency and accuracy of drug dosages. This can be challenging due to the variability in 3D printing processes and the complexity of ensuring uniformity in printed medications.
3. *Consistency in Testing*: The lack of uniform testing procedures for evaluating 3D-printed pharmaceuticals adds complexity to their regulatory approval. Standardized testing methods are not yet fully established for 3D-printed drugs.

This means there's no consensus on how to best assess the dissolution rates, stability, and pharmacokinetics of these novel drug forms.

4. *Collaborative Efforts*: It's essential for industry players, regulatory bodies, and healthcare practitioners to work together to overcome these regulatory obstacles. Effective collaboration is needed to address these regulatory challenges. For instance, pharmaceutical companies must work closely with device manufacturers to ensure that 3D printers are capable of producing drugs that meet regulatory standards.
5. *Engagement with Regulators*: Proactive discussions with regulatory authorities are vital to navigate the complex regulatory environment and ensure innovation in drug production while safeguarding quality and patient safety. Navigating these challenges requires a concerted effort to develop appropriate regulations and foster collaboration across the pharmaceutical industry. Proactive engagement with regulatory bodies like the FDA is crucial. An example of this would be participating in pilot programs or guidance development initiatives to help shape the future regulatory landscape for 3D-printed pharmaceuticals.

These examples illustrate the multifaceted nature of the regulatory challenges associated with FDM-printed pharmaceutical products. Addressing these issues will require ongoing dialogue between all stakeholders involved, as well as a willingness to adapt and evolve regulatory standards as the technology progresses.

11.6.3 Strategies for Navigating Regulatory Pathways

1. *Choosing Appropriate Materials*: Option for materials that meet the regulatory criteria for safety and effectiveness. This involves selecting materials that are safe for patient use and suitable for drug production. The selection of materials is critical. For instance, when selecting a polymer for drug printing, it must not only be able to produce the desired drug release profile but also be biocompatible and meet the regulatory requirements for contact with humans.
2. *Validating the Printing Process*: Develop a detailed validation plan to prove that the FDM 3D printing process is reliable and produces products that match the required standards consistently. Validation involves demonstrating that the FDM 3D printing process can consistently produce the same quality of product. This might include showing that the printer can reliably create layers of medication with the correct dosage and that these layers bond correctly without altering the drug's efficacy.
3. *Implementing Quality Measures*: Put in place thorough quality measures at every stage of production, from initial material selection to the final post-processing steps, to ensure the final product is safe and effective. Quality measures could include setting up in-line monitoring systems to check the quality of products as they are printed, as well as rigorous post-printing testing to ensure that each batch meets the necessary specifications.

4. *Continuous Regulatory Dialogue*: Engage regularly with regulatory authorities like the FDA to keep up-to-date with the latest regulations and contribute to the development of new guidelines. This means staying engaged with regulatory bodies through meetings, conferences, and comment periods on new guidance documents. It's about being proactive in understanding and shaping the regulatory landscape.
5. *Adhering to Regulatory Guidelines*: Follow the guidelines and reports provided by regulatory agencies, such as the FDA's Guidance Agenda, which outlines specific requirements for 3D printing in drug manufacturing. Companies must ensure they are following all current guidelines, which may involve adapting their processes as new guidance is released. For example, if new guidelines are issued regarding the sterility of printed products, companies must adjust their processes to comply.
6. *Monitoring Post-Approval Performance*: After receiving regulatory approval, continue to track the product's performance in real-world settings to ensure it remains compliant and safe for use. By employing these approaches, pharmaceutical companies can effectively manage the regulatory requirements for FDM 3D-printed drugs and ensure a smooth path to market introduction. After a product is approved and on the market, companies should have systems in place to monitor its performance. This could involve tracking adverse event reports or conducting post-market studies to ensure that the product continues to meet safety and efficacy standards. These strategies represent a comprehensive approach to navigating the regulatory pathways for FDM-printed pharmaceutical products. They emphasize the importance of preparation, compliance, and ongoing engagement with regulatory processes.

11.7 Case Studies and Applications

11.7.1 Examples of FDM 3D Printing Applications in Pharmaceuticals

1. *Tissues and Organs*: FDM can be used to create complex structures that mimic human tissues and organs, which can be used for research or transplantation.
2. *Customized Prosthetics*: Prosthetics made using FDM can be tailored to fit the unique anatomy of a patient, improving comfort and functionality.
3. *Personalized Drug Delivery Systems*: FDM allows for the creation of drug delivery devices that can release medications at controlled rates, dissolve quickly in the mouth, or stay in the stomach for extended periods. This customization can lead to improved patient adherence and better therapeutic outcomes.
4. *Pharmaceutical Devices*: With FDM, devices such as inhalers, pumps, or implants can be manufactured to meet specific patient needs, potentially improving the efficacy of treatments. These applications highlight the potential of FDM 3D printing to provide personalized healthcare products that cater to individual patient needs.

11.7.2 Case Studies Highlighting Successful Implementation and Outcomes

1. *Customized Medications*: FDM 3D printing is revolutionizing the pharmaceutical field by enabling the creation of bespoke medications. This technique allows for intricate drug designs that are customized to meet each patient's unique therapeutic requirements. For instance, Aprecia Pharmaceuticals developed Spritam, an anti-epileptic drug that utilizes 3D printing to produce a porous formulation that dissolves quickly with a sip of water, enhancing ease of administration for patients who struggle with swallowing pills [46].
2. *Heat-Sensitive Drug Processing*: Innovative approaches in FDM 3D printing have been developed to handle heat-sensitive medications. By crafting specialized filaments that preserve the integrity of the drug during the printing process, medications that would otherwise be compromised by heat can now be effectively incorporated into printed dosage forms. An example includes the use of low-temperature melting polymers as carriers for heat-sensitive drugs, ensuring they remain stable and effective.
3. *Drug Development Acceleration*: The agility of FDM 3D printing accelerates drug development by facilitating swift prototyping and evaluation of novel formulations and delivery mechanisms. This rapid iteration process is crucial in the pharmaceutical industry's race to bring new treatments to market.
4. *Transdermal Systems*: FDM 3D printing is being explored for producing transdermal systems like microneedle arrays. These arrays can painlessly penetrate the skin to deliver medication directly into the bloodstream, bypassing the digestive system. A notable application is the development of microneedle flu vaccines, which could potentially increase vaccination rates due to their ease of use and reduced discomfort compared to traditional needles.
5. *Targeted Cancer Therapies*: Research in FDM 3D printing has also extended to creating patches for targeted cancer therapy. By adjusting the porosity of these patches, scientists can control the release rate of anti-cancer drugs, aiming for precise treatment delivery to tumor sites while minimizing systemic side effects. These advancements showcase FDM 3D printing's potential in crafting personalized treatment options and enhancing drug delivery methods, marking significant strides in patient-centered care and pharmaceutical innovation.

11.7.3 Future Trends and Emerging Applications

1. *Tailored Drug Production*: The future of FDM 3D printing in pharmaceuticals is gearing towards hyper-personalized medicine. This means drugs could be custom-made to fit a patient's specific health profile, potentially improving treatment efficacy and reducing adverse effects. For example, the University of Nottingham has been working on 3D printing personalized tablets that could combine a patient's entire medication regimen into a single daily pill.

2. *On-Site Medication Printing*: Hospitals might soon be equipped with 3D printers capable of producing drugs as needed, which could revolutionize emergency care by providing immediate access to life-saving medications. This is particularly beneficial for producing orphan drugs for rare diseases, which are often not kept in stock due to low demand.
3. *Advanced Drug Release Mechanisms*: With FDM 3D printing, it's possible to engineer sophisticated drug delivery systems that control how and when medication is released into the body. A research group at MIT has developed a 3D-printed pill that can release drugs for several days or weeks after ingestion, which could be particularly useful for treating chronic conditions [47].
4. *Biological Printing*: The field of bioprinting is burgeoning, with researchers exploring ways to print living tissues for drug testing or even organ transplants. Organovo, for instance, has been pioneering the 3D printing of functional human tissues that could be used for medical research and therapeutic applications.
5. *Regulatory Evolution*: As FDM 3D printing technology progresses, regulatory agencies are expected to develop more detailed guidelines to ensure the safety and efficacy of printed pharmaceuticals. This will pave the way for broader adoption of this technology in drug development and healthcare.

These trends highlight the transformative potential of FDM 3D printing in reshaping pharmaceutical manufacturing and personalized medicine.

11.8 Future Directions and Innovations

1. *Innovative Material Development*: The pharmaceutical industry is exploring new polymeric materials for 3D printing that could revolutionize drug delivery by enhancing drug stability and efficacy. For instance, researchers are investigating biocompatible polymers that can dissolve at controlled rates for targeted drug release.
2. *Personalized Implants*: The future of medicine includes 3D-printed implants tailored to individual patients, which could release therapeutic agents directly to the affected area. An example is the development of spinal implants that can be loaded with pain medication to provide localized relief after surgery.
3. *Advanced Printlets*: These are not just ordinary tablets; they are customizable in every aspect, from dosage to release profile, thanks to FDM 3D printing. A notable example is Aprecia Pharmaceuticals' Spritam®, the first FDA-approved 3D-printed drug that dissolves quickly with a sip of liquid, designed for patients with epilepsy.
4. *Digital Drug Manufacturing*: The convergence of digital design with pharmaceutical manufacturing promises a more agile production process. This could mean rapid prototyping of drug formulations, allowing for quick responses to epidemic outbreaks with tailored medications.

5. *Pharmaceutical Production Transformation*: As FDM 3D printing matures, it's set to enable complex drug formulations that were previously impossible, such as multi-drug capsules with staged release timings for combination therapies.

These future directions indicate a shift towards more personalized, efficient, and innovative pharmaceutical solutions.

11.8.1 Advancements in FDM Printing Technology

1. *Enhanced Durability and Efficiency*: The latest FDM 3D printers have been engineered to produce components that are not only stronger but also created at a quicker pace. For instance, Stratasys' Fortus 450mc can print high-strength parts suitable for functional prototyping and production tooling [48].
2. *Expanded Printing Dimensions*: The advent of larger print beds has revolutionized the scale at which objects can be printed, enabling the construction of bigger and more intricate designs. The BigRep ONE, for example, boasts a massive build volume, allowing for life-size prints.
3. *Material Innovation*: FDM technology now accommodates a broader array of materials, including metals and ceramics, broadening its utility beyond traditional polymers. Markforged is a leader in this area with their Metal X printer that can print industrial-grade metal parts.
4. *Eco-Friendly Practices*: The push towards eco-friendly 3D printing is leading to the development of printers and filaments that are more environmentally sustainable. Companies like 3D Systems offer biodegradable materials like PLA, which are derived from renewable resources.
5. *Architectural Complexity*: Cutting-edge FDM printers can fabricate complex fiber structures with precise control over their functional properties. This is exemplified by the work done at MIT's Media Lab, where researchers have printed fiber preforms that can sense, store energy, and even compute.

These advancements are propelling FDM 3D printing into new realms of possibility across diverse sectors.

The Advancements in FDM 3D Printing Technology

1. *High-Performance Thermoplastics*: The use of high-performance thermoplastics like PEEK (polyether ether ketone) and ULTEM™ is becoming more common in FDM printing [47]. These materials are known for their excellent mechanical properties and resistance to high temperatures, making them ideal for aerospace and medical applications.
2. *Multi-Material Printing*: Some FDM printers now offer the capability to print with multiple materials in a single print job, allowing for parts with varying properties like rigidity and flexibility. The Ultimaker S5 is an example of a printer that can handle multiple materials, offering great versatility.

3. *Precision and Resolution*: The precision of FDM printers has significantly improved, with some machines capable of layer resolutions as fine as 50 µm. The Prusa i3 MK3S+ is renowned for its exceptional layer resolution and print quality [49].
4. *Wireless Connectivity and Automation*: Modern FDM printers often come equipped with wireless connectivity and automation features that streamline the printing process. For instance, the MakerBot Replicator+ can be controlled remotely via an app, making the printing process more convenient and efficient.

These examples demonstrate how FDM 3D printing technology continues to evolve, pushing the boundaries of what can be achieved in manufacturing and design.

11.8.2 Opportunities for Overcoming Current Challenges

Exploring solutions to address FDM 3D printing's current hurdles presents several promising avenues:

1. *Enhancing Print Fidelity*: Initiatives like OMNI3D's webinars offer guidance on refining the detail and exactness of printed items, which is essential for sectors demanding superior print standards.
2. *Advancing Large-Scale Printing*: Innovations in large-scale 3D printing are tackling the difficulties associated with creating and prototyping sizable components, cutting down on time and costs linked to assembly and large-scale tool production.
3. *Streamlining with Software*: Tools such as Fabpilot are revolutionizing FDM printing by providing comprehensive software solutions for file correction, organization, and printer management, facilitating large-scale operations.
4. *Improving Material Standards*: Efforts to enhance filament integrity are crucial. Strategies are being devised to combat challenges like variable filament sizes, humidity retention, or contamination that can mar print quality.
5. *Knowledge Sharing*: An increase in educational materials is aiding users in navigating and resolving prevalent FDM printing issues, thereby improving overall print success. These strategies are instrumental in advancing the capabilities of FDM 3D printing, making it a more robust and versatile tool for a myriad of uses.

11.8.3 Potential Impact on the Pharmaceutical Industry and Healthcare Landscape

FDM 3D printing is poised to revolutionize both the pharmaceutical sector and healthcare services:

1. *Customized Therapeutics*: This technology facilitates the production of drugs tailored to the specific needs of patients, enhancing the efficacy of treatments.

2. *Intricate Medication Structures*: It enables the crafting of complex medication structures and flexible dosing options, improving how medications are administered.
3. *Accelerated Drug Development*: 3D printing can speed up the creation of new medications, shortening the time they take to reach the market and potentially reducing development costs.
4. *Sustainability in Production*: The method promises less waste generation in drug manufacturing, leading to more eco-friendly practices.
5. *Healthcare Application*: The integration of this technology into diverse medical environments, such as hospitals and pharmacies, could improve medical service delivery.
6. *Innovative Delivery Mechanisms*: FDM 3D printing is at the forefront of developing new drug delivery mechanisms, tissue engineering solutions, and prosthetic organ creation.

These advancements are just a glimpse into the future, as continuous improvements in 3D printing technology herald new possibilities for enhancing patient care and drug development processes.

11.9 Conclusion

FDM 3D printing is emerging as a transformative force in drug production, heralding a new era of personalized medicine with its capacity for creating bespoke drug formulations. This innovative approach promises to slash manufacturing costs by minimizing the reliance on specialized machinery. It also introduces groundbreaking methods for constructing complex medication structures and combined drug therapies, offering precise control over their release. Moreover, it aligns with sustainable practices by potentially reducing waste, marking a significant step forward in eco-friendly pharmaceutical manufacturing. As FDM 3D printing technology advances, it stands to significantly improve healthcare outcomes and revolutionize the pharmaceutical landscape.

In conclusion, FDM 3D printing is set to be a game-changer in the pharmaceutical industry by enabling:

1. *Personalized Medicine*: Customized drug formulations tailored to individual patient needs.
2. *Cost Efficiency*: Reduction in manufacturing costs through less need for specialized equipment.
3. *Innovative Manufacturing*: Creation of complex drug structures and multi-drug combinations with precise control over release mechanisms.
4. *Sustainability*: Potential for more eco-friendly production with reduced waste.

As this technology continues to evolve, it promises to enhance the quality of healthcare delivery and open up new possibilities in drug development and manufacturing.

11.9.1 Summary of Key Findings and Insights

FDM 3D printing is set to revolutionize pharmaceutical manufacturing by offering unprecedented personalization in drug production, aligning treatments more closely with individual patient profiles for enhanced efficacy. This cutting-edge technology not only promises substantial cost savings by streamlining production and reducing material waste but also fosters innovation through the development of complex drug forms and advanced delivery systems. Embracing sustainability, FDM 3D printing is anticipated to lead the way in eco-conscious manufacturing processes, marking a significant leap forward in the pursuit of patient-centric and environmentally responsible pharmaceutical practices.

11.9.2 Recommendations for Future Research and Development

Future research and development in the realm of FDM 3D printing for pharmaceuticals should prioritize the exploration of innovative materials that enhance both the printing process and drug delivery. Efforts should be directed towards perfecting the FDM technique to achieve greater accuracy and consistency in medication production. Establishing robust regulatory standards will be crucial to ensure the safety and effectiveness of 3D printed drugs. Additionally, identifying viable commercialization avenues will be very important to bringing laboratory successes to the pharmaceutical market, with an emphasis on meeting consumer demands and ensuring scalability.

11.9.3 Closing Remarks

It has been a pleasure discussing the exciting field of FDM 3D printing in pharmaceuticals, and this technology holds great promise for the future of medicine, offering personalized treatments and innovative drug delivery systems. As research and development continue to advance, we can look forward to significant contributions to healthcare from FDM 3D printing.

References

1. Cailleaux S, Sanchez-Ballester NM, Gueche YA, Bataille B, Soulairol I. Fused deposition Modeling (FDM), the new asset for the production of tailored medicines. J Contr Release. 2021;330:821–41. https://doi.org/10.1016/j.jconrel.2020.10.056.
2. Abdelhamid M, Koutsamanis I, Corzo C, Maisriemler M, Ocampo AB, Slama E, Alva C, Lochmann D, Reyer S, Freichel T, Salar-Behzadi S, Spoerk M. Filament-based 3D-printing of placebo dosage forms using brittle lipid-based excipients. Int J Pharm. 2022;624:1–12.
3. Siemiński P. Chapter 7 – Introduction to fused deposition modeling. In: Pou J, Riveiro A, Davim JP, editors. Handbooks in advanced manufacturing, additive manufacturing. Elsevier; 2021. p. 217–75. https://doi.org/10.1016/B978-0-12-818411-0.00008-2.

4. Daminabo SC, Goel S, Grammatikos SA, Nezhad HY, Thakur VK. Fused deposition modeling-based additive manufacturing (3D printing): techniques for polymer material systems. Mater Today Chem. 2020;16:100248. https://doi.org/10.1016/j.mtchem.2020.100248.
5. Montez M, Willis K, Rendler H, Marshall C, Rubio E, Rajak DK, Rahman MH, Menezes PL. Fused deposition modeling (FDM): processes, material properties, and applications. In: Kumar P, Misra M, Menezes PL, editors. Tribology of additively manufactured materials. Elsevier; 2022. p. 137–63. https://doi.org/10.1016/B978-0-12-821328-5.00005-6.
6. Wasti S, Adhikari S. Use of biomaterials for 3D printing by fused deposition modeling technique. A Review Front Chem. 2020;8:315. https://doi.org/10.3389/fchem.2020.00315.
7. Korte C, Quodbach J. Formulation development and process analysis of drug-loaded filaments manufactured via hot-melt extrusion for 3D-printing of medicines. Pharm Dev Technol. 2018;23(10):1117–27. https://doi.org/10.1080/10837450.2018.1433208.
8. Dumpa N, Butreddy A, Wang H, Komanduri N, Bandari S, Repka MA. 3D printing in personalized drug delivery: an overview of hot-melt extrusion-based fused deposition modeling. Int J Pharm. 2021;600:120501.
9. Araújo MRP, Sa-Barreto LL, Gratieri T, Gelfuso GM, Cunha-Filho M. The digital pharmacies era: how 3D printing technology using fused deposition modeling can become a reality. Pharmaceutics. 2019;11(3):128. https://doi.org/10.3390/pharmaceutics11030128.
10. Mohammed A, Elshaer A, Sareh P, Elsayed M, Hassanin H. Additive manufacturing technologies for drug delivery applications. Int J Pharm. 2020;580:119245. https://doi.org/10.1016/j.ijpharm.2020.119245.
11. Wang H, Vemula SK, Bandari S, Repka MA. Preparation of core-shell controlled release tablets using direct powder extrusion 3D printing techniques. J Drug Deliv Sci Technol. 2023;88:104896. https://doi.org/10.1016/j.jddst.2023.104896.
12. Than YM, Titapiwatanakun V. Tailoring immediate release FDM 3D printed tablets using a quality by design (QbD) approach. Int J Pharm. 2021;599:120402. https://doi.org/10.1016/j.ijpharm.2021.120402.
13. Agnello F, Finocchiaro S, Laudani C, Legnazzi M, Mauro MS, Rochira C, Scalia L, Capodanno D. A review of polypills for the prevention of atherosclerotic cardiovascular disease. Am Heart J. 2023;266:74–85. https://doi.org/10.1016/j.ahj.2023.08.012.
14. Anaya BJ, Cerda JR, D'Atri RM, Yuste I, Luciano FC, Kara A, Ruiz HK, Ballesteros MP, Serrano DR. Engineering of 3D printed personalized polypills for the treatment of the metabolic syndrome. Int J Pharm. 2023;642:123194. https://doi.org/10.1016/j.ijpharm.2023.123194.
15. Al-Litani K, Ali T, Martinez PR, Buanz A. 3D printed implantable drug delivery devices for women's health: formulation challenges and regulatory perspective. Adv Drug Deliv Rev. 2023;198:114859. https://doi.org/10.1016/j.addr.2023.114859.
16. Cano-Vicent A, Tambuwala MM, Hassan SS, Barh D, Aljabali AAA, Birkett M, Arjunan A, Serrano-Aroca Á. Fused deposition modelling: current status, methodology, applications and future prospects. Addit Manuf. 2021;47:102378. https://doi.org/10.1016/j.addma.2021.102378.
17. Kristiawan R, Imaduddin F, Ariawan D, Ubaidillah A, Z. A review on the fused deposition modeling (FDM) 3D printing: filament processing, materials, and printing parameters. Open Eng. 2021;11(1):639–49. https://doi.org/10.1515/eng-2021-0063.
18. Kumaresan R, Samykano M, Kadirgama K, Harun WSW, Rahman P, Dr M, Mustafizur. Fused deposition modeling: process, materials, parameters, properties, and applications. Int J Adv Manuf Technol. 2022;120:1531–70. https://doi.org/10.1007/s00170-022-08860-7.
19. Lee WC, Wei CC, Chung SC. Development of a hybrid rapid prototyping system using low-cost fused deposition modeling and five-axis machining. J Mater Process Technol. 2014;214(11):2366–74.
20. Valino AD, Dizon JRC, Espera AH, Chen Q, Messman J, Advincula RC. Advances in 3D printing of thermoplastic polymer composites and nanocomposites. Prog Polym Sci. 2019;98:101162. https://doi.org/10.1016/j.progpolymsci.2019.101162.
21. Kiendl J, Gao C. Controlling toughness and strength of FDM 3D-printed PLA components through the raster layup. Compos Part B. 2020;180:107562. https://doi.org/10.1016/j.compositesb.2019.107562.

22. Pérez M, Medina-Sánchez G, García-Collado A, Gupta M, Carou D. Surface quality enhancement of fused deposition modeling (FDM) printed samples based on the selection of critical printing parameters. Materials (Basel). 2018;11(8):1382. https://doi.org/10.3390/ma11081382.
23. Forster AM. Materials testing standards for additive manufacturing of polymer materials: state of the art and standards applicability. In: White L, editor. Additive manufacturing materials: standards, testing and applicability. Nova Science Publishers, Inc.; 2015. p. 67–123.
24. Manzanares Palenzuela CL, Novotný F, Krupička P, Sofer Z, Pumera M. 3D-printed graphene/polylactic acid electrodes promise high sensitivity in electroanalysis. Anal Chem. 2018;90(9):5753–7. https://doi.org/10.1021/acs.analchem.8b00561.
25. Chohan JS, Singh R, Boparai KS. Parametric optimization of fused deposition modeling and vapor smoothing processes for surface finishing of biomedical implant replicas. Measurement. 2016;94:602–13.
26. Nikolova MP, Chavali MS. Recent advances in biomaterials for 3D scaffolds: a review. Bioactive Mater. 2019;4:271–92. https://doi.org/10.1016/j.bioactmat.2019.07.001.
27. Campo EA. Polymeric materials and properties. In: Campo EA, editor. Plastics design library, selection of polymeric materials. William Andrew Publishing; 2008. p. 1–39. https://doi.org/10.1016/B978-081551551-7.50003-6.
28. Mĺkva M, Prajová V, Yakimovich B, Korshunov A, Tyurin I. Standardization–one of the tools of continuous improvement. Proc Eng. 2016;149:329–32. https://doi.org/10.1016/j.proeng.2016.06.674.
29. da Silva D, Kaduri M, Poley M, Adir O, Krinsky N, Shainsky-Roitman J, Schroeder A. Biocompatibility, biodegradation, and excretion of polylactic acid (PLA) in medical implants and theranostic systems. Chem Eng J. 2018;340:9–14. https://doi.org/10.1016/j.cej.2018.01.010.
30. Doshi M, Mahale A, Singh SK, Deshmukh S. Printing parameters and materials affecting mechanical properties of FDM-3D printed parts: perspective and prospects. Mater Today Proc. 2022;50(5):2269–75. https://doi.org/10.1016/j.matpr.2021.10.003.
31. Couţi N, Porfire A, Iovanov R, Crişan AG, Iurian S, Casian T, Tomuţă I. Polyvinyl alcohol, a versatile excipient for pharmaceutical 3D printing. Polymers (Basel). 2024;16(4):517. https://doi.org/10.3390/polym16040517.
32. Mamo HB, Adamiak M, Kunwar A. 3D printed biomedical devices and their applications: a review on state-of-the-art technologies, existing challenges, and future perspectives. J Mech Behav Biomed Mater. 2023;143:105930. https://doi.org/10.1016/j.jmbbm.2023.105930.
33. Attia MS, Elshahat A, Hamdy A, Fathi AM, Emad-Eldin M, Ghazy FS, Chopra H, Ibrahim TM. Soluplus® as a solubilizing excipient for poorly water-soluble drugs: recent advances in formulation strategies and pharmaceutical product features. J Drug Deliv Sci Technol. 2023;84:104519. https://doi.org/10.1016/j.jddst.2023.104519.
34. Salehi S, Boddohi S. Design and optimization of kollicoat® IR based mucoadhesive buccal film for co-delivery of rizatriptan benzoate and propranolol hydrochloride. Mater Sci Eng C. 2019;97:230–44. https://doi.org/10.1016/j.msec.2018.12.036.
35. Jagtap P, Tagad R. A brief review on Kollidon. J Drug Deliv Therap. 2019;9:493–500. https://doi.org/10.22270/jddt.v9i2.2539.
36. Cheung Ma W, Liang Goh G, Meera Priyadarshini B, Yee Yeong W. 3D printing and 3D-printed electronics: applications and future trends in smart drug delivery devices. Int J Bioprint. 2023;9(4):725. https://doi.org/10.18063/ijb.725.
37. Pivar M, Gregor-Svetec D, Muck D. Effect of printing process parameters on the shape transformation capability of 3D printed structures. Polymers (Basel). 2021;14(1):117. https://doi.org/10.3390/polym14010117.
38. Mustapha AN, Zhang Y, Zhang Z, Ding Y, Yuan Q, Li Y. Taguchi and ANOVA analysis for the optimization of the microencapsulation of a volatile phase change material. J Mater Res Technol. 2021;11:667–80. https://doi.org/10.1016/j.jmrt.2021.01.025.
39. Hamzaçebi C. Taguchi method as a robust design tool. In: Li P, Pereira PAR, Navas H, editors. Quality control – intelligent manufacturing, robust design and charts. IntechOpen; 2020. https://doi.org/10.5772/intechopen.94908.

40. McCall J. Genetic algorithms for modelling and optimisation. J Comput Appl Math. 2005;184(1):205–22. https://doi.org/10.1016/j.cam.2004.07.034.
41. Aly P, Mohsen C. Comparison of the accuracy of three-dimensional printed casts, digital, and conventional casts: an in vitro study. Eur J Dent. 2020;14(2):189–93. https://doi.org/10.1055/s-0040-1705243.
42. Pawar K, Gore R, Palekar S. A review on approval process and regulation of medical devices as per US FDA and CDSCO. Int J Drug Regul Aff. 2023;11:61–70. https://doi.org/10.22270/ijdra.v11i1.586.
43. Marinopoulos T, Li S, Silberschmidt VV. Structural integrity of 3D-printed prosthetic sockets: experimental study for paediatric applications. J Mater Res Technol. 2023;24:2734–42. https://doi.org/10.1016/j.jmrt.2023.03.192.
44. Chavan Y, Paul K, Kolekar N. Food safety and hygiene: current policies, quality standards, and scope of artificial intelligence. In: Chakraborty R, Mathur P, Roy S, editors. Food production, diversity, and safety under climate change. Springer; 2024. p. 61–70. https://doi.org/10.1007/978-3-031-51647-4_26.
45. Jain P, Kathuria H, Dubey NK. Advances in 3D bioprinting of tissues/organs for regenerative medicine and in-vitro models. Biomaterials. 2022;287:121639. https://doi.org/10.1016/j.biomaterials.2022.121639.
46. Eisenstein M. First 3D-printed pill. Nat Biotechnol. 2015;33:1014. https://doi.org/10.1038/nbt1015-1014a.
47. Mohammed AA, Algahtani MS, Ahmad MZ, Ahmad J, Kotta S. 3D printing in medicine: technology overview and drug delivery applications. Ann 3D Print Med. 2021;4:100037. https://doi.org/10.1016/j.stlm.2021.100037.
48. Stratasys Fortus 450mc. Retrieved from https://www.stratasys.com/en/3d-printers/printer-catalog/fdm-printers/fortus-450mc/.
49. Hu Z, He J, Chen W, Liu W, Ding J, He C, Wang S, Ning F, Li X. High-performance carbon fiber reinforced polyether-ether-ketone composite pellets 3D-printed via screw-extrusion additive manufacturing. Compos Sci Technol. 2024;246:110362. https://doi.org/10.1016/j.compscitech.2023.110362.

Case Studies and Success Stories in FDM 3D Printing for Pharmaceuticals

12

Dinesh Kumar, Rajni Tanwar, Kavita Bahmani, Sumit Kumar, Rahul Pal, and Kuldeep Vinchurkar

Abstract

Fused deposition modeling (FDM) 3D printing has significantly impacted pharmaceutical drug delivery and medicine personalization. Case studies and success stories demonstrate its wide applications and promising achievements in the pharmaceutical industry. Examples include Aprecia Pharmaceuticals' FDA-approved ZipDose® tablets and the University of Michigan's personalized dose form studies. Collaborations between Aprecia Pharmaceuticals and Cycle Pharmaceuticals have driven the development of Printlets by FabRx and advanced drug delivery systems. FDM printing has improved patient treatment adherence and medication effectiveness, enabling on-demand pharmaceutical manufacture and drug delivery device prototypes. It has also helped build new medication delivery devices and complex in-vitro drug testing models. This technology has the potential to revolutionize medication discovery, production, and personalized treatment.

D. Kumar (✉) · R. Tanwar · R. Pal
School of Pharmacy, Desh Bhagat University, Mandi Gobindgarh, Punjab, India
e-mail: ap4.pharmacy@deshbhagatuniversity.in

K. Bahmani
Department of Pharmaceutical Sciences, Guru Jambeshwar University of Science and Technology, Hisar, Haryana, India

S. Kumar
Central University of Haryana, Mahendergarh, Haryana, India

K. Vinchurkar
Department of Pharmaceutics, Sandip Institute of Pharmaceutical Sciences (SIPS), Affiliated To Savitribai Phule Pune University (SPPU, Pune), Nashik, Maharashtra, India

K. Vinchurkar, S. Mane (eds.), *Innovations in Drug Manufacturing*,
https://doi.org/10.1007/978-981-96-9075-6_12

Keywords

FDM 3D printing · Case studies · Personalized medicine · Drug delivery

12.1 Introduction

An innovative manufacturing process that builds three-dimensional objects layer by layer on a computer-aided design platform is known as three-dimensional printing (3DP). Originally created for use in manufacturing, 3D printing has lately shown great promise as a technology. The pharmaceutical industry's manufacturing process for prescription products has been significantly altered as a result of the emergence of 3D printing. This has significantly facilitated the conversion of non-digitalized medical products into digital 3D content [1–3]. The integration of physical and digital production in the pharmaceutical industry has led to the development of various 3D medical products, with 3D printing technology being a significant technological revolution in process innovation in this area [4–6]. 3D printing is a technology that is specifically designed to develop formulations that are customized to meet the unique requirements of each patient. Administration dose accuracy is one of the most critical factors in targeted drug delivery. At present, the industry adheres to a one-size-fits-all approach; however, traditional mass production of doses can be replaced by patient-specific dosage formulation [7].

The demand for customized devices and technological innovation is the primary factor contributing to the expansion of personalized medicine. This is accomplished by fabricating customized prostheses and small series of concentrations that are individually selected. Three-dimensional printing (3DP) is a potent and revolutionary method in the pharmaceutical and biomedical market, utilized for the engineering of tissues and organs, the development of novel dosage forms, the exacting production of devices, and the modeling of diseases. 3DP's applications are constantly expanding as a swiftly evolving field of technology, art, and science. The International Standard Organization defines 3DP as the process of fabricating objects by deposition of a material using a print head or nozzle [8].

3D printing involves designing a 3D object using computer-aided design software, optimizing geometry, exporting the model to a common file format, importing the file to the software, and generating printed layers. The height of the printed layer significantly influences the object's quality and printing time. The object is then fabricated by applying or solidifying material layers for durability and precision. The 3D printing process is represented in Fig. 12.1 [9].

3D printing enables the development of customized treatments that are tailored to the unique therapeutic or individual requirements of each patient. Patients can now choose formulation types from a catalogue, allowing them to select factors like flavor, texture, color, shape, and size. This improves adherence to medications, enhances patient autonomy, and encourages engagement with treatment pathways [10]. In order to improve treatment effectiveness and decrease the risk of unwanted

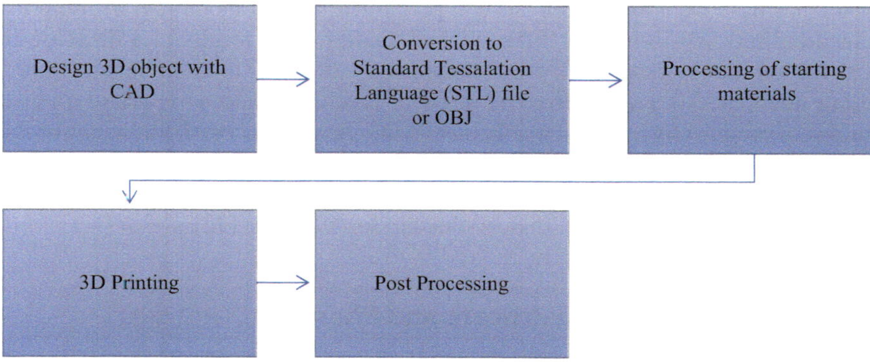

Fig. 12.1 Procedure of 3D printing. (Samiei N. [9]. A schematic representation of different processing steps involved in fabrication of 3D printing objects. https://rdcu.be/dRkn7. Accessed 10 July 2024)

effects caused by improper dosing, 3D-printed polyprintlets may be used to provide exact or flexible doses of numerous medications [11, 12]. Because traditional mass-produced formulations may not be suited for pediatric populations owing to problems like insufficient palatability or improper concentrations, personalized pharmaceutical manufacture provides many advantages [13, 14].

Numerous studies have focused on creating child-friendly 3D-printed formulations, including chocolate-based and digestible options [15, 16]. Using placebo printlets made using four different 3D printing technologies – digital light processing (DLP), SLA, SLS, SSE, and FDM – Januskaite et al. examined the visual preferences of youngsters ranging from 4 to 11 years old in 2020. In terms of aesthetic appeal, the survey ranked DLP printlets first, followed by SLS, FDM, and SSE. When told that the SSE printlet could be chewed, most kids (79%) switched to that option, suggesting that they prefer that kind of dose form [17].

In 2019, a clinical study at the University of Santiago de Compostela in Spain used a 3D printer to create personalized therapies for maple syrup urine disease in children aged 3–16. Specifically, the purpose of the research was to investigate the severe metabolic disease that prevents the body from digesting certain amino acids, which results in the buildup of hazardous substances in the blood and urine. The technology could be beneficial for elderly populations or those on complex dosing regimens with high tablet burden.

Research has demonstrated that polypharmacy can result in non-adherence and perplexity among patients, which increases the likelihood of dosing errors [18, 19].

3D printing is a fast prototyping technique that may be used to assess individual or small batches of different versions of pharmaceutical products throughout the development of preclinical and clinical formulations. This may accelerate the evaluation of the impact of formulation compositions on crucial quality characteristics, such as medicine performance in laboratory and animal models. 3D-printed medicines have been assessed in several preclinical animal models, expediting the transition into first-in-human (FIH) clinical studies. This results in a decrease in both the duration and expenses of development as compared to traditional manufacturing methods. 3D printing may be used in preclinical and early-phase clinical studies to produce tiny, customizable therapeutic items as needed, allowing for the evaluation of their safety and effectiveness [20–22]. Studies have effectively used 3D printing to produce drugs with restricted therapeutic indices, such as warfarin, levothyroxine, and tacrolimus, in dose-flexible formulations [23].

12.2 3D Printing in Healthcare and Pharma

The pharmaceutical sector's most prospective implementation of 3DP is the customization of dosage forms, which enables the development of personalized medication regimens. This is accomplished by modifying the release profiles of the dosage forms, adjusting the concentrations and their combinations, or fabricating them to meet the needs of patients and special patient populations. Several formulations are customized using 3DP technology to ensure that the optimal dose is administered to the patient, as the therapeutic dose varies based on the body weight and age of the children. The quantity of liquid API dispensed is adjusted in Oro dispersible film (ODF) formulations to achieve this. The medications can be further customized by modifying the geometry and dimensions of these ODFs. Furthermore, the dosage intensity in other dosage forms can be adjusted to accommodate the patient's needs. For instance, a study employed HME and FDM to print theophylline tablets in a range of 60–300 mg by adjusting the printing scale [24, 25].

In recent years, attempts have been made to divide tablets by hand or with a splitter in order to attain the intended dose range. Nevertheless, it has been demonstrated to be ineffective due to the fact that divided tablets do not adhere to the pharmacopeial standards. Additionally, the combination and encapsulation of two distinct medications has been facilitated by the development of personalized 3DP granules or mini-printlets. The 3DP process is the most patient-centric manufacturing technique as a result of the quintessential reasons that enable the customization of medication doses, thereby ensuring the utmost safety and efficacy for patients [26].

3D printing advancements have revolutionized medicine creation, personalized implants, and prostheses. Spritam©, the initial 3D-printed product, has earned attention for its 3D-printed dosage forms, including tablets and capsules. Additionally, 3D printing is being used to create personalized implants tailored to fit specific anatomical dimensions, while 4D printing, which incorporates the element of time, is being investigated for applications like implants that can change shape within the body. These developments hold promise for various medical and healthcare applications, including tissue engineering, organ-on-chip technologies, and more.

12.3 3D Printing of Personalized Medicines

The printing materials' medication loading and quality attributes must be considered while 3D printing medicinal inks. FDM printing requires a flexible filament that can be extruded and loaded with a steady medicine dose to create solid dosage forms. The filament melts in the printer's extrusion head and may be layered to produce the design. The quality of 3D-printed solid dosage forms depends on medication stability during the procedure, while the production of sufficient units depends on printing time. Oral solid dose forms take 7–15 minutes to print, significantly less than industrial tablet presses, but may cost more than generic compressed pills due to their higher production time. Although FDM printers are cheaper, maintaining the quality and disinfection of printed medications may be difficult. The M3DIMAKER is the only GMP-compliant medication 3D printer available for under EUR 80,000. FabRx prints blister packaging to reduce cross-contamination. Pharmaceutical-grade excipients with clear audit trails are needed to make drugs or drug-loaded filaments, restricting manufacturing methods. Regulatory agencies and ethical committees have little experience with these items, and 3D-printed solid dosage forms may fail pharmacopoeia tests like disintegration. Health workers must be trained in 3D printing technology to assure quality printed drugs. Successful clinical translation of this technology requires appropriate point-of-care training. Some of the examples of 3D technologies used for personalized medicines are illustrated in Fig. 12.2 [27, 28].

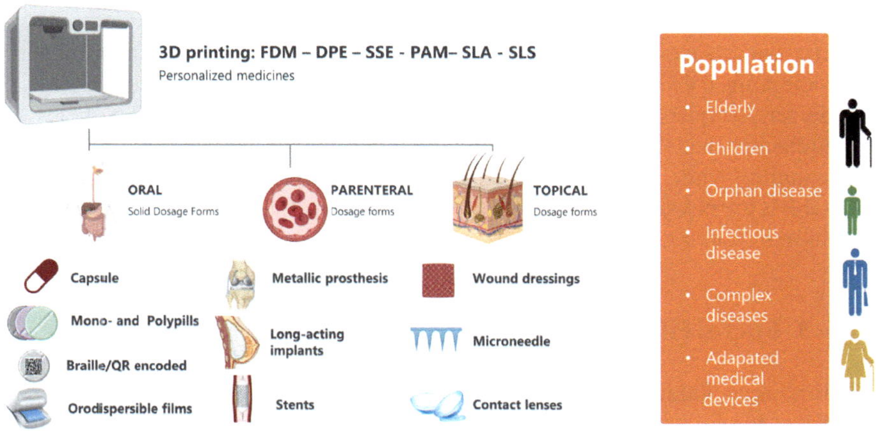

Fig. 12.2 Advanced 3D technologies for personalized medicines. (Serrano et al. [27]. Application of 3D printing technologies to manufacture personalized medicines. Digital image. https://www.mdpi.com/2077292. Accessed 19 July 2024)

12.3.1 Tablets

Powder binder jetting is the only 3D printing technique now used at the industrial scale for commercial purposes.

Aprecia Labs uses this technique to produce Spritam, a 1000 mg oral dispersible tablet that contains levetiracetam. The tablet is fabricated by combining a powdered substrate with a liquid adhesive, causing them to adhere to one another. The tablet is printed directly into containers, eliminating the requirement for dosage forms or the recirculation of unprinted powder. The automated zip dosage assembly method removes the tablet's outer shell and cap, enabling fast swallowing and effectiveness [28].

12.3.2 Polypills

Polypills are individualized solid pharmaceutical formulations that consolidate many drugs into a solitary tablet while modifying the dosage and release characteristics. They are commonly used for treating metabolic syndrome, infectious diseases, and pain. FDM is the top 3D printing technique for manufacturing polypills due to its ease of implementation, no need for postprocessing, and suitable characteristics for tensile strength and drug release profile modification [29].

Polypills for Parkinson's disease have been made utilizing hot-melt extrusion and FDM techniques, including three medications: levodopa, benserazide, and pramipexole. These pills may have four or more Active Pharmaceutical Ingredients (APIs), such as lisinopril and amlodipine for treating hypertension, indapamide as a diuretic, and rosuvastatin for managing dyslipidemia. Filaments were manufactured by combining PVA and sorbitol, with distilled water serving as a temporary co-plasticizer. A triphasic polypill has been created for people with type 2 diabetes and hypertension, including captopril, glipizide, and nifedipine. Captopril is excreted via mannitol, while glipizide and nifedipine are absorbed via a hydrophilic matrix. The tablets are physically segregated by a layer consisting of croscarmellose sodium and sodium starch glycolate [30].

12.3.3 Buccal Films

3D printing techniques are effective in producing oral dispersible films, especially beneficial for patients with deglutition issues. The technique of single-screw extrusion (SSE) is used to produce films in a sequential manner using maltodextrin, sorbitol, and hydroxyethyl cellulose as the materials. QR codes and data matrices may be used to validate solid dosage forms, allowing for precise track and trace measurement management. Additionally, Braille and Moon patterns may be printed to facilitate tablet identification [31, 32].

3D-printed tablets have shown promise in manufacturing medications for uncommon orphan illnesses such as maple syrup urine disease, which involves supplementing isoleucine and valine in children's treatment. These tablets show lower variability and higher patient acceptability compared to conventional capsules. This suggests the potential of 3D printing in creating personalized solid dosage forms for rare metabolic disorders. Pharmaceutical businesses are now allocating resources towards the development of 3D printing technologies. One such company, Triastek, located in China, is actively involved in a clinical study aimed at 3D printing a specific oral medicine for ulcerative colitis that targets the colon. Nevertheless, the majority of current studies are focused upon the advancement of customized prostheses and medical equipment [33].

12.3.4 Implants

Biodegradable polymers such as PLA, PGA, PVA, and PCL have the ability to be used in the production of durable implants and stents. These synthetic polymers have a prolonged breakdown period inside the human body compared to natural polymers. FDM 3D printing has effectively produced a range of APIs, including hormones, cytostatics, anesthetics, and antimicrobials. Implants made from PVA and PLA, created using 3D printing technology, remained intact for a period of 300 days. Personalized vaginal rings, made from PLA, PCL and polysorbate 80, exhibited extended release properties. Additionally, 3D-printed scaffolds designed for breast cancer treatment demonstrated continuous release of cytostatic medicines for more than 30 days. Antimicrobials may be applied to biodegradable stents to hinder infection and minimize adverse effects after surgery [34].

12.4 3D Printing Applications in Biopharmaceuticals

The expanding biopharmaceutical sector is revolutionizing the use of 3D printing in tissue engineering, namely in the context of organ-on-chip (PAM) applications. Peptides and proteins are used for the purpose of regenerating cartilage and bone. However, the integration of these substances with cell-based scaffolds has shown enhancements in the creation of both cartilage and bone tissues. Cartilage healing has been facilitated by constructing bilayer porous scaffolds using Gel MA hydrogels, whereas subchondral regeneration has been achieved using hydroxyapatite. PLA scaffolds have been improved by applying a coating of BMP-2-derived peptides that are linked to dopamine, resulting in increased bone formation [35, 36].

Hydrogels, formed by a non-thermal process, use water as the only medium. The design of peptide hydrogels centers on modifying the amphiphilic balance of the backbone sequence, which enables the gelation process to occur naturally. Interactions such as hydrogen bonding, electrostatic interactions, and aromatic stacking induce the folding of proteins into their native conformations, leading to the formation of secondary structures such as α-helices, β-sheets, and hairpin motifs [37, 38].

Researchers are now working on creating solid dosage forms utilizing 3D printing technology that include biopharmaceuticals. One example is a tablet designed to treat ulcerative colitis by releasing the medication in the ileo-colonic region. Research used polymeric microneedle patches fabricated using stereolithography (SLA) to improve the transdermal administration of insulin. The microneedles had dimensions of 1 mm in length and 1 mm in diameter. To reduce toxicity, a biocompatible Class I resin was used. The process of post-printing included immersing the object in isopropyl alcohol and exposing it to UV light in order to eliminate any remaining unpolymerized resin. Insulin exhibited complete and immediate release for a duration of more than 30 minutes after its application to pig skin. Multiunit implants, created by 3D printing using polycaprolactone, lauric acid, and melanin, allow for the regulated administration of protein drugs through remote light activation. The implants exhibited encouraging outcomes in an in vivo model of a diabetic mouse, effectively reducing blood glucose levels over many days [39].

12.4.1 Nanomedicines

Nanomedicines are being produced using 3D printing technologies; however, the concentration of nanoparticles is critical due to the possibility of aggregations and defects. The presence of nanoparticle attractions and Van der Waals-induced aggregations poses a hurdle when trying to integrate nanoparticles with high drug-loading capacity into a polymer matrix. Particle homogeneity may be enhanced through preprocessing procedures such as ultrasound, surfactants, and ball milling. The hydrogel contains polymeric PCL nanocapsules, which were combined with redispersible 3D-printed solid dosage forms. These dosage forms contained polyphenols, namely, curcumin and resveratrol. However, the release of all active components was not fully achieved, which was a difficult obstacle to overcome. Curcumin, a compound encapsulated inside liposomes, was also deposited into tissue scaffolds created using 3D printing technology. This resulted in significant cytotoxicity against osteosarcoma and the promotion of osteoblast viability [40].

12.5 FDM Technology in Pharmaceuticals

Various preparations, including 3D-printed tablets, aripiprazole oral dispersion films, and controlled-release formulations, have been extensively prepared using FDM technology. The preliminary investigation assessed the level of approval among patients for 3D-printed tablets with different forms and sizes. The findings suggested that smaller, circular pills were more enjoyable to consume. In 2015, Goyanes et al. used FDM technology to fabricate multilayer capsules and double capsules, with caffeine and paracetamol as prototype medications. The FDM technique has been used in transdermal medicine administration as well. Goyanes et al. created personalized nasal covers specifically designed for treating acne, while

Muwaffak et al. used 3D printing technology to produce wound dressings shaped like the nose and ear. In vitro tests showed that 3D-printed films have increased disintegration rates. FDM technology has also been used in the realm of transdermal medicine administration, leading to the creation of personalized nose shields and wound dressings. Figure 12.3 shows some of the tablets prepared by FDM technology in different sizes and 3D-printed samples [41].

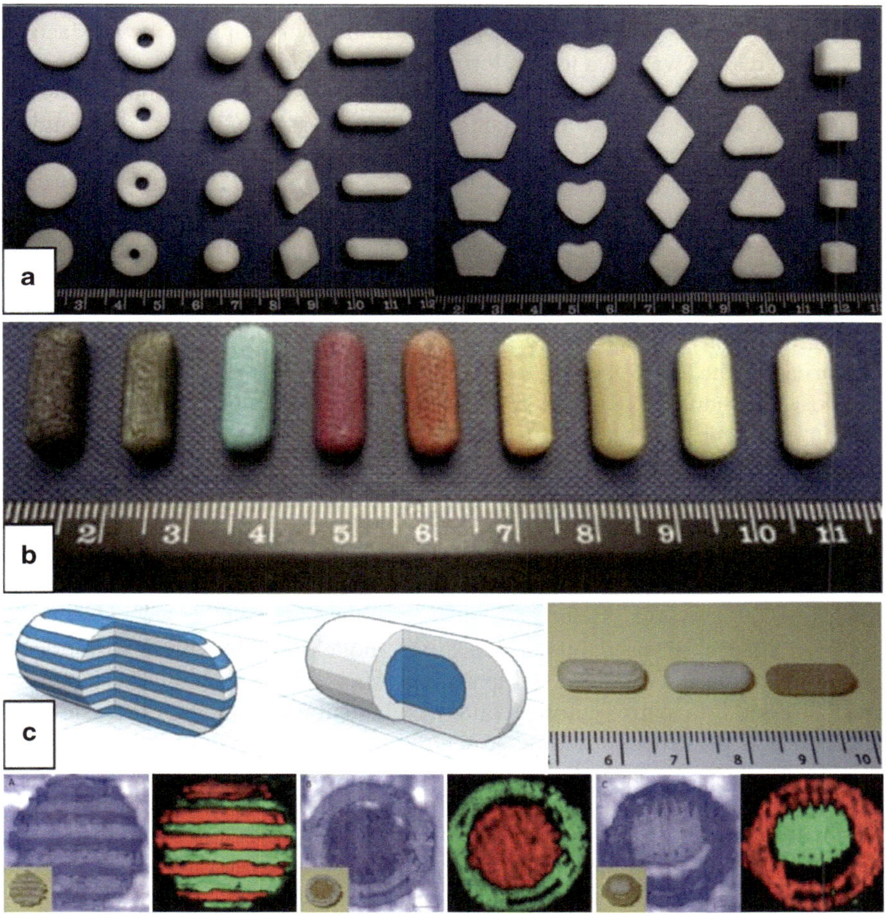

Fig. 12.3 Photographs showcasing a wide range of tablets created using FDM technology: (**a**) Photographs depicting a variety of 3D-printed devices in different shapes and sizes. (**b**) Section showcases images of 3D-printed grains in capsule shape, exhibiting a range of hues. (**c**) The photographs include 3-D-printed samples, white light images, 2-dimensional Raman mapping images, as well as images of sectioned multilayer devices and sectioned DuoCaplet models. (Wang et al. [42]. Images of various types of tablets prepared by FDM technology: (**a**) Images of 3D-printed tablets with different shapes and sizes; (**b**) images of 3D-printed tablets in capsule form with different colors; (**c**) sectioned multilayer device and sectioned DuoCaplet (caplet in caplet) model images, 3D-printed preparations, and white light and 2-dimensional Raman mapping images. Digital image. https://www.mdpi.com/2094830. Accessed 22 July 2024)

12.6 FDM Technology for Oral Personalized Dosage Form by Passive Diffusion Method

Passive diffusion was used as a loading technique for filaments printed using FDM technology in clinical settings to fabricate personalized oral medicines. The researchers developed a pre-screening tool that utilizes Hansen Solubility Parameters (HSP) and HSP distances (Ra) to determine the optimal combination of drug, solvent, and filament for achieving high drug loading rates. Surface irregularity and stiffness greatly enhance passive diffusion. A Support Vector Machine (SVM) regression was used to develop a prediction model for medication loading. The findings demonstrate a strong association between the roughness average (Ra) and the rigidity of the filament, as well as the ability of a model Biopharmaceutics Classification System (BCS) Class II medication, nifedipine (NFD), to diffuse. An approximate drug dose of 3% by weight was achieved. The dissolving and chemical stability of 3D-printed granules generated using PVA-derived filament showed promising results. The research suggests that combining FDM (fused deposition modeling) with passive diffusion in clinical settings may be easily achieved to create customized drugs that are customized to meet individual requirements [43].

Spritam®, the FDA-approved first 3D-printed pill, is powered by Aprecia's ZipDose® Technology platform. This novel approach employs three-dimensional printing to generate a porous formulation that dissolves with a liquid drink, thereby delivering a high drug dosage of up to 1000 mg in a single dose. The platform, which was created using 3DP technology from the Massachusetts Institute of Technology, employs a layer-by-layer powder bed fusion system. The first layer contains the active pharmaceutical ingredient and excipients, while succeeding layers contain a binder liquid, ensuring optimal integration and aggregation [44].

Xuyu Chai et al. used fusion deposition modeling 3D printing to fabricate intragastric sustained-release tablets containing domperidone. These tablets were inserted into hydroxypropyl cellulose filament using hot melt extrusion and subsequently printed into hollow-structured tablets. Skowyra et al. have shown that fused deposition modeling is capable of printing PVA filaments with extended drug release of prednisolone for a period of up to 24 h following oral administration. This technology is also effective for 4-ASA and 5-aminosalicylic acid (5-ASA). Nevertheless, the high temperature necessary for operation can degrade a significant number of pharmaceutical excipients and active medications. Pietrzak et al. used hot melt extrusion with fused deposition modeling (3D printing) to expand the range of polymers and enhance medication dosing. They effectively proved that it is possible to print theophylline caplets with both immediate and prolonged release capabilities, with a pharmacological payload of 50% [26, 45].

12.7 3D Printing in Hospitals

3D printing, also known as additive manufacturing (AM), is a commonly used prototype technique in hospitals for creating therapeutic, diagnostic, and instructional tools. It is more adaptable than conventional fabrication technologies and provides a flexible alternative for low production quantities, despite its limited mass-production capacity. 3D printing has the ability to create a wide range of items and gadgets without the additional costs and time required by conventional technologies. Additionally, it has the ability to create patient-specific structures that are tailored to the individual anatomy and treatment of a patient. This makes it very important for creating customized surgical instruments, anatomical models, implants, research tools, and on-demand components in the medical industry [46].

The 3D printing facility at a hospital has the capacity to build novel clinical and research prospects, immediately address unforeseen needs, and provide fresh therapeutic chances. During the COVID-19 epidemic, hospitals and small enterprises used 3D printing to produce essential supplies, including nasopharyngeal diagnostic probes, face shields, and viral filter adapters. 3D printing is an essential tool for hospitals to enhance their ability to adapt to both routine clinical operations and emergency situations, hence improving their operational resilience and healthcare infrastructure. The system provides advanced healthcare solutions that may be used in both typical and atypical clinical circumstances, as well as research and development and hospital support services [47, 48].

12.7.1 Standard Clinical Cases [49–51]

Clinical applications, including custom-made or patient-specific devices, should have standard operating procedures outlining the ordering, fabrication, post-processing, sterilization, delivery, and usage of prints.

12.7.1.1 Anatomical Models

Anatomical models created via 3D printing are extensively used in hospitals to aid in preoperative planning and provide guidance during surgical procedures. They enhance the localization of tumors, decrease the duration and expenses of operating room procedures, increase surgeons' confidence, and improve patient outcomes. An example of this is the use of a three-dimensional pelvic model, which provides a visual representation of the tumor's spatial connection to adjacent bones, nerves, arteries, and veins. This approach saves time and minimizes the risk of problems.

12.7.1.2 Surgical Instruments

Dental surgical instruments are used in the field of medicine to divide and represent the unique anatomical features of patients for reconstructive surgeries. The dental implant drilling sites and depths are aligned using biocompatible resin and press-fit metal bushings. Alternative landmarks may be used, and 3D modeling software is employed to generate the suitable model. Upon completion, the guides enhance the efficiency of operations by optimizing factors such as drill location, angle, and depth. This enables the clinician to adhere to a digitally prepared surgical technique.

12.7.1.3 Boluses of Radiation Treatment

High-energy radiation treatment in cancer patients necessitates delivering precise doses either at the skin surface or with low penetration depth. Bolusing is used; nevertheless, conventional sheets often result in the presence of voids. The use of 3D printing technology for the production of boluses enables the scanning of patients and minimizes the presence of air spaces. An instance may be seen in a situation involving nasal cancer, where the use of a 3D-printed bolus ensured accurate administration of the prescribed dosage to the affected area while simultaneously minimizing the radiation exposure to surrounding tissues such as the brain.

12.7.1.4 Brachytherapy Applicators

Brachytherapy is an essential therapeutic modality for rectal and vaginal/cervical malignancies, including the administration of concentrated radiation directly to the affected area. Conventional applicators provide many methods of therapy but do not have the ability to be adjusted according to the individual needs of each patient. 3D printing enables customization of applicator dimensions, form, and needle path to accommodate variations in anatomy or atypical physiology. A 3D-printed vaginal brachytherapy applicator is designed with customized lumens to ensure accurate placement of the radiation source and a patient-specific anatomical design. The primary implement, collets, and set screw are produced by 3D printing using an SLA printer, using biocompatible resin [52].

12.7.2 Nonstandard Clinical Cases

Clinical applications, often unforeseen or unique situations, are non-standard cases with no defined workflow and do not frequently repeat. These applications can also include educational tools for healthcare providers in training. Unconventional uses of anatomical models, tools, and guides might vary from uncommon heart problems in infants to assisting in the separation of twins. These applications may need different specifications, purposes, or additional steps to be completed, even if they have similarities with traditional procedures.

12.7.3 Research and Development

Hospital R&D and training involve various applications, including training, testing, experimentation, and prototyping. 3D printing is crucial for these applications, ranging from simple mounts to full anatomical models. The use of 3D printing technology in radiation oncology and medical physics is quickly progressing for the purpose of creating imaging phantoms, which are used for testing, quality assurance, and plan verification. Customized CT or MR phantoms are produced by adjusting their parameters, even if commercially supplied phantoms are expensive and not widely accessible.

12.7.4 Hospital Support Services

This category encompasses apps that specifically address the operational requirements of hospitals, excluding medical equipment or applications actively involved in clinical care. Smaller hospitals worldwide are increasingly using these support services, even though they were originally designed for larger research facilities [53].

12.8 FDM-Based Bioprinting of Implant Transplantation Devices and Prosthetics

Particularly in the bioprinting of tissues and organs for transplantation, the function of additive manufacturing technique (AMT) in personalized medicine is essential. FDM-based 3DP layers living cells to engineer tissue in accordance with a blueprint. Bone, heart, skin, and tracheal grafts have been manufactured using bioprinting [54, 55].

AMTs are essential in the field of biomedicine for the development of prosthetics, which enables the creation of engineered and personalized extremities. Orthopedic obstacles are effectively resolved through the efficient generation of customized prostheses through three-dimensional printing. Studies have employed 3D printing to develop modular prostheses for the femur and joint, which have led to a painless recovery and optimal weight-bearing capacity. The procedure typically commences with medical imaging, segmentation, 3D scanning, and 3D modeling [56–58].

12.9 Integration of Solid Dispersion with FDM Additive Manufacturing

API-polymer admixture is essential for the implementation of solid dispersion technology and FDM. A linked technology has the capacity to combine the advantages of both approaches into a unified solution. Currently, the solid dispersion technique is being researched as a means to get API-loaded filament for FDM additive manufacturing. Although not widely acknowledged, this technology has the capacity to expand the scope of APIs that may be compared to FDM. Methods such as hot melt extrusion (HME), melting or fusion, solvent evaporation, supercritical fluid, lyophilization, and electrospinning can be used to create solid dispersions. These dispersions can include substances like polyvinylpyrrolidone (PVP), polyethylene glycol (PEG), hydroxypropyl cellulose (HPC), hydroxypropyl methylcellulose acetyl succinate (HMPC-AS), and hydroxypropyl methylcellulose (HPMC). Studies have shown that the solubility of pharmaceuticals may be increased by carefully choosing dispersants in the correct proportions. For instance, the process of griseofulvin dissolving from PVP solid dispersions was improved by a factor of 11 when using a drug/carrier ratio of 1:20. The market for goods such as fenofibrate, duloxetine, and vemurafenib showcases the capacity of solid dispersions to improve the solubility of drugs [59].

12.10 Conclusion

Fused deposition modeling (FDM) 3D printing is revolutionizing the pharmaceutical sector by enabling customized treatment, enhancing therapeutic results, and increasing patient adherence. The technique has the ability to create complex drug formulations, such as multi-drug tablets with controlled release profiles. Additionally, its fast prototyping capabilities have greatly decreased the time and expenses involved in bringing novel formulations to the market. Easy-to-ingest dosage forms are advantageous for certain patient populations, including pediatric and geriatric patients, as they enhance medication adherence and comfort. Deploying FDM printers in remote locations has opened new avenues for on-demand manufacturing, providing essential medicines in underserved areas and enhancing global health equity. However, technical issues such as material limitations and print quality require ongoing research and collaboration between industry stakeholders and regulatory bodies. The future of FDM 3D printing in pharmaceuticals has great promise, since it signifies a shift towards customized, efficient, and easily available treatment.

References

1. Hsiao W-K, Lorber B, Reitsamer H, Khinast J. 3D printing of oral drugs: a new reality or hype? Expert Opin Drug Deliv. 2017;15(1):1–4. https://doi.org/10.1080/17425247.2017.1371698.
2. Scoutaris N, Ross S, Douroumis D. Current trends on medical and pharmaceutical applications of inkjet printing technology. Pharm Res. 2016;33:1799–816.
3. Zhang J, Vo AQ, Feng X, Bandari S, Repka MA. Pharmaceutical additive manufacturing: a novel tool for complex and personalized drug delivery systems. AAPS PharmSciTech. 2018;19:3388–402.
4. Awad A, Trenfield SJ, Gaisford S, Basit AW. 3D printed medicines: a new branch of digital healthcare. Int J Pharm. 2018;548(1):586–96.
5. Konta AA, García-Piña M, Serrano DR. Personalised 3D printed medicines: which techniques and polymers are more successful? Bioengineering. 2017;4(4):79.
6. Shafiee A, Atala A. Printing technologies for medical applications. Trends Mol Med. 2016;22(3):254–65.
7. Pawar R, Pawar A. 3D printing of pharmaceuticals: approach from bench scale to commercial development. Futur J Pharm Sci. 2022;8(1):48.

8. Jamróz W, Szafraniec J, Kurek M, Jachowicz R. 3D printing in pharmaceutical and medical applications–recent achievements and challenges. Pharm Res. 2018;35:1–22.
9. Samiei N. Recent trends on applications of 3D printing technology on the design and manufacture of pharmaceutical oral formulation: a mini review. Beni-Suef Univ J Basic Appl Sci. 2020;9:1–12.
10. Trenfield SJ, Awad A, Goyanes A, Gaisford S, Basit AW. 3D printing pharmaceuticals: drug development to frontline care. Trends Pharmacol Sci. 2018;39(5):440–51.
11. Robles-Martinez P, Xu X, Trenfield SJ, et al. 3D printing of a multi-layered polypill containing six drugs using a novel stereolithographic method. Pharmaceutics. 2019a;11:274. https://doi.org/10.3390/pharmaceutics11060274.
12. Gioumouxouzis CI, Baklavaridis A, Katsamenis OL, Markopoulou CK, Bouropoulos N, Tzetzis D, Fatouros DG. A 3D printed bilayer oral solid dosage form combining metformin for prolonged and glimepiride for immediate drug delivery. Eur J Pharm Sci. 2018;120:40–52.
13. Tagami T, Ito E, Kida R, Hirose K, Noda T, Ozeki T. 3D printing of gummy drug formulations composed of gelatin and an HPMC-based hydrogel for pediatric use. Int J Pharm. 2021;594:120118.
14. Breitkreutz J, Boos J. Paediatric and geriatric drug delivery. Expert Opin Drug Deliv. 2007;4(1):37–45.
15. Aita E, Ilias JR, Breitkreutz J, Quodbach J. 3D-printing with precise layer-wise dose adjustments for paediatric use via pressure-assisted microsyringe printing. Eur J Pharm Biopharm. 2020;157:59–65.
16. Karavasili C, Gkaragkounis A, Moschakis T, Ritzoulis C, Fatouros DG. Pediatric-friendly chocolate-based dosage forms for the oral administration of both hydrophilic and lipophilic drugs fabricated with extrusion-based 3D printing. Eur J Pharm Sci. 2020;147:105291.
17. Januskaite P, Xiaoyan X, Ranmal SR, Gaisford S, Basit AW, Tuleu C, Goyanes A. I spy with my little eye: a paediatric visual preferences survey of 3D printed tablets. Pharmaceutics. 2020;12(11):1100.
18. Goyanes A, Madla CM, Umerji A, Piñeiro GD, Montero JMG, Diaz MJL, Barcia MG, et al. Automated therapy preparation of isoleucine formulations using 3D printing for the treatment of MSUD: first single-centre, prospective, crossover study in patients. Int J Pharm. 2019;567:118497.
19. Maher RL, Hanlon J, Hajjar ER. Clinical consequences of polypharmacy in elderly. Expert Opin Drug Saf. 2014;13(1):57–65.
20. Seoane-Viaño I, Trenfield SJ, Basit AW, Goyanes A. Translating 3D printed pharmaceuticals: from hype to real-world clinical applications. Adv Drug Deliv Rev. 2021a;174:553–75.
21. Goyanes A, Fernández-Ferreiro A, Majeed A, Gomez-Lado N, Awad A, Luaces-Rodríguez A, Gaisford S, Aguiar P, Basit AW. PET/CT imaging of 3D printed devices in the gastrointestinal tract of rodents. Int J Pharm. 2018;536(1):158–64.
22. Shin S, Kim TH, Jeong SW, Chung SE, Lee DY, Kim D-H, Shin BS. Development of a gastroretentive delivery system for acyclovir by 3D printing technology and its in vivo pharmacokinetic evaluation in beagle dogs. PLoS One. 2019;14(5):e0216875.
23. Seoane-Viaño I, Ong JJ, Luzardo-Álvarez A, González-Barcia M, Basit AW, Otero-Espinar FJ, Goyanes A. 3D printed tacrolimus suppositories for the treatment of ulcerative colitis. Asian J Pharm Sci. 2021b;16(1):11.
24. Varghese R, Sood P, Salvi S, Karsiya J, Kumar D. 3D printing in the pharmaceutical sector: advances and evidences. Sens Int. 2022;3:100177.
25. Keerthi ML, Shireesh Kiran R, V. Uma Maheshwar Rao, Aparna Sannapu, A. Geetha Dutt, and K. Sai Krishna. Pharmaceutical mini-tablets, its advantages, formulation possibilities and general evaluation aspects: a review. Int J Pharm Sci Rev Res. 2014;28(1):214–21.
26. Pietrzak K, Isreb A, Alhnan MA. A flexible-dose dispenser for immediate and extended release 3D printed tablets. Eur J Pharm Biopharm. 2015;96:380–7.

27. Serrano DR, Kara A, Yuste I, Luciano FC, Ongoren B, Anaya BJ, Molina G, et al. 3D printing technologies in personalized medicine, nanomedicines, and biopharmaceuticals. Pharmaceutics. 2023;15(2):313.
28. Ayyoubi S, Cerda JR, Fernández-García R, Knief P, Lalatsa A, Healy AM, Serrano DR. 3D printed spherical mini-tablets: geometry versus composition effects in controlling dissolution from personalised solid dosage forms. Int J Pharm. 2021;597:120336.
29. Windolf H, Chamberlain R, Breitkreutz J, Quodbach J. 3D printed mini-floating-Polypill for Parkinson's disease: combination of levodopa, benserazide, and pramipexole in various dosing for personalized therapy. Pharmaceutics. 2022;14(5):931.
30. Robles-Martinez P, Xiaoyan X, Trenfield SJ, Awad A, Goyanes A, Telford R, Basit AW, Gaisford S. 3D printing of a multi-layered polypill containing six drugs using a novel stereolithographic method. Pharmaceutics. 2019b;11(6):274.
31. Russi L, Gaudio C. 3D printed multicompartmental capsules for a progressive drug release. Ann 3D Print Med. 2021;3:100026.
32. Elbl J, Gajdziok J, Kolarczyk J. 3D printing of multilayered orodispersible films with in-process drying. Int J Pharm. 2020;575:118883.
33. Goh O, Goh WJ, Lim SH, Hoo GS, Liew R, Ng TM. Preferences of healthcare professionals on 3D-printed tablets: a pilot study. Pharmaceutics. 2022;14(7):1521.
34. Liu Y, Du T, Qiao A, Mu Y, Yang H. Zinc-based biodegradable materials for orthopaedic internal fixation. J Funct Biomater. 2022;13:164.
35. Qiao X, Yang Y, Huang R, Shi X, Chen H, Wang J, Chen Y, Tan Y, Tan Z. E-jet 3D-printed scaffolds as sustained multi-drug delivery vehicles in breast cancer therapy. Pharm Res. 2019;36:1–16.
36. Xu H, Wang C, Liu C, Li J, Peng Z, Guo J, Zhu L. Stem cell-seeded 3D-printed scaffolds combined with self-assembling peptides for bone defect repair. Tissue Eng Part A. 2022;28:111–24.
37. Murphy RD, Garcia RV, Heise A, Hawker CJ. Peptides as 3D printable feedstocks: design strategies and emerging applications. Prog Polym Sci. 2022;124:101487.
38. Song X, Li X, Wang F, Wang L, Lv L, Xie Q, Zhang X, Shao X. Bioinspired protein/peptide loaded 3D printed PLGA scaffold promotes bone regeneration. Front Bioeng Biotechnol. 2022;10:832727.
39. Uddin MJ, Scoutaris N, Economidou SN, Giraud C, Chowdhry BZ, Donnelly RF, Douroumis D. 3D printed microneedles for anticancer therapy of skin tumours. Mater Sci Eng C. 2020;107:110248.
40. Fisusi FA, Siew A, Chooi KW, Okubanjo O, Garrett N, Lalatsa K, Serrano D, et al. Lomustine nanoparticles enable both bone marrow sparing and high brain drug levels – a strategy for brain cancer treatments. Pharm Res. 2016;33:1289–303.
41. Syrlybayev D, Zharylkassyn B, Seisekulova A, Akhmetov M, Perveen A, Talamona D. Optimisation of strength properties of FDM printed parts – a critical review. Polymers. 2021;13(10):1587.
42. Wang S, Chen X, Han X, Hong X, Li X, Zhang H, Li M, Wang Z, Zheng A. A review of 3D printing technology in pharmaceutics: technology and applications, now and future. Pharmaceutics. 2023;15(2):416.
43. Cerda JR, Arifi T, Ayyoubi S, Knief P, Ballesteros MP, Keeble W, Barbu E, Healy AM, Lalatsa A, Serrano DR. Personalised 3D printed medicines: optimising material properties for successful passive diffusion loading of filaments for fused deposition modelling of solid dosage forms. Pharmaceutics. 2020;12(4):345.
44. Jose PA, Peter Christoper GV. 3D printing of pharmaceuticals–a potential technology in developing personalized medicine. Asian J Pharm Res Dev. 2018;6(3):46–54.
45. Skowyra J, Pietrzak K, Alhnan MA. Fabrication of extended-release patient-tailored prednisolone tablets via fused deposition modelling (FDM) 3D printing. Eur J Pharm Sci. 2015;68:11–7.
46. Tack P, Victor J, Gemmel P, Annemans L. 3D-printing techniques in a medical setting: a systematic literature review. Biomed Eng Online. 2016;15:1–21.

47. Ganapathy A, Chen D, Elumalai A, Albers B, Tappa K, Jammalamadaka U, Hoegger MJ, Ballard DH. Guide for starting or optimizing a 3D printing clinical service. Methods. 2022;206:41–52.
48. Ravi P, Burch MB, Farahani S, Chepelev LL, Yang D, Ali A, Joyce JR, et al. Utility and costs during the initial year of 3D printing in an academic hospital. J Am Coll Radiol. 2023;20(2):193–204.
49. Ballard DH, Mills P, Duszak R Jr, Weisman JA, Rybicki FJ, Woodard PK. Medical 3D printing cost-savings in orthopedic and maxillofacial surgery: cost analysis of operating room time saved with 3D printed anatomic models and surgical guides. Acad Radiol. 2020;27(8):1103–13.
50. Hellman S, Frisch P, Platzman A, Booth P. 3D printing in a hospital: centralized clinical implementation and applications for comprehensive care. Digit Health. 2023;9:20552076231221899.
51. Inserra A, Borro L, Spada M, Frediani S, Secinaro A. Advanced 3D modeling and printing for the surgical planning of a successful case of thoraco-omphalopagus conjoined twins separation. Front Physiol. 2020;11:566766.
52. Pratt EC, Skubal M, Larney BM, Causa-Andrieu P, Das S, Sawan P, Araji A, et al. Prospective testing of clinical Cerenkov luminescence imaging against standard-of-care nuclear imaging for tumour location. Nat Biomed Eng. 2022;6(5):559–68.
53. Sta Agueda JRH, Chen Q, Maalihan RD, Ren J, da Silva ÍGM, Dugos NP, Caldona EB, Advincula RC. 3D printing of biomedically relevant polymer materials and biocompatibility. MRS Commun. 2021;11(2):197–212.
54. Akmal JS, Salmi M, Mäkitie A, Björkstrand R, Partanen J. Implementation of industrial additive manufacturing: intelligent implants and drug delivery systems. J Funct Biomater. 2018;9(3):41.
55. Ventola CL. Medical applications for 3D printing: current and projected uses. Pharm Ther. 2014;39:704–11.
56. Salmi M. Additive manufacturing processes in medical applications. Materials. 2021;14(1):191.
57. Rosicky J, Grygar A, Chapcak P, Bouma T, Rosicky J. Application of 3D scanning in prosthetic and orthotic clinical practice. In: *Proceedings of the 7th international conference on 3D body scanning technologies*. Lugano, Switzerland, 30 November–1 December 2016. Hometrica Consulting—Dr. Nicola D'Apuzzo; 2016, pp. 88–97.
58. Akilbekova D, Mektepbayeva D. Patient specific in situ 3D printing. In: Kalaskar DM, editor. *3D printing in medicine*. Woodhead Publishing; 2017. p. 91–113.
59. Khalid GM, Billa N. Solid dispersion formulations by FDM 3D printing – a review. Pharmaceutics. 2022;14(4):690.

Future Prospective and Emerging Technologies in 3D Printing of Pharmaceuticals

13

Amrita Thakur, Neeta Rai, Kushagra Nagori,
Hemant Ramchandra Badwaik, Kartik Tularam Nakhate,
and Ayushman Roy

Abstract

The utilization of 3D printing in medicine has brought about profound changes, particularly in pharmaceuticals and dosage form design, offering cost-effective solutions. Techniques like stereolithography, hot melt extrusion, and bioprinting have revolutionized pharmaceutical production, enabling tailored treatment approaches. This technology facilitates personalized drug development and manufacturing, enhancing the efficacy of active pharmaceutical ingredients. Notably, 3D printing allows the evaluation of formulations using bio-printed organs, a significant advancement in pharmaceutical research. Moreover, medical devices such as pacemakers and dental implants benefit from 3D printing's precision and customization. This chapter provides an in-depth exploration of 3D printing's evolution, current applications, and future prospects, including advancements like 4D and 5D printing. Through detailed discussions, it aims to shed light on the transformative potential of 3D printing in medicine, from drug development to biomedical device manufacturing.

A. Thakur (✉) · N. Rai
Department of Pharmaceutics, Vishwakarma University, Pune, Maharashtra, India

K. Nagori
Rungta College of Pharmaceutical Sciences and Research, Bhilai, Chhattisgarh, India

H. R. Badwaik
Shri Shankaracharya Institute of Pharmaceutical Sciences and Research, Bhilai, India

K. T. Nakhate
Shri Vile Parle Kelavani Mandal's Institute of Pharmacy, Dhule, Maharashtra, India

A. Roy
Faculty of Pharmacy, Kalinga University, Naya Raipur, Chhattisgarh, India

K. Vinchurkar, S. Mane (eds.), *Innovations in Drug Manufacturing*,
https://doi.org/10.1007/978-981-96-9075-6_13

Keywords

3D printing · Stereolithography · Hot melt extrusion · Bioprinting · 4D–5D printing

13.1 Advanced 3D Printing Technologies

A new concept in the pharmaceutical sector has been introduced, which is called the 3D printing technique, or additive manufacturing (AM), solid-free technology, or rapid prototyping. This technique, according to the American Society for Testing Material (ASTM), uses a print head, nozzle, or another printing technology [1]. As we know, traditional dosage forms have been found to have limitations, which mainly involve failing to fulfill individual patients' requirements. Therefore, the 3D technique has been developed to address this problem and upgrade the conventional pharmaceutical formulation [2]. The 3D technique can be grouped into different techniques, which include bioprinting, digital light processing (DLP), extrusion-based fused deposition modeling (FDM), hot-melt extrusion (HME), inkjet-based 3DP, selective laser sintering (SLS), semi-solid extrusion (SSE), and stereolithography (SLA) [2]. These techniques are economical, easy to use, and facilitate on-demand printing of the pharmaceutical dosage forms [3]. A significant change in people's perceptions has been observed towards personalized medicine [4]. According to Pharmaceutical Point, 3D printing can be defined as a layer-by-layer creation of the dosage form using digital blueprints. In the early 1990s, a method was developed for layer-by-layer fabrication of solid structures [5].

The 3D printing uses computer-aided design (CAD) for depositing a single layer of the fed substrate on the platform. The base of the object is yielded when the printer nozzle ejects the fed substrate on an x–y plane. Thereafter, the printer head navigates along the z-axis depending upon the blueprint instructions to eject the liquid binder into the printer base till the required thickness is achieved. Clinging to the instructions transmitted by the CAD file on the computer, the whole process repeats multiple times till the desired dosage form is not achieved. The completion of the fabrication process is achieved when post-printing treatment, i.e., removal of the unbound substrate, is done.

Hence, the 3D printing technique enables highly reproducible dosage forms with a collection of materials and complex drug release kinetics [6]. A huge number of dosage forms, medical devices, and bio-printed scaffolds have been developed using the basic principle of the 3D technique [7]. Moreover, 3D printing techniques are used for preparing biosensors that help to measure the levels of glucose, lactate, sweat, etc. In addition to this, some wearable smart bandages also include the use of 3D-printed biosensors that measure oxygen saturation levels and electrocardiography (ECG) [8]. Figure 13.1 describes the different techniques and classifications of 3D printing techniques.

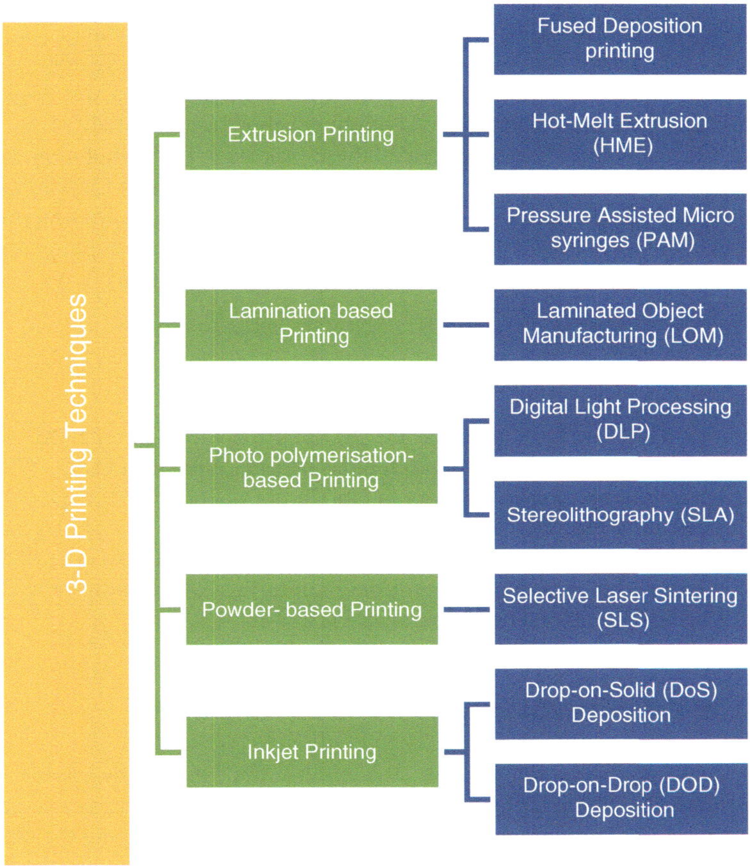

Fig. 13.1 Different 3D printing techniques and classification

13.2 Integration of Artificial Intelligence (AI) and Machine Learning

The growing interest in 3D printing technology for the manufacturing of personalized medicines and medical devices has gained keen interest within the health industry. However, it was observed that the procedure to develop these 3D printing formulations is time-consuming. Therefore, researchers now are actively searching for ways to utilize machine learning and AI for the utilization of formulation development along with 3D printing. For this, a balanced database for machine learning is very important to optimally predict the formulation to be developed.

Pattern recognition from large and complex datasets can be done by using machine learning, which is one of the applications of artificial learning. The studies showed that the AI/ML-based formulations have been getting more approval from the US Food and Drug Administration (FDA) in recent years at a very high speed [9]. HME and FDM are the forms of 3D printing techniques, and studies have shown that five ML techniques have accelerated these processes for formulation development. This study was performed by researchers from University College London. They utilize a dataset comprising 614 drug-loaded formulations by keeping three parameters – processing temperature (extrusion temperature and printing temperature), feedstock characteristics, and printability – in consideration.

13.2.1 Use of Machine Learning in 3D Printing

The integration of artificial intelligence (AI) and machine learning (ML) in 3D printing has opened new possibilities for the pharmaceutical industry. While 3D printing itself has proven revolutionary in fabricating customized drug products and medical devices, the introduction of AI and ML enhances the precision, efficiency, and scalability of these processes. These technologies contribute to optimized drug design, automated processes, and real-time monitoring, which altogether advance the pharmaceutical manufacturing paradigm [10].

13.2.2 AI-Enhanced Drug Design and Development

AI has shown immense potential in streamlining drug design by analyzing vast amounts of data and predicting outcomes more efficiently than traditional methods. In the context of 3D printing, AI algorithms can assist in optimizing the structural design of printed drug forms. For instance, AI-driven design processes allow for the customization of drug release profiles by predicting how specific geometries of a printed drug will behave in the human body. By analyzing patient-specific data such as metabolism and disease progression, AI models can design drug forms that offer personalized treatments [11].

Moreover, AI enhances the selection of materials for 3D printing. The traditional trial-and-error approach in selecting the right excipients or polymers for drug delivery can be replaced with AI-driven predictive models. These models evaluate the physical and chemical properties of potential materials to identify the best candidates for achieving desired release profiles or ensuring compatibility with active pharmaceutical ingredients (APIs) [12].

13.2.3 Optimizing the 3D Printing Process with AI and ML

AI and ML algorithms play a crucial role in optimizing the 3D printing process itself. One area where this integration has proven transformative is in error detection and correction during the printing process. AI algorithms can analyze data from sensors embedded in 3D printers to monitor for inconsistencies in layer deposition, temperature fluctuations, or structural defects. This real-time analysis allows for immediate adjustments, ensuring that the final product meets the required quality standards [13].

Additionally, AI-driven process control systems help in minimizing material wastage and improving energy efficiency. For example, ML algorithms can predict the optimal print settings (such as speed, temperature, and layer thickness) to achieve the best possible outcome, reducing the time required for manual fine-tuning of parameters [14]. This efficiency is particularly beneficial in pharmaceutical applications where precision and reproducibility are critical for patient safety.

13.2.4 AI-Powered Automation in Pharmaceutical 3D Printing

The pharmaceutical industry is increasingly exploring AI-powered automation to handle the complex and delicate processes involved in 3D printing drug formulations. Autonomous 3D printing systems, controlled by AI, are capable of monitoring and adjusting various parameters without human intervention. This level of automation not only increases throughput but also reduces human error, which is vital in the manufacturing of personalized medicines. For instance, AI systems can automatically adjust print parameters based on real-time feedback from the printer or the surrounding environment, ensuring optimal conditions for producing high-quality drug products. Additionally, automated systems can track multiple variables simultaneously—such as humidity, temperature, and material viscosity—allowing for more precise control of the printing environment [15].

13.3 Smartphone-Based 3D Printing Solutions

The advent of smartphone-based 3D printing solutions has revolutionized accessibility and portability in additive manufacturing. In recent years, smartphones have evolved from communication devices to powerful computational tools capable of supporting sophisticated technologies such as 3D printing. This development opens up exciting opportunities for the pharmaceutical industry, particularly in the areas of on-demand, portable, and personalized drug manufacturing. The concept of smartphone-driven 3D printing aligns with the growing demand for personalized medicine and decentralized production models, which can bring pharmaceutical manufacturing closer to the point of care [16].

13.3.1 The Emergence of Smartphone-Based 3D Printers

Smartphone-based 3D printing leverages the high-resolution cameras and powerful processors of modern smartphones to perform tasks that would traditionally require dedicated desktop systems. With the integration of custom apps, smartphones can control the movement of 3D printing platforms, provide light sources for resin curing (in the case of stereolithography), or interface with cloud-based servers for file storage and processing [17]. Several smartphone-driven 3D printing technologies have already been introduced into the market, including mobile-based 3D printing kits that allow users to print small-scale objects using their smartphone's screen and a light-sensitive resin [18]. In pharmaceutical applications, the portability and simplicity of smartphone-based 3D printing are particularly advantageous. This technology has the potential to allow patients, healthcare providers, or even pharmacists to print drug formulations in remote or resource-limited settings. With appropriate regulatory oversight, these systems could ensure the availability of essential medications in areas with limited access to pharmaceutical products [19].

13.3.2 On-Demand Drug Manufacturing

One of the most promising applications of smartphone-based 3D printing in the pharmaceutical industry is on-demand drug manufacturing. This approach enables the production of medications at the point of care, tailored to the individual needs of patients. With smartphone-based 3D printing, healthcare professionals can produce patient-specific dosage forms quickly, allowing for adjustments in drug concentration, release profiles, or even the combination of multiple active pharmaceutical ingredients (APIs) in a single dose. This is particularly useful for patients who require personalized dosages, such as children, the elderly, or those with rare diseases [20]. For example, a smartphone-controlled 3D printer can be programmed to fabricate orodispersible tablets (ODTs) with precise dosage amounts for patients who have difficulty swallowing conventional pills. Moreover, healthcare providers in rural or underserved areas can use smartphone-based 3D printers to create medications on-site, reducing the need for transportation and storage of large quantities of drugs [21].

13.3.3 Advancements in Materials for Smartphone-Based 3D Printing

Smartphone-based 3D printing solutions have primarily focused on producing small-scale objects, but advances in materials science are making it possible to print pharmaceutical-grade products. Researchers are developing biocompatible and drug-loaded printing materials that are suitable for use in smartphones. Polymers such as polycaprolactone (PCL) and polylactic acid (PLA), which are already used in medical applications, can be adapted for smartphone-based 3D printers, allowing for the safe production of drug delivery systems [22]. Furthermore, new light-curable resins are being developed that can be activated using the light emitted by smartphone screens. These resins can be impregnated with active pharmaceutical ingredients, enabling the creation of drug-laden structures. The ability to incorporate APIs directly into 3D printing materials opens the door to producing complex dosage forms such as multi-layered tablets with varied release profiles or transdermal drug delivery patches [23].

13.3.4 Challenges and Limitations

Despite its potential, smartphone-based 3D printing for pharmaceutical applications faces several challenges. The first is the limited build volume, as the size of objects that can be printed is constrained by the dimensions of the smartphone screen. While this may be sufficient for small-scale applications such as drug tablets or microneedle patches, larger pharmaceutical products or medical devices may require more advanced hardware. Additionally, smartphone-based 3D printing is still relatively slow compared to conventional 3D printing technologies, which may limit its feasibility for mass production [24]. Another challenge is ensuring the quality and consistency of the printed drug products. In pharmaceutical manufacturing, the quality of the final product is critical to ensure patient safety. Variability in print resolution, environmental conditions, and material properties can affect the consistency of the printed medications. As smartphone-based 3D printing evolves, regulatory frameworks will need to be established to ensure that products meet rigorous quality standards [25].

13.3.5 Future Prospects of Smartphone-Based 3D Printing in Pharmaceuticals

The future of smartphone-based 3D printing in pharmaceuticals is promising, especially with ongoing advancements in mobile technology and materials science. As smartphones continue to improve in terms of processing power, camera resolution, and battery life, the capabilities of smartphone-based 3D printing systems will expand. Moreover, the development of more sophisticated apps that can handle the complexities of pharmaceutical manufacturing will further streamline the process, making it more accessible to healthcare professionals and patients alike [25]. Looking forward, one exciting possibility is the integration of smartphone-based 3D printing with telemedicine. Patients in remote areas could consult with healthcare providers via telehealth platforms, and based on the consultation, a 3D-printed medication could be fabricated directly in the patient's home or local clinic using a smartphone-driven printer. This scenario represents a significant leap toward personalized and decentralized healthcare [26].

13.4 4D and 5D Printing Innovations

3D printing technology, despite its transformative impact on the pharmaceutical industry, is evolving further to meet the increasing demand for advanced drug delivery systems and personalized healthcare solutions. The advent of 4D and 5D printing technologies represents the next frontier in additive manufacturing, promising more dynamic, adaptable, and complex structures that can respond to external stimuli. These innovations have profound implications for the future of pharmaceutical development, offering new possibilities for creating "smart" drug delivery systems, tissue engineering, and personalized medicine.

13.4.1 The Concept of 4D Printing in Pharmaceuticals

While 3D printing involves creating static objects, 4D printing introduces the element of time as the fourth dimension. In 4D printing, materials are designed to change shape, structure, or function over time in response to external environmental stimuli such as temperature, moisture, pH, or light. These stimuli-responsive materials allow for the creation of dynamic drug delivery systems that can adapt to the body's conditions or external triggers, providing a more controlled and efficient method of drug administration [27]. In the pharmaceutical industry, 4D printing offers the potential to design drug delivery devices that change form or release patterns after they are administered. For example, a drug capsule printed with 4D materials could swell in response to changes in the body's pH levels, allowing for timed or site-specific release of medication. This ability to change shape or function over time makes 4D printing ideal for developing novel dosage forms, particularly in the fields of personalized medicine and controlled drug delivery [28]. 4D printing also presents opportunities for creating biocompatible scaffolds in tissue engineering, which can change shape as tissues regenerate. These adaptive structures provide more effective support for cell growth and tissue repair, making 4D printing an invaluable tool in regenerative medicine [29].

13.4.2 Materials for 4D Printing in Drug Delivery

The success of 4D printing in pharmaceutical applications depends on the development of stimuli-responsive or "smart" materials, also known as shape-memory polymers (SMPs). These materials can return to a predefined shape when exposed to specific external stimuli. In drug delivery, SMPs can be designed to encapsulate active pharmaceutical ingredients (APIs) and release them in response to stimuli such as body temperature, enzyme activity, or environmental changes in the gastrointestinal tract [30]. Hydrogels are another type of material commonly used in 4D printing due to their ability to swell and contract in response to moisture or pH changes. Hydrogels can be loaded with drugs and printed into various shapes that respond to the body's internal environment, enabling controlled drug release over time. This can be particularly useful for conditions that require long-term treatment, such as cancer or diabetes, where medication needs to be administered in precise doses over extended periods [31].

13.4.3 Applications of 4D Printing in Personalized Medicine

The ability of 4D printing to create dynamic, adaptable structures aligns perfectly with the growing trend toward personalized medicine. As treatments increasingly shift from a "one-size-fits-all" approach to individualized therapies, 4D printing allows for the customization of drug delivery devices that can respond to the specific needs of each patient. For instance, a 4D-printed implant could release medication in response to changes in a patient's body temperature or inflammatory markers, providing a tailored approach to treatment that adjusts to the patient's physiological condition [32]. This adaptability is particularly useful in the treatment of complex, chronic conditions where patients require medications that respond to fluctuating symptoms or disease progression. By utilizing 4D printing, pharmaceutical manufacturers can create systems that not only deliver the correct dosage of medication but also adjust its release profile in real time according to the patient's needs [33].

13.4.4 The Promise of 5D Printing in Pharmaceuticals

While 4D printing focuses on the incorporation of time and stimuli-responsive materials, 5D printing introduces the concept of adding extra axes to the printing process. In traditional 3D printing, objects are created layer by layer along three axes (x, y, and z). 5D printing, on the other hand, uses additional degrees of freedom by incorporating rotation of the printing platform and the print head. This allows for more complex geometries and higher structural integrity of printed objects [34]. For the pharmaceutical industry, 5D printing opens the door to creating more intricate and robust drug delivery systems that could not be achieved with traditional 3D printing methods. For example, 5D printing allows for the fabrication of complex drug-eluting stents or implants that can withstand the mechanical forces exerted by the human body, making them more durable and efficient for long-term drug delivery [35].

13.4.5 4D–5D Printing: Future Directions

The future of 4D and 5D printing in pharmaceuticals is promising, with applications extending far beyond drug delivery systems. One of the most exciting prospects is the potential for creating multifunctional devices that can not only deliver medication but also monitor patient health in real time. For example, a 4D-printed medical device could change shape in response to physiological changes and send data to healthcare providers, allowing for more proactive treatment management [36]. Additionally, combining 4D and 5D printing technologies with bioprinting holds potential for creating dynamic, patient-specific tissues or organs that can adapt and respond to the body's natural processes. This could revolutionize the fields of regenerative medicine and organ transplantation by providing customizable, adaptive solutions for patients with tissue damage or organ failure [37]. As research into 4D and 5D printing continues to grow, the pharmaceutical industry will likely see an expansion of these technologies into areas such as wound healing, tissue regeneration, and personalized therapeutics. However, significant challenges remain, particularly regarding the development of new materials, scalability of the printing process, and regulatory approval for clinical applications [27].

13.5 Personalized Medicine and Patient-Specific Dosage Forms

Personalized medicine, an approach that tailors medical treatment to the individual characteristics of each patient, is rapidly becoming a major focus in healthcare. The use of 3D printing in personalized medicine offers a unique opportunity to manufacture patient-specific dosage forms, allowing for custom drug formulations that are specifically designed to meet the therapeutic needs of individual patients. This customization can involve adjusting drug dosages, release profiles, or the combination of multiple active pharmaceutical ingredients (APIs) to address specific health conditions. With 3D printing, personalized medicine is poised to revolutionize pharmaceutical care by ensuring that patients receive the most effective treatment based on their unique genetic makeup, physiology, and lifestyle.

13.5.1 The Role of 3D Printing in Personalized Medicine

Traditional pharmaceutical manufacturing processes have been designed for mass production, where uniform drug formulations are produced in large quantities to treat broad populations. However, this "one-size-fits-all" approach often fails to address the diverse therapeutic needs of individual patients. Variations in age, body weight, metabolism, and genetics can significantly impact how a patient responds to a given medication. By using 3D printing, pharmaceutical companies can manufacture personalized medications on demand, ensuring that each patient receives the optimal dosage and drug combination [38]. The flexibility of 3D printing enables the production of dosage forms that are tailored to individual requirements. For instance, pediatric or geriatric patients, who often require lower dosages or easier-to-administer formulations, can benefit from 3D-printed tablets or capsules with customized sizes, shapes, and drug concentrations. Additionally, patients with complex medical conditions requiring multiple medications can receive personalized dosage forms that combine several APIs into a single, easy-to-take pill [39].

13.5.2 Advantages of Patient-Specific Dosage Forms

The ability to tailor drug formulations offers several advantages, particularly for patient populations with unique medical needs. Patient-specific dosage forms can improve treatment outcomes by ensuring that medications are administered in the right dose and at the right time, reducing the risk of adverse drug reactions and improving adherence to prescribed therapies. This is especially important in the treatment of chronic diseases, where the long-term management of drug regimens is crucial to maintaining patient health [40]. 3D printing also enables the development of dosage forms with complex release profiles. For example, 3D-printed tablets can be engineered with multiple layers that release drugs at different rates, providing sustained or delayed drug release according to the patient's needs. This can enhance therapeutic efficacy and improve patient compliance by reducing the frequency of drug administration. Furthermore, the ability to combine multiple medications into a single pill simplifies the treatment process for patients who would otherwise need to manage multiple prescriptions [41].

13.5.3 Applications of 3D Printing in Pediatric and Geriatric Medicine

Personalized medicine is particularly beneficial for pediatric and geriatric patients, who often have difficulty adhering to standard drug regimens. Children, for example, frequently require lower doses of medication, but standard tablets or capsules may not be available in the correct dosage. Using 3D printing, pharmaceutical manufacturers can create smaller, child-friendly tablets that contain the precise amount of active ingredient needed for pediatric patients. Moreover, 3D printing can be used to produce chewable, flavored, or fast-dissolving tablets that are easier for children to take [42]. For elderly patients, who may struggle with swallowing large tablets or capsules, 3D printing allows for the creation of orodispersible tablets (ODTs) that dissolve quickly in the mouth, requiring no water for administration. Additionally, elderly patients often have multiple chronic conditions that require polypharmacy, or the use of multiple medications simultaneously. By combining several drugs into a single, personalized dosage form, 3D printing can reduce pill burden and simplify medication management for older adults.

13.5.4 Pharmacogenomics and 3D Printing

Pharmacogenomics, the study of how genes affect a person's response to drugs, is a key component of personalized medicine. Genetic differences can influence how a patient metabolizes certain medications, which can affect drug efficacy and the risk of side effects. 3D printing offers the potential to integrate pharmacogenomic data into drug manufacturing, enabling the production of personalized medications that are tailored to a patient's genetic profile [43]. For example, patients with genetic variations that affect drug metabolism can receive 3D-printed dosage forms that are adjusted to account for these differences. This can help prevent adverse drug reactions and ensure that patients receive the most effective treatment based on their genetic makeup. The ability to incorporate pharmacogenomic information into drug formulations represents a significant advancement in the field of personalized medicine and paves the way for more targeted and individualized therapies [44].

13.5.5 Challenges and Regulatory Considerations

While the use of 3D printing in personalized medicine holds great promise, there are several challenges that need to be addressed before it can become a widespread practice. One of the primary challenges is ensuring the quality and consistency of 3D-printed dosage forms. Pharmaceutical manufacturing is highly regulated to ensure that drug products are safe, effective, and of high quality. The introduction of 3D printing technologies into drug manufacturing will require new regulatory frameworks to ensure that personalized medications meet the same rigorous standards as traditionally manufactured drugs [45]. Additionally, the cost and complexity of 3D printing technology may present barriers to its widespread adoption in clinical practice. While the technology is rapidly advancing, the equipment and materials needed for 3D printing can be expensive, making it difficult for smaller healthcare facilities to implement. However, as the technology continues to evolve and become more affordable, it is likely that 3D printing will play an increasingly important role in personalized medicine [46].

13.5.6 Future Prospects of 3D Printing in Personalized Medicine

As the field of personalized medicine continues to grow, 3D printing is expected to play a central role in the development of customized drug formulations. With ongoing advances in 3D printing technology and materials science, the potential for creating more complex, patient-specific dosage forms will continue to expand. In the future, it is possible that patients will have access to on-demand, personalized medications that are tailored to their unique genetic profiles, medical histories, and treatment needs [47]. Moreover, the integration of artificial intelligence and machine learning with 3D printing technology could further enhance the ability to create personalized dosage forms. By analyzing patient data, AI algorithms can help predict the most effective drug formulations for individual patients, allowing for the production of customized medications that optimize treatment outcomes [48].

13.6 Bioprinting and Organ-on-a-Chip Technologies

The convergence of bioprinting and organ-on-a-chip technologies represents a revolutionary shift in pharmaceutical development, regenerative medicine, and drug testing. These innovations enable the fabrication of complex biological structures and functional tissue models, potentially transforming the ways in which scientists study human physiology and develop new treatments. While bioprinting involves the 3D printing of cells and biomaterials to create living tissues, organ-on-a-chip technology utilizes microfluidic systems to mimic the functions of human organs on a small, chip-like device. Together, these technologies are driving the future of personalized medicine, drug screening, and even organ transplantation. Bioprinting, a subset of 3D printing, uses bioinks made from living cells and biomaterials to create tissue-like structures that replicate the form and function of human organs. The process of bioprinting typically involves layer-by-layer deposition of bioinks, followed by cellular assembly, maturation, and tissue formation. This approach allows for precise control over the composition, architecture, and mechanical properties of the printed structures, enabling the creation of tissues that closely resemble those found in the human body [49]. Bioprinting holds enormous potential for regenerative medicine, where the ultimate goal is to create functional tissues and organs for transplantation. In addition to organ transplantation, bioprinted tissues can be used for personalized drug testing, where patient-specific tissue models can be created to predict how an individual's body will respond to a particular drug. This approach eliminates the need for animal models, improving the accuracy and efficiency of drug testing [50].

13.6.1 Applications of Bioprinting in Drug Development

One of the most promising applications of bioprinting is in the field of drug development. Traditionally, drug discovery and testing have relied on animal models and 2D cell cultures, which often fail to accurately predict how a drug will behave in the human body. Bioprinted tissues, however, provide a more accurate and physiologically relevant platform for drug testing, as they can mimic the 3D structure and function of human tissues. For example, bioprinted liver tissues have been used to assess the toxicity of drugs, as the liver is responsible for metabolizing many pharmaceuticals. By printing functional liver tissue, researchers can study how different drugs are metabolized and identify potential toxic effects before clinical trials [51]. Similarly, bioprinted skin tissue has been used for testing topical drugs and cosmetics, providing a more ethical and accurate alternative to animal testing [52].

13.6.2 Organ-on-a-Chip Technology: Mimicking Human Organs

While bioprinting focuses on creating 3D tissue structures, organ-on-a-chip (OoC) technology takes a different approach by using microfluidic devices to replicate the physiological functions of entire organs. Organ-on-a-chip devices consist of small, transparent chips with tiny channels and compartments that contain living cells. These cells are cultured in a way that mimics the structure and function of human organs, such as the lung, liver, heart, or kidney. One of the key advantages of organ-on-a-chip technology is its ability to simulate the dynamic environment of living organs. The microfluidic channels allow for the controlled flow of fluids, such as blood or nutrients, which is critical for maintaining cell viability and function. By replicating the mechanical forces and biochemical signals found in the body, organ-on-a-chip devices provide a more realistic model for studying human physiology and disease [53].

13.6.3 Integration of Bioprinting and Organ-on-a-Chip

While bioprinting and organ-on-a-chip technologies are powerful on their own, the integration of these two approaches holds even greater potential. By combining the structural complexity of bioprinted tissues with the functional capabilities of organ-on-a-chip devices, researchers can create highly sophisticated models of human organs for drug testing, disease modeling, and regenerative medicine. For example, bioprinted cardiac tissue could be integrated into a heart-on-a-chip device to study how the heart responds to different drugs or environmental conditions. Similarly, bioprinted neural tissue could be incorporated into a brain-on-a-chip platform to investigate neurological diseases such as Alzheimer's or Parkinson's. This combination of technologies enables the creation of complex, multi-organ systems that more accurately represent the interactions between different organs in the human body [54].

13.6.4 Personalized Medicine and Disease Modeling

Bioprinting and organ-on-a-chip technologies are expected to play a central role in the future of personalized medicine. By using a patient's own cells, researchers can bioprint tissues that are genetically and physiologically identical to the patient's own body. These personalized tissue models can then be used to test how a patient will respond to specific drugs, allowing for the development of customized treatments that are tailored to the individual's unique biology [55]. In addition to personalized drug testing, bioprinting and organ-on-a-chip technologies are being used to model a wide range of diseases. For example, bioprinted cancer tissues have been developed to study tumor growth and response to chemotherapy, while liver-on-a-chip devices have been used to model liver diseases such as hepatitis and cirrhosis. These models provide valuable insights into disease mechanisms and enable the development of more targeted and effective therapies [56].

13.6.5 Challenges and Future Prospects

Despite the enormous potential of bioprinting and organ-on-a-chip technologies, several challenges remain. One of the primary challenges is the complexity of replicating the full functionality of human organs. While researchers have made significant progress in creating bioprinted tissues and organ-on-a-chip devices, these models are still relatively simple compared to the intricacy of real human organs. Achieving the full complexity of organs, including their vascularization, innervation, and immune responses, remains a major challenge [57]. Additionally, the scalability of these technologies is a significant hurdle. Bioprinting functional organs for transplantation is still in its early stages, and it may take many years before this technology is ready for widespread clinical use. Organ-on-a-chip devices, while promising for drug testing, also face challenges in terms of standardization and integration into existing pharmaceutical workflows. Nonetheless, the future prospects of bioprinting and organ-on-a-chip technologies are highly promising. As these technologies continue to evolve, they are likely to play an increasingly important role in drug development, personalized medicine, and regenerative therapies. The ability to create patient-specific tissues and organs could revolutionize the treatment of a wide range of diseases, from cancer to heart disease to neurodegenerative disorders [58].

13.7 Nanomedicine Applications and Drug Delivery Systems

Nanomedicine, which involves the use of nanoscale materials for medical purposes, has emerged as one of the most transformative areas of biomedical research. By manipulating materials at the nanometer scale, scientists are developing novel drug delivery systems that can target specific tissues, cross biological barriers, and release drugs in a controlled manner. When integrated with 3D printing technology, nanomedicine offers exciting opportunities to create personalized and highly efficient drug delivery systems. These innovations have the potential to improve the efficacy of therapies, minimize side effects, and enable the development of entirely new therapeutic approaches for treating complex diseases such as cancer, cardiovascular disorders, and neurological conditions.

13.7.1 Nanomedicine and Its Advantages in Drug Delivery

Nanomedicine involves the design, development, and application of nanoscale materials, such as nanoparticles, liposomes, dendrimers, and nanotubes, for therapeutic purposes. The use of nanomaterials in drug delivery offers several advantages, including improved solubility of poorly water-soluble drugs, increased drug stability, enhanced targeting of specific tissues, and controlled drug release. By delivering drugs at the nanoscale, it becomes possible to achieve therapeutic concentrations in diseased tissues while minimizing exposure to healthy tissues, thus reducing potential side effects [59]. A key advantage of nanomedicine is its ability to overcome biological barriers, such as the blood-brain barrier (BBB), which traditionally limits the delivery of drugs to the brain. Nanoparticles can be engineered to cross these barriers and deliver drugs directly to the site of disease. This is particularly important in treating neurological disorders such as Alzheimer's and Parkinson's disease, where effective drug delivery to the brain remains a significant challenge [60].

13.7.2 Integration of Nanomedicine with 3D Printing

The integration of nanomedicine with 3D printing has opened up new possibilities for creating personalized drug delivery systems. 3D printing allows for the precise fabrication of drug delivery devices that can be tailored to the unique needs of individual patients. When combined with nanomaterials, these devices can be designed to release drugs in a controlled manner, ensuring optimal therapeutic outcomes. For example, 3D-printed scaffolds loaded with nanoparticles can be used for localized drug delivery in tissue engineering applications. These scaffolds can be implanted at the site of injury or disease, where they slowly release drugs over time to promote healing or prevent infection. Similarly, 3D-printed implants can be combined with nanomaterials to create personalized drug delivery systems that release anticancer drugs directly into tumors, minimizing the exposure of healthy tissues to toxic chemotherapy agents [61].

13.7.3 Nanoparticle-Based Drug Delivery Systems

Nanoparticles are one of the most widely used nanomaterials in drug delivery systems due to their ability to encapsulate drugs, protect them from degradation, and target specific tissues. These systems can be designed to release drugs in response to specific stimuli, such as changes in pH, temperature, or enzymatic activity, ensuring that the drug is released only when and where it is needed. Lipid-based nanoparticles, such as liposomes and solid lipid nanoparticles, have been successfully used for delivering a wide range of drugs, including anticancer agents, antibiotics, and vaccines. Liposomal drug delivery systems, for example, have been used to improve the therapeutic index of anticancer drugs like doxorubicin by reducing their toxicity and enhancing their accumulation in tumors [62]. Polymeric nanoparticles offer another promising approach to drug delivery, as they can be engineered to release drugs in a sustained or controlled manner over time. These nanoparticles can be functionalized with targeting ligands that bind to specific receptors on the surface of diseased cells, allowing for highly selective drug delivery [63].

13.7.4 Nanomedicine in Targeted Cancer Therapy

One of the most important applications of nanomedicine is in the field of oncology, where it is being used to develop targeted drug delivery systems for cancer therapy. Traditional cancer treatments, such as chemotherapy, often cause significant damage to healthy tissues, leading to severe side effects. Nanoparticle-based drug delivery systems can improve the selectivity of cancer therapies by targeting the delivery of chemotherapeutic agents directly to tumor cells. Nanoparticles can be functionalized with antibodies, peptides, or small molecules that recognize and bind to specific markers on the surface of cancer cells. Once bound, the nanoparticles are taken up by the cancer cells, where they release their drug payload in a controlled manner.

This targeted approach reduces the systemic toxicity of chemotherapy and enhances its efficacy by ensuring that higher concentrations of the drug reach the tumor site [64]. Gold nanoparticles (AuNPs) are particularly useful in cancer therapy due to their ability to absorb light and convert it into heat, a process known as photothermal therapy. By attaching anticancer drugs to gold nanoparticles, researchers can use light to trigger the release of the drug and simultaneously destroy cancer cells through localized heating [65].

13.7.5 Nanomedicine for Neurological Disorders

Nanomedicine also holds great promise for the treatment of neurological disorders, where the ability to deliver drugs across the blood-brain barrier (BBB) is critical. Nanoparticles can be engineered to cross the BBB and deliver drugs directly to the brain, providing a potential solution for treating conditions such as Alzheimer's disease, Parkinson's disease, and brain tumors. For example, nanoparticles made from biodegradable polymers, such as poly(lactic-co-glycolic acid) (PLGA), can be loaded with neuroprotective drugs and delivered to the brain to slow the progression of neurodegenerative diseases. Additionally, nanoparticles functionalized with targeting ligands can bind to receptors on the surface of brain endothelial cells, facilitating their transport across the BBB [66].

13.7.6 Nanomedicine in Vaccines and Immunotherapy

Nanomedicine is also playing an increasingly important role in the development of vaccines and immunotherapies. Nanoparticles can be used as vaccine delivery platforms, where they protect antigens from degradation, enhance their immunogenicity, and facilitate their uptake by immune cells. This approach has been used to develop more effective vaccines for diseases such as influenza, HIV, and cancer [67]. In cancer immunotherapy, nanoparticles are being used to deliver immune checkpoint inhibitors and other immunomodulatory agents that enhance the body's immune response to cancer cells. By targeting the delivery of these agents to the tumor microenvironment, nanomedicine can improve the efficacy of cancer immunotherapies and reduce their associated toxicities [68].

13.7.7 Challenges and Future Directions

Despite the significant progress in nanomedicine, several challenges remain. One of the main challenges is the "scalability" of nanoparticle-based drug delivery systems, as the production of uniform and well-characterized nanoparticles on a large scale can be difficult. Additionally, the "safety" of nanomaterials needs to be thoroughly evaluated, as nanoparticles may interact with biological systems in unpredictable ways, potentially leading to toxicity. Another challenge is the "regulatory" landscape for nanomedicine, which is still evolving. The unique properties of nanomaterials present challenges for regulatory agencies in terms of defining standards for safety, efficacy, and quality control. However, as nanomedicine continues to advance, it is expected that regulatory frameworks will adapt to ensure the safe and effective use of these technologies in clinical practice [69]. Looking to the future, the integration of nanomedicine with other emerging technologies, such as artificial intelligence (AI) and 3D printing, is expected to further revolutionize drug delivery. AI can be used to design and optimize nanoparticles with specific properties, while 3D printing can be used to create personalized drug delivery systems that incorporate nanomaterials. These innovations are likely to lead to the development of more effective, personalized treatments for a wide range of diseases [70].

13.8 Conclusion

The future of 3D printing in pharmaceuticals is poised to revolutionize the industry, offering unprecedented customization, efficiency, and innovation in drug development and production. This technology promises to address current limitations in conventional pharmaceutical manufacturing by enabling the creation of personalized medications tailored to individual patient needs. The potential to fabricate complex drug formulations with precise control over dosage, release profiles, and multi-drug combinations opens new avenues for treating chronic diseases and enhancing therapeutic outcomes. Emerging technologies in 3D printing, such as bioprinting and the use of novel materials, are further expanding the possibilities for pharmaceutical applications. Bioprinting, for instance, could pave the way for printing tissues and organs, significantly impacting regenerative medicine and drug testing. The integration of smart materials and nanotechnology into 3D printing holds promise for developing advanced drug delivery systems with controlled release mechanisms and targeted therapy. The incorporation of machine learning (ML) and artificial intelligence (AI) is set to further accelerate the advancements in the 3D printing of pharmaceuticals. ML and AI can optimize the design and production processes by predicting the best formulations, improving precision in drug dosing, and ensuring quality control. These technologies can also analyze vast datasets to discover new drug compounds and predict patient-specific responses, thereby enhancing the personalization of treatments. However, to fully realize the potential of 3D printing in pharmaceuticals, several challenges must be addressed. These include ensuring the scalability and reproducibility of printed products, establishing stringent regulatory frameworks, and conducting comprehensive clinical trials to validate the safety and efficacy of 3D-printed medications. Collaboration between industry, academia, and regulatory bodies will be crucial in overcoming these hurdles and driving the adoption of 3D printing technologies in mainstream pharmaceutical practice. In conclusion, the future prospects and emerging technologies in 3D printing of pharmaceuticals herald a transformative era in healthcare, where personalized medicine becomes a reality and innovative therapeutic solutions are within reach. As research and development continue to advance, 3D printing, augmented by ML and AI, is set to play a pivotal role in shaping the future landscape of pharmaceutical manufacturing and patient care.

References

1. Mancilla-De-La-Cruz J, Rodriguez-Salvador M, Ruiz-Cantu L. The next pharmaceutical path: determining technology evolution in drug delivery products fabricated with additive manufacturing. Foresight STI Gov. 2020;14(3):55–70. https://doi.org/10.17323/2500-2597.2020.3.55.70.
2. Lim SH, Kathuria H, Tan JJY, Kang L. 3D printed drug delivery and testing systems: a passing fad or the future? Adv Drug Deliv Rev. 2018;132:139–68. https://doi.org/10.1016/J.ADDR.2018.05.006.
3. Sadée W, Dai Z. Pharmacogenetics/genomics and personalized medicine. Hum Mol Genet. 2005;14(2):R207–14. https://doi.org/10.1093/HMG/DDI261.
4. Jamróz W, Szafraniec-Szczęsny J, Kurek M, Jachowicz R. 3D printing in pharmaceutical and medical applications: recent achievements and challenges. Pharm Res. 2018;35(9):176. https://doi.org/10.1007/S11095-018-2454-X.
5. Norman JR, Madurawe D, Moore CMV, Khan MA, Khairuzzaman A. A new chapter in pharmaceutical manufacturing: 3D-printed drug products. Adv Drug Deliv Rev. 2017;108:39–50. https://doi.org/10.1016/J.ADDR.2016.03.001.
6. Ursan I, Chiu L, Pierce A. Three-dimensional drug printing: a structured review. J Am Pharm Assoc. 2013;53(2):136–44. https://doi.org/10.1331/JAPHA.2013.12217.
7. Kotta S, Nair A, Alsabeelah N. 3D printing technology in drug delivery: recent progress and application. Curr Pharm Des. 2018;24(42):5039–48. https://doi.org/10.2174/1381612825666181206123828.
8. Kalkal A, Kumar S, Kumar P, Pradhan R, Willander M, Packirisamy G, Kumar S, Malhotra BD. Recent advances in 3D printing technologies for wearable (bio)sensors. Addit Manuf. 2021;46:102088. https://doi.org/10.1016/J.ADDMA.2021.102088.
9. Benjamens S, Dhunnoo P, Meskó B. The state of artificial intelligence-based FDA-approved medical devices and algorithms: an online database. NPJ Digit Med. 2020;3:118. https://www.nature.com/articles/s41746-020-00324-0 (Accessed 29 July 2024)
10. Norman J, Madurawe RD, Moore CM, Khan MA, Khairuzzaman A. A new chapter in pharmaceutical manufacturing: 3D-printed drug products. Adv Drug Deliv Rev. 2017c;108:39–50.
11. Li X, He J, Ji H. Machine learning algorithms for pharmaceutical 3D printing: challenges and prospects. J Pharm Sci. 2020;109(6):1567–80.
12. Zhang YS, Yao Y, Zhou X, Wang W. Bioprinting and organ-on-a-chip: engineered microenvironments for studying tissue development and disease. Trends Biotechnol. 2021;39(4):335–44.
13. Ligon SC, Liska R, Stampfl J, Gurr M, Mülhaupt R. Polymers for 3D printing and customized additive manufacturing. Chem Rev. 2017;117(15):10212–90.
14. Rajput SS, Sood AK, Ahluwalia V. Machine learning techniques for optimizing 3D printing processes. Addit Manuf. 2019;29:100776.
15. Gibson I, Rosen DW, Stucker B. Additive manufacturing technologies: 3D printing, rapid prototyping, and direct digital manufacturing. Springer; 2021.
16. Limaye RJ, Kumar A, Pillai MM. A review on 3D printing in healthcare: a new era in pharmaceuticals. Int J Pharm Sci Res. 2018;9(4):1504–16.
17. Gallegos LM, Horn TJ, Choi J, Kim S. Smartphone-driven 3D printing: a new approach to decentralized manufacturing. Addit Manuf. 2020;34:101283.
18. Mueller B, Vurpillot S, Schmid R, et al. Mobile 3D printing with smartphones: new opportunities in decentralized manufacturing. J Manuf Sci Eng. 2021;143(6):064503.
19. Gupta R, Rani P, Choudhary A. 3D printing in pharmaceuticals: current trends and future directions. J Pharm Bioallied Sci. 2019;11(2):98–102.

20. Norman J, Madurawe RD, Moore CM, Khan MA, Khairuzzaman A. A new chapter in pharmaceutical manufacturing: 3D-printed drug products. Adv Drug Deliv Rev. 2017;108:39–50.
21. Santilán G, Acuña E, Ruíz D, Hernández H. 3D printing for drug delivery: from concept to clinic. Adv Drug Deliv Rev. 2021;174:307–32.
22. Kalaskar DM. 3D printing in medicine. Woodhead Publishing. Series in Biomaterials; 2017. p. 101–45.
23. Tan DK, Maniruzzaman M, Nokhodchi A, et al. Mobile 3D printing for point-of-care manufacturing in healthcare. Expert Opin Drug Deliv. 2020;17(11):1579–95.
24. Wang X, Jiang X, Zhang Y. Smartphone-based 3D printing technologies: a future direction for on-demand healthcare manufacturing. J Med Syst. 2020;44(8):145.
25. Goyanes A, Martínez PR, Buanz A, et al. Smartphone-based 3D printing of personalized drug delivery systems. Int J Pharm. 2021;597:120283.
26. Wei L, Zhao Y, Gao F. The future of personalized medicine: smartphone-driven 3D printing and telemedicine. Bioeng Transl Med. 2018;3(1):106–14.
27. Momeni F, Liu X, Ni J. A review of 4D printing. Mater Des. 2017;122:42–79.
28. Tibbits S. 4D printing: multi-material shape change. Archit Des. 2018;88(4):116–21.
29. Hussein KH, Park KM, Yang S. 4D bioprinting: technologies and challenges in tissue engineering. Acta Biomater. 2019;101:1–16.
30. Gandhi A, Paul A, Sen SO. Stimuli-responsive materials for 4D printing in pharmaceuticals. Int J Pharm. 2020;585:119498.
31. Faber JA, Arrieta AF, Studart AR. Bioinspired 4D printing. Nat Rev Mater. 2019;4(6):318–35.
32. Ashammakhi N, Hasan A, Kaivosoja E. The future of 4D printing in pharmaceutical sciences and its potential impact on healthcare. J Control Release. 2019;295:144–58.
33. Jeon O, Alt DS, Pan H. 4D printing technology to engineer bioinspired structures for pharmaceutical applications. J Control Release. 2020;321:130–40.
34. Pietrzak K, Majewska J, Ziółkowski G. 5D printing: new horizons in pharmaceuticals. Adv Drug Deliv Rev. 2020;156:23–36.
35. Farkas A, Wang T, He Y. 5D printing in pharmaceuticals: a review of applications and future prospects. J Pharm Sci. 2021;110(7):2527–40.
36. Zhao Q, Qi HJ, Xie T. Recent progress in shape memory polymer: new behaviors, enabling materials, and mechanistic understanding. Prog Polym Sci. 2020;62:86–113.
37. Duan B, Kapetanovic E, Jin Y. 4D bioprinting for personalized and dynamic tissue engineering. Adv Funct Mater. 2019;29(36):1903754.
38. Alomari M, Mohamed FH, Basit AW. Personalised medicine through 3D printing: hypothesis, fact or reality? Int J Pharm. 2015;494(2):581–93.
39. Goyanes A, Buanz ABM, Basit AW, Gaisford S. 3D printing of medicines: engineering novel oral devices with unique design and drug release characteristics. Mol Pharm. 2017;12(11):4071–80.
40. Prasad LK, Smyth H, Barrow DA. 3D printing and personalised medicines: additive manufacturing technologies to address the needs of older patients. Adv Drug Deliv Rev. 2019;151:85–93.
41. Sun Y, Yang W, Tan X. Application of 3D printing in oral solid dosage forms: a review. J Pharm Sci. 2020;109(4):1246–1255.
42. Cern A, Read ES, Mehta K. 3D printing of personalised medicines for paediatrics. J Pharm Sci. 2019;108(1):78–81.
43. Amin R, Barakat R, Asaad A. Pharmacogenomics: a bridge to personalized medicine in pharmaceutical care. Front Pharmacol. 2019;10:267.
44. Khaled SA, Burley JC, Alexander MR. Personalized 3D printed medicines for better patient care: an update. Curr Pharm Des. 2021;27(15):1672–81.
45. Melocchi A, Loreti G, Del Curto MD. Regulatory challenges and technical requirements for pharmaceutical 3D printing. J Control Release. 2021;334:164–77.
46. Norman J, Madurawe RD, Khan MA. 3D printing in pharmaceutical and medical applications: recent advances and challenges. Adv Drug Deliv Rev. 2017a;108:39–50.

47. Goyanes A, Martinez PR, Gaisford S. Advances in 3D printing for pharmaceuticals. J 3D Print Med. 2021;5(2):73–91.
48. Domínguez-Robles J, Romero-Granados R, Perrot A. Artificial intelligence and 3D printing in personalized drug development. Adv Drug Deliv Rev. 2020;165:153–66.
49. Murphy SV, Atala A. 3D bioprinting of tissues and organs. Nat Biotechnol. 2014;32(8):773–85.
50. Mandrycky C, Wang Z, Kim K, Kim DH. 3D bioprinting for engineering complex tissues. Biotechnol Adv. 2016;34(4):422–34.
51. Buchanan CF, Voigt JD, Szafran S. Bioprinting human liver tissue models for drug discovery and toxicity testing. Biotechnol Adv. 2021;51:107772.
52. Nguyen D, Hägg DA, Forsman A, Ekholm E, Shalaly ND, Enejder A. Cartilage tissue engineering by the 3D bioprinting of cells, bioinks, and scaffolds. J Tissue Eng Regen Med. 2021;11(2):144–55.
53. Huh D, Hamilton GA, Ingber DE. From 3D cell culture to organs-on-chips. Trends Cell Biol. 2013;21(12):745–54.
54. Zhang YS, Aleman J, Shin SR, Kilic T, Kim D, Mousavi Shaegh SA. Multispecies organ-on-a-chip systems with integrated sensors for flexible user-defined biology. Nat Commun. 2016;8(1):1–12.
55. Wang X, Ao Q, Tian X, Fan J, Wei Y, Hou W, Bai S. 3D bioprinting technologies for hard tissue and organ engineering. Materials. 2018;11(8):1499.
56. Zhang H, Zhao Y, Yang F. Artificial intelligence in 3D printing: revolutionizing pharmaceutical manufacturing. Int J Pharm. 2021b;598:120267.
57. Dvir T, Timko BP, Kohane DS, Langer R. Nanotechnological strategies for engineering complex tissues. Nat Nanotechnol. 2021;6(1):13–22.
58. Kang HW, Lee SJ, Ko IK, Kengla C, Yoo JJ, Atala A. A 3D bioprinting system to produce human-scale tissue constructs with structural integrity. Nat Biotechnol. 2020;34(3):312–9.
59. Torchilin VP. Multifunctional, stimuli-sensitive nanoparticulate systems for drug delivery. Nat Rev Drug Discov. 2014;13(11):813–27.
60. Pardridge WM. Drug transport across the blood-brain barrier. J Cereb Blood Flow Metab. 2020;32(11):1959–72.
61. Langer R. Nanotechnology in drug delivery and tissue engineering: from discovery to applications. Nano Lett. 2018;18(1):1–6.
62. Allen TM, Cullis PR. Liposomal drug delivery systems: from concept to clinical applications. Adv Drug Deliv Rev. 2013;65(1):36–48.
63. Danhier F, Feron O, Préat V. To exploit the tumor microenvironment: passive and active tumor targeting of nanocarriers for anti-cancer drug delivery. J Control Release. 2012;161(2):229–42.
64. Davis ME, Chen Z, Shin DM. Nanoparticle therapeutics: an emerging treatment modality for cancer. Nat Rev Drug Discov. 2008;7(9):771–82.
65. Huang X, Jain PK, El-Sayed IH, El-Sayed MA. Gold nanoparticles: interesting optical properties and recent applications in cancer diagnostics and therapy. Nanomedicine. 2010;2(5):681–93.
66. Saraiva C, Praça C, Ferreira R, Santos T, Ferreira L, Bernardino L. Nanoparticle-mediated brain drug delivery: overcoming blood–brain barrier to treat neurodegenerative diseases. J Control Release. 2016;235:34–47.
67. Wang J, Chen Y, Yang Y, Xiao F, Wu Y. Nanomedicine applications in the treatment of cancer: focus on drug delivery, immune modulation, and nanotoxicity evaluation. J Drug Target. 2019;27(6):1–15.
68. Zhang Y, Deng Y, Tong J. Emerging trends of nanomedicine in cancer immunotherapy. Biomater Sci. 2018;6(1):1437–47.
69. Mitragotri S, Lahann J. Physical approaches to biomaterial design. Nat Mater. 2017;8(1):15–23.
70. Mout R, Moyano DF, Rana S, Rotello VM. Surface functionalization of nanoparticles for nanomedicine. Chem Soc Rev. 2017;41(7):2539–44.

Global Collaboration and Partnership in Advancing FDM 3D Printing

14

Disha Sharma, Anuradha Derashri, Akanksha Dwivedi, V. H. Bhaskar, and Kuldeep Vinchurkar

Abstract

Pharmaceutical FDM 3D printing (3DP) is revolutionizing the drug manufacturing industry globally by offering flexibility in design, dosing adjustments, rapid prototyping, and precise drug release control. The technology enables personalized pharmaceuticals, reduces development time, and transforms drug design and manufacturing processes. With its simplicity, cost-effectiveness, and strength, FDM technology is widely adopted in pharmaceuticals.

Currently, the 3D-printed drug industry is at an early stage, mainly concentrated in Europe, the United States, and China, focusing on large-scale production and personalized drug delivery. While no regulatory guidelines exist yet, various countries are recognizing the potential of 3D printing in pharmaceuticals and are working towards establishing regulatory standards.

Collaboration and partnerships on a global scale to advance FDM 3D printing in pharmaceuticals could lead to breakthroughs in personalized medicine, improved drug delivery, and enhanced patient care worldwide. The technology can establish scientific standards in the pharmaceutical field, driving innovation in drug development models. Efforts are ongoing to navigate unique registration paths for 3D-printed preparations, address intellectual property rights, and adapt drug regulations to this innovative technology.

D. Sharma · A. Derashri (✉) · V. H. Bhaskar
LSHGCT's Gahlot Institute of Pharmacy, Navi Mumbai, Maharashtra, India

A. Dwivedi
Acropolis Institute of Pharmaceutical Education and Research, Indore, Madhya Pradesh, India

K. Vinchurkar
Department of Pharmaceutics, Sandip Institute of Pharmaceutical Sciences (SIPS), Affiliated To Savitribai Phule Pune University (SPPU, Pune), Nashik, Maharashtra, India

K. Vinchurkar, S. Mane (eds.), *Innovations in Drug Manufacturing*, https://doi.org/10.1007/978-981-96-9075-6_14

The promising future of the 3D-printed drug industry hinges on continuous efforts to promote intelligent and personalized drug preparation technologies through innovation and collaboration across diverse expertise and resources.

Keywords

FDM · 3DP · Regulatory standards · Personalized medicine · Dosing adjustment

14.1 Overview

In the previous few decades, additive manufacturing has seen tremendous growth in impact because of the growing need for customized medical and pharmaceutical equipment. One of the most potent and innovative tools available now, 3D printing is well-used in the expansion of tissues, sickness modeling, and the exact production of custom dosage forms [34]. The most recent developments include customized and implantable dosage forms, all-purpose drug distribution structures with accelerated release properties, anatomically correct implantation and phantoms, and cell-based resources for regenerative treatment [7]. Personalized medicine is becoming more and more popular in the medical field these days. The "one size fits all" concept of mainstream pharmaceutical therapy requires that the majority of patients receive the same medication at the same doses and delivery times [21].

Three-dimensional printing, or 3D printing, is a novel form of production for pharmaceutical and biological applications. Components can be placed layer by layer using fused deposition modeling (FDM), an inexpensive extrusion-based 3D printing technology that produces solid structures. Fused deposition modeling (FDM) is a new and flexible manufacturing practice for creating customized drug delivery devices with precise prescription doses and controlled drug release characteristics [35].

In the field of medical disciplines, fused deposition modeling (FDM) is the most frequently assessed 3D printing method since it uses moderately simpler and less luxurious gear, offers a wide range of excipient options, and is easy to produce dosage forms—even with complex geometries—that are well-accepted by patients. In the FDM process, a heated, drug-loaded polymer thread is extruded through a nozzle tip and formed into the desired geometry onto an assembly plate. One possible hazard with this form of printing is that the drugs might be placed in extremely elevated temperatures during material extrusion and printing [6]. In a recent study, we showed that the thermal decomposition of 4-aminosalicylic acid during the print process using FDM exceeded 50%, emphasizing the necessity to lower the manufacturing temperatures for medications that are thermally fluctuated [31].

Currently, conventional industrial methods cannot produce patient-specific oral medicinal formulations. Using 3D printing, and more specifically fused deposition modeling (FDM), offers an intriguing opportunity to tailor oral medication administration. Three FDM approaches have been stated: "Impregnation-FDM," "Hot Melt Extrusion combined with FDM," and "Print-fill." These procedures resulted in the invention of 47 active compounds, five families of excipients with various applications, and thermoplastic polymers that served as the primary ingredient. Solutions are being developed to address the in-elevation printing heats that were initially preventing the use of thermosensitive chemicals with this method of printing. Additionally, preliminary storage experiments reveal that many prints are moisture sensitive [10]. For the treatment of rare diseases and specific populations requiring modified dosages or release kinetics, FDM seems to be a good fit. Healthcare regulatory agencies should be involved in future clinical trials using FDM. Future attempts should focus on implementing a quality strategy like "Quality by Design" to gain clearance from organizations and support the development of this technology for producers [40].

In 2009, the patent for fused deposition modeling (FDM) technology became available. The process involves inserting a malleable filament into the boiler plate. Figure 14.1 illustrates how the filament interacts to soften to a semi-solid state and is extruded into thin layers on the bed. The printer model determines whether the bed or heated head moves throughout extrusion, which facilitates precise layer placement. Heat during layer deposition promotes molecular bonding with the prior film [4]. This method produces complicated products from digital designs, eliminating the need for molds or traditional manufacturing procedures. There are currently no established GMP guidelines regarding medical printing using FDM or pharmaceutical filament manufacture [48].

The exploratory investigative services major goal is to conduct systematic research to determine how FDM technology might be used to produce highly customized oral medicines. As a result, a brief introduction of the 3D printers, software, and raw materials used in pharma FDM is provided, with an emphasis on how FDM

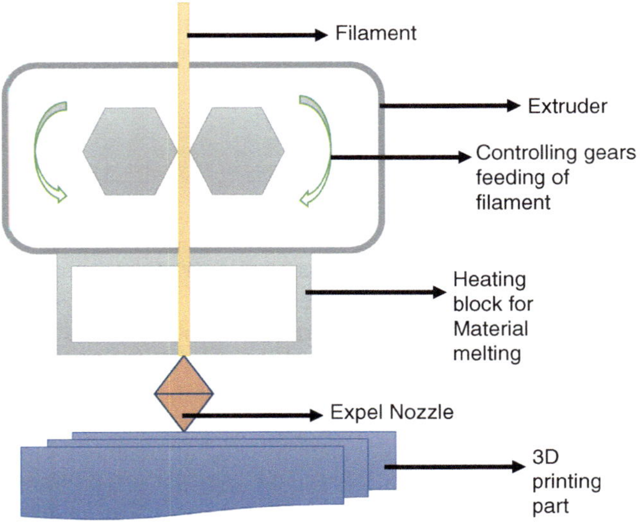

Fig. 14.1 3D printing FDM model

might improve dose and release kinetics matching. The scoping investigation's major goal is to conduct a systematic study to determine how FDM technology might be used to produce highly personalized oral medicines. As a result, a concise introduction of the 3D tools, software, and raw materials used in medical FDM is provided, with an emphasis on how FDM might improve dose and release kinetics [19].

The technique of three-dimensional printing (3DP) is currently used to create many different types of medications; therefore, it is apparent that this unique manufacturing method (ET) has an opportunity to revolutionize the field of personalized medicine (PM). 3DP enables the combination of numerous APIs in a single formulation, as well as the fabrication of dosage forms with various geometries, sophisticated topologies, or strata with varying distribution profiles [47]. In addition, it is simpler to obtain dosages that can be modified to meet the necessities of every patient, accounting for variations in substance resistance and metabolic processes, especially for active ingredients having a brief period of therapeutic effect. Furthermore, 3DP can conceal tastes, improving patient adherence—a difficult task when it comes to pediatric medications [44].

The arena of additive construct, or AM, continues to expand, and the use of 3D printing makes it possible to generate multifaceted and portable assemblies that would be challenging to produce using existing techniques [50]. It is evident that over decades, 3D printing has primarily been used in experimental manufacturing, and its use in actual production is still in its infancy.

As FDM develops into a cutting-edge production method, numerous sectors have higher expectations, and those expectations are satisfied. Printer manufacturers like Ultimaker, German RepRap, Stratasys, XYZprinting, Markforged, Zortax, and Dagoma are continually employed to recover their imprinters, while software companies like Siemens PLM Software, Dassault, and Autodesk organizations are mounting unique CAD programmes to work with the novel printing devices. Despite an entire decade of advancements, there are still many problems with printing for declaration of quality and consistency in FDM, which are brought on by hidden flaws or inconsistencies in printable goods [11].

14.1.1 Background

During 1983, when Chuck Hull, a co-founder of 3D Systems, invented the first three-dimensional printer, the area of manufacturing with additives advanced significantly. In the following years, this sort of technology gained prominence and became more widely available at reduced prices. The emphasis turned to new materials and applications in the late 1990s and early 2000s, and additive manufacturing technology saw an increase in use in industries like robotics, healthcare, and aviation. Due to its exceptional accuracy and precision in creating complicated structures, 3D printing technology is much sought after nowadays. Furthermore, new methods like bioprinting and 4D printing have created new opportunities in the medical industry [25].

Because the process of additive manufacturing is at its peak and has dealt with numerous obstacles, it is now possible to create 3D models of a wide range of materials, including metals, thermoplastics, hydrogels, extracellular matrix chemicals, pottery, and composites with fiber reinforcement, polymers, concrete materials, and sometimes shape-memory alloys, also known as smart components. Furthermore, modern technology has thankfully ushered in a new era of mass customization, giving customers more options for the finished product based on their preferences. In addition, 3D printing companies can be located closer to their clients or even in their homes for private use, which enables greater adaptability and adaptability in manufacturing processes in addition to better quality control. Moreover, the requirement for international shipping has been greatly diminished by the application of 3D printing technology, saving time and energy [15]. Aside from its many uses, 3D printing has transformed a number of medical specialties, including surgery, orthopedics, and even organ transplantation. This technology has enabled accurate surgical instruction, customized surgical procedures, prosthetics sculpted to fit an individual's unique anatomy, three-dimensional tissues, and even full working organs and organisms. Since expertise makes it possible to create replacement organs that are tailored to each patient individually, it has demonstrated significant promise in helping to meet the growing need for organ transplantation. Beyond the field of medicine, printing in three dimensions finds extensive use in nearly every industry. This adaptable technology can be used to create everything from clothing and toys to intricate airplane components and even whole rockets and turbines. There are numerous uses for fused deposition modeling (FDM), a practical print technique in the medical field. Thermoplastic filaments that have been heated to a semi-solid state are then blown out and deposited layer by layer in FDM. As the successive layers are placed on top of one another, not only will they cool and solidify, but they will additionally form a molecular link with the heating filament. The technique only works with thermoplastic materials, although it offers excellent material layer bonding. As of right now, this sort of equipment is employed in the manufacturing of occlusal appliances and in pharmaceutical applications, such as controlled-release medication administration systems. Fused deposition modeling has little use in dentistry, despite its usefulness in a variety of different medical situations [28]. Charles Hull introduced the notion of additive manufacturing (AM), rapid prototyping (RP), and solid-freeform technology. Hull started working on photopolymer-based thermoplastic devices at Ultra Violet Products in California in the early 1980s after graduating from the College of Colorado with a B.S. in engineering physics. Hull was driven to improve prototype development procedures because of their long manufacturing time (1–2 months) and high likelihood of design flaws that needed to be fixed through multiple rounds of development. After being granted the first invention in 1986 for stereolithography, Hull went on to acquire numerous other inventions related to the technique.

Hull and 3D Systems was the company that created the first 3D printer, known as the "Stereolithography Apparatus," as well as the SLA-250, the first commercial 3D printer offered to the general population. After fused deposition modeling (FDM) became known and subsequently patented by Stratasys in 1990, thanks to Hull's and

Scott Crump's research, the advent of 3D printing was poised to revolutionize both production and education.

In 1993, MIT researchers Michael Cima and Emanuel Sachs received a patent for the first "3D printer," a device capable of printing materials such as plastic, metal, and ceramic pieces. Six Solidscape and Objet Geometries (which merged with Stratasys), Z business, and DTM Company (which teamed with 3D Systems) are among the other enterprises that have created commercialized 3D printers [45].

Industrial applications for the technology of 3D printing can be found in the motorized and aerospace subdivisions, wherever it is utilized for printing prototypes of automobile and aircraft parts. Structural models are printed for the architectural field, and consumer goods companies like Black & Decker and Trek use them to develop prototypes. Rapid growth is being observed in the usage of 3D printing for defense in both public and private domains. For example, there have been documented applications in the manufacturing of security gear and gun prototypes. Meanwhile, in the early 2000s, the utilization of 3D printing was employed in the therapeutic field to produce dental implants and prosthetics. The uses have also surfaced in the culinary and fashion industries.

The utilization of 3D production in academic environments is currently limited to biomedical and engineering purposes, despite its enormous possibilities in the field of chemical science. This article attempts to outline and contrast the most common printing techniques as well as talk about some of the recent developments in chemistry and other fields of study and education that make use of 3D printing technology [20].

Fused deposition modeling, or FDM, is one of the most popular methods of manufacturing for rapid prototyping today. It was invented by Scott Crump, the founder of Stratasys. FDM creates a three-dimensional model by extruding thermoplastic materials and depositing the semi-molten ingredients on a stage-by–stage basis. The component needed to create three-dimensional models, polymeric filaments, is transported by two rollers to the extruder's nozzle tip attached to the printer heads. Temperature-control devices heat the filaments to a semi-molten state. As the head of the printer proceeds horizontally along the layout of each determined cross-sectional layer, the semi-melted components emerge from the spray nozzle and combine in the right locations. After that, the stage descends, and another layer is applied in the same manner. Layer by layer, these operations are repeated to create a three-dimensional structure [38]. Typically, the internal frameworks are printed level by level after the part's shape has been produced. The slicing software's inherent characteristics result in surface defects such as chordal and staircase effects from this specific technique.

Heterogeneities in filament input width and density could lead to internal problems since they affect how the substance comes out through the printer needle. FDM's ability to build items composed of various materials by printing and then modifying the print material is one of its primary advantages since it gives users greater oversight around the construction of equipment for testing [12]. Additionally, standard materials like polystyrene, glass-reinforced polymers, metal, ceramics, and bioresorbable materials can all be printed as three-dimensional models using fused deposition modeling (FDM). The particulate is frequently utilized in a filament procedure by mixing metal or ceramic powders with a binder [2, 33].

14.1.2 Principle of FDM 3D Printing Technique

Because of the foundations of the technology of additive manufacturing or pharmaceutical three-dimensional printing, this method is ideal for the automated production of granular pediatric medicines. Compared to liquid medications, solid medications provide a number of advantages for treating pediatric patients. They exhibit great dosage accuracy, strong microbiological stability, superior chemical and physical stability, and controlled release qualities. Doses can only be adjusted gradually within predetermined limits when using standard production techniques. Pharmaceuticals may now be manufactured with exact and completely adjustable dosages thanks to 3D printing. There are many challenges faced by 3D printing, but it has several advantages in practical life, as shown in Fig. 14.2. Forms for medications are created using a computer-aided design (CAD) package and published coating through coating in a predetermined shape. It is theoretically possible to print in any size or shape [37].

In fused deposit modeling (FDM), additionally referred to as the extrusion of materials, the additive manufacturing technique employs polymers as the starting point (filaments). Usually, the material being printed is pushed through the 3D printer's nozzle after being heated to a melted condition. The sprayer bounce can change in three degrees of freedom (DoF) according to the code called G-code directions to position the sprayed polymer on the building plate. The fundamental idea behind the technique of FDM is shown in the conceptual figure (Fig. 14.1). As you may have seen, the equipment feeds filament into the extruder and nozzle

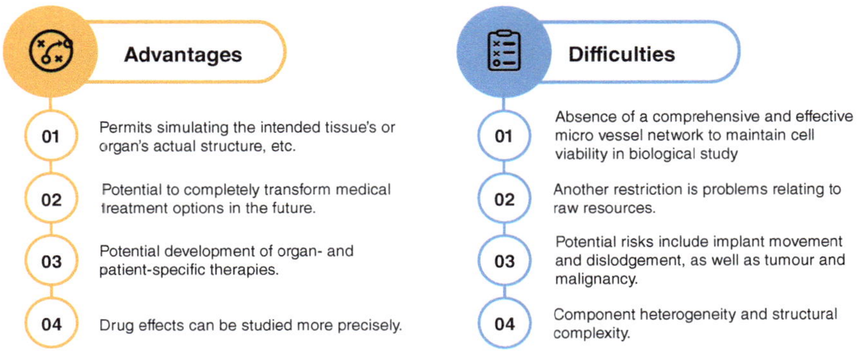

Fig. 14.2 Advantages and difficulties in 3D printing model formation

Table 14.1 Comparison between different 3D printing [8, 9, 13, 18, 46]

Method	Principle	Materials used
Stereolithography (SLA)	Identification of the photoresin coating and its curing by UV	Adhesive or acrylic-like resins with proprietary photo designers, support material: Polyethylene glycols/ propylene, glycerine, and acrylate (all combined together).
Inkjet	Powder-liquid binding; photoresins can be printed inkjet using Polyjet technology, a mix of SLA and inkjet.	Plaster powder fragments (50–100 μm in diameter) resemble photoresins.
Selective laser sintering (SLS)	Particles of powder heated by a laser	Nylon, powdered PC, ABS, PVC, metals, ceramic powders, resin, and polyester.
Fused deposition modeling (FDM)	Thermoplastic molten extruded	Wax balances, PC, ABS, PS,, metals/ ceramics (with binder), nylon
Laminated object manufacturing (LOM)	Utilizing a laser or razor to reduce hot, adhesive-coated sheet material	Metal sheets, paper, cellulose adhesive-coated polymer

continuously by rotating its two breakers in conflicting guidelines. This material will be added to the construction plate layer by layer until the desired shape and measurements are reached [30]. During the procedure, the machine's nozzle moves forward and backward in accordance with the geographic coordinates of the CAD model employed in the G-code files until the element has the right dimension and shape. Certain FDM systems (3D printers) can use multiple-state extruded nozzles for installing compositions of gradient ingredients. Various printers for 3D printing are designed for different types of thermoplastic filament, as the filament's properties largely impact the level of detail and efficacy of the extrusion. The vast majority of low-cost FDM three-dimensional printers can only produce a single kind of thermoplastic material, polylactic acid (PLA), and it's especially prevalent [43]. Table 14.1 compares 3D printing methods and explains how FDM differs from various other methods for creating 3D objects.

14.2 Innovative Global Regulatory Agencies to Address FDM 3D Printing Technology

The enormous future potential of 3D printing, especially in the aftermath of the COVID-19 epidemic, prompted the development of personalized therapeutic devices (MDs) and revolutionized the healthcare industry. This study seeks to offer a summary of the current state of additive manufacturing and the potential that is now being investigated following the introduction of the new medical equipment regulation (MDR) in the EU. The early-phase implementation of the qualitative by design (QbD) quality control system is a significant advancement in MD advancement. Not only does this underscore the current challenges associated with 3D bioprinting in particular, but it could additionally guarantee that MD innovation is successfully completed by putting into practice a regulatory-backed QbD idea. Medical creation of devices can be targeted to accelerate by using a quality-by-design (QbD) technical and crisis management approach that considers the requirements of patients, the biomedical sector, and regulatory organizations [51]. A quality-by-design (QbD) scientific and risk analysis approach ensures that the manufacturing of medical devices is accelerated in a targeted manner by taking into account the requirements of patients, the biomedical community, and regulatory bodies.

The regulators are focusing on the 3D printing process and its numerous underlying mechanisms in order to revolutionize the manufacturing and use of dosage forms; however, it has raised a number of concerns about the supervision and performance evaluation of commercially printed 3D-printed products both before and after they become readily accessible to purchase [17]. In 2017, the Food and Drug Administration (FDA) issued its final guidance on the technical issues for regulating printed medical devices using 3D printer, focusing on the gadget's conception, production, and usage. The recommendations provide preliminary legal standards for the use of health products manufactured with a printer that prints in three dimensions. However, as some products—especially ones that are customized for a patient—may require a separate evaluation of their effectiveness as well as their safety, these notions may not be applicable to all 3D-printed therapeutic strategies.

Despite the FDA's approval of the originally printed tablets [32], there currently exist no rules or regulations governing 3D-printed medications. The pharmaceutical industry's advances in printing will also provide unique challenges. These include the necessity to research the foundations underlying different printing advances, assess the efficacy of pharmaceuticals printed in three dimensions, analyze the distribution of planning in vivo and in vitro, and monitor the quality of three-dimensional formulations. Fortunately, the FDA's Office of Testing and Research is convening meetings to discover solutions to these issues. Furthermore, an increasing number of professionals are calling for research in this field. If applicable regulatory requirements are reinforced, printing technology in pharmaceutical formulations could transition from theoretical study to practical implementation [17].

Both technological and regulatory obstacles are presented by 3D production skills in the highly regulated therapeutic business. Pharmaceutical companies are frequently reluctant to embrace new technologies without comprehensive validation data because of the strict quality and risk management procedures that regulatory authorities have imposed. The industry's dependence on tried-and-true manufacturing techniques and the absence of a strong regulatory framework—which specifically addresses the special requirements of 3D printing—complicate this cautious approach. The current standards focus more on manufacturing process validation than on individual production line components since they were created with traditional manufacturing processes in mind. There is a lack of precise regulatory advice because of the reference regulatory authorities' limited knowledge and paperwork about new production technologies like 3D printing [39].

The necessity for regulatory improvements to keep up with technical innovations is expanding as technology advances. This entails setting guidelines for the certification of 3D printing machinery, procedure endorsement, and excellent regulatory procedures particular to the expertise's use in the manufacturing of pharmaceuticals. Regulating organizations are starting to create frameworks that take into account the unique characteristics of 3D printing in order to solve these issues. For example, more comprehensive criteria for 3D printing in pharmaceutical production may be derived from the FDA's recommendations on technical concerns for additively created medical equipment. The pharmaceutical industry's capacity to successfully negotiate various regulatory environments, protect patient safety, and promote technological advancement will determine the direction of 3D printing in the decades to come [27].

Therefore, cooperation between providers, technology experts, and regulatory bodies would be required to establish a framework for regulation that allows the safe and efficient integration of 3D printing into pharmaceutical development, producing goods, and academic operations.

For the pharmaceutical business to remain innovative, regulatory agencies must support new technology. Technological advancements such as 3D printing are accelerated by regulatory backing, which also guarantees that their commercialization is consistent with public health objectives. Regulators may preserve patient safety and progress science by reducing possible dangers connected with new technology through the provision of clear standards and procedures. Such regulatory validation is necessary to preserve the truthfulness and effectiveness of the therapeutic manufacturing procedure [14].

Physical quality faults (bending, layer shifting, z-layer separation, etc.) are expected in the background of 3D-printed medicines, likewise, and pose excellent control difficulties. The current state of technology and quality control measures might not be enough to stop these kinds of errors, which emphasizes the crucial role regulatory bodies play in enforcing laws that strike a balance between technology's limitations, its performance, and the safety and effectiveness of pharmaceutical products. In order for the pharmaceutical industry to properly utilize cutting-edge technology like 3D printing and eventually enhance outcomes for patients, regulatory monitoring is necessary [3].

There is a pressing need to create regulatory standards for 3D-printed preparations, as no regulatory agency has yet released rules for themselves. Presumably, when 3D printing expertise develops and investigators do more work, it will eventually be able to offer the pharmaceutical business a set of scientific standards encompassing theory, manufacture, and laws [49].

The last three decades have seen the development of 3D printing technology. It's only lately been widely accessible and reasonably priced enough for people in general to use. It's a way to turn computer designs into actual sculptures. It is now simple to access all the supplies, software tools, and repositories for sharing and downloading designs required to produce printed products. Currently, Michigan Technological University is building an open library of optical device components that are 3D printed. At the moment, polylactic acid and acrylonitrile butadiene styrene are the components that 3D printers utilize most frequently. Generally speaking, 3D printers work by building objects from multiple thin layers of material. Typically, multiple thin layers of material are used to make objects using 3D printers [24]. Depending on whether a fused deposition modeling, stereolithography, or selective laser sintering printer is being utilized, different material selection and layer bonding processes apply.

SLS is a type of 3D printing for materials that use custom powders. A residue is shaped into an appropriate form using a laser, which is also used to bind newly deposited powder layers together. The outermost layer of material is subsequently reinforced by shot peening. Parts made of metal, wax, nylon, ceramic, or composite materials can be printed using this type of technology. Although they are more expensive, SLS machines with post-curing procedures produce extremely accurate models with flawless surfaces [23].

In terms of operation, FDM and inkjet printers are comparable. Using a quick prototype technique known as "layered manufacturing," it deposits the melted plastic lines in layers onto the surface using printer heads.

14.2.1 Type of Collaborations in Global Market

Industries such as manufacturing have been using 3D printing for decades, mostly to create product prototypes. For the purpose of creating molds and models, several businesses utilize huge, quick 3D printers known as "rapid prototyping machines." For business use, there are tons of .stl files accessible. A large number of these printed products are interchangeable with conventionally manufactured products.

There are now businesses using 3D printing for commercial medical uses. Among them are Organovo, a business that creates living human tissue via 3D printing, Helisys, and Ultimaker. Currently, nonetheless, 3D printing has little effect on medicine. Currently, the $700 million three-dimensional printing market has only $11 million (1.6%) allocated to medical applications [29].

14.2.1.1 Commercial Collaboration

Technology for 3D printing is becoming easier to use and less expensive so that customers may afford it. Downloading software from internet databases of 3D printing designs has become more widely available, partly because of its growing applicability and declining price. Anything may now be printed, including jewelry, firearms, clothes, and auto parts.

The public has had access to two freely available 3D printers until 2006: RepRap (www.reprap.org/wiki/RepRap) and Fab@Home (www.fabathome.org). The entry hurdle for those looking to investigate and create novel concepts for 3D printing has been significantly reduced by the ready accessibility of these types of open-source machines [20].

The democratization of the creation and production of products is another advantageous aspect of three-dimensional printing. The range of materials that can be used for 3D printing is expanding, and the cost of those materials is also decreasing. This makes it possible for more people, especially those in the medical field, to design and create unique items for their own use or for commercial purposes using just a 3D printer and their creativity.

The properties of data packages for 3D printing also provide an unprecedented opportunity for researchers to collaborate with one another. Six Researchers can use downloadable. Files from freely available repositories instead of attempting to duplicate the settings described in scholarly publications [33]. Commercial tissue engineering scaffolds have only been launched by a small number of companies. The widely recognized manufacturer of 3D-printable healthcare products with FDA approval, Organogenesis Inc., recently announced GINTUITTM, a 2012-certified biological engineering product for oral soft tissue regeneration. It is a combination of gene therapy and therapy with a cell product that has been commercialized and contains fibroblasts and keratinocytes in bovine collagen. Another well-known supplier, Stryker, introduced the titanium lumbar posterior cage, Tritanium® LP, in 2016. Titanium alloy and plenty of porous DMLS technology are used in the construction of the timber cage. The permeable interior surfaces of the timber backbone promote blood flow and development of bones [16].

14.2.1.2 Vaccine, Medication, and Prosthetic Limbs

The printed beads using 3D printer known as VaxBeads, which stand for multiple immunizations, took first place in the Printers for Peace contest held by Michigan Technological University. Patients are supposed to wear these tiny beads as a bracelet, acting as a kind of visual health record. The patient's date of birth, identification number, and monogram are all included on each VaxBead strand. It was recently suggested that such "beads" further symbolize patient prescription drugs, including dosage information, in order to expand on this concept [1]). Consumers in developing countries frequently don't know the true name and dosage of the medications they take because of inaccurate documentation or missing official records.

Time, a total publication, featured "Not Impossible," an investigative company that specializes in resolving complex medical issues with inexpensive, freely available methods, in April 2012. In the war-torn Sudan, "Not Impossible" has begun employing 3D printing technology to create high-tech, low-cost prosthetic limbs with controlled fingers. Together with Mick Ebeling, co-founder and chief operating officer of "Not Impossible," American surgeon Dr. Tom Catena has made significant contributions to the medical care of people in developing nations. The two have established a research facility at a nearby hospital that uses consumer-grade 3D printers to create affordable artificial limbs, making them straightforward and readily available for anybody who needs one. This project is a significant step forward towards delivering good healthcare to citizens in inferior countries suffering from terrible illnesses [36]. Furthermore, 3D printing may be effective in treating gangrene or severe diabetes that requires amputation.

14.2.1.3 Drug Transport

Administering drugs will undoubtedly change as 3D printing finds greater application in medical fields. Not only may medications be printed with individual doses, but they can also have many layers of both immediate and sustained release, which lets the dosage profile be changed. This enables more individualized treatment plans and might help patients using high-dose drugs cut down on the number of tablets they must take. Systems for perfectly fitting a patient's anatomy with 3D-printed medication distribution are also being developed. The breadth of subjects addressed in this introduction shows how profoundly 3D printing technology is changing medicine. Actually, there are already so many different possibilities for 3D production in medication that it is practically hard to conduct a thorough and exhaustive analysis of them all. A variety of contemporary investigations have concentrated on a particular area, such as the review of 3D printing based on medical imaging by Mehndiratta et al., the research of bioprinting for tissues and systems by Pati et al., and the evaluation of three-dimensional publishing in surgery by Martelli et al. This evaluation will look at developments in each one of the software programs we've mentioned above over the last 3 years (from 2014 to the present) to show the current situation of the discipline at the moment [42].

14.2.1.4 Personalized 3D-Printed Medicines

3D Printed Medications Like Spritam®

The FDA authorized Spritam® (Aprecia Pharmaceuticals, East Windsor, NJ, USA), the very first medicine to be 3D printed, in 2015. Spritam® contains the antiepileptic API levetiracetam. Its soluble and porous matrix composition allowed for a significant solubilization time savings without sacrificing pharmacological efficacy over that of traditional pills.

Aprecia Pharmaceuticals marks Spritam® with the ZipDose technology, which is based on the layer-by-layer manufacturing method of powder bed fusing. The active ingredient and every excipient obligatory to brand the matrix drug make up the major coating. A binder liquid is then applied to ensure flawless aggregation and integration between each succeeding layer that is uniform. The result is an orally dispersible tablet that dissolves quickly in barely any alcohol and has a dosage capability of almost 1000 mg of API. The development demonstrates how technological advances can be used to create customized forms of administration with characteristics that can't be obtained by compression or other traditional methods of production.

Polypill

A "polypill" is a solitary dose that comprises multiple medications. The elderly population benefits greatly from this idea since they are more likely to experience various illnesses and, consequently, multiple therapies. The development of the revolutionary dose of multi-active solid form recognized as a polypill has been made possible by the application of 3D extrusion printing. With the help of this innovative technique, five different medications with predetermined release patterns were successfully integrated into separate compartments. With the integration of many customized tablets, this advancement streamlines complex drug regimens, offering a promising solution for patients managing multiple prescriptions. Because of the technology's flexibility, drug combinations and release patterns can be commissioned to meet the precise needs of every patient.

Featuring compartments for pravastatin, atenolol, ramipril, hydrochlorothiazide, aspirin, and extended-release, the polypill project was concentrated on circulatory system management. XRPD and ATR-FTIR techniques were used to confirm that there were no adverse reactions between the medicine and its excipient and that the 3D printing process had not changed the medicament's properties. This accomplishment confirms that a complex polypill with unique geometries was successfully created using 3D banishment production, demonstrating the polypill's aptitude to efficiently distribute several active components via varied release mechanisms. This significant achievement has great potential to enhance patient compliance and customize dosages in the handy single-tablet shape, especially for both the avoidance and management of cardiovascular disorders [41].

Similar research was done by Khaled, who employed 3D extrusion-based manufacturing as a novel method of producing multi-active tablets with precisely organized statement designs for three unrelated prescriptions. A "polypill," created using a 3D preservative procedure, combines intricate drug schedules into a solitary, adaptable pill. The tablet has an osmotic captopril pump in addition to sustained-release glipizide and nifedipine chambers. This combination may be useful in the treatment of hypertensive diabetes. In this work, extrusion at room temperature is employed for analysis, utilizing standard pharmaceutical excipients. The US Pharmacopoeia (USP) dissolving test is used to monitor drug release, and procedures like X-ray powder diffraction (XRPD) and amplified entire reflection-Fourier transformation ultraviolet (ATR-FTIR) are employed to evaluate pharmaceutical-excipient mixtures. The captopril compartment behaves like an osmotic pump, according to the results, releasing the drug in a zero-order manner [26].

14.3 Challenges and New Trends

Since 3D printing can be used to customize medications, systems, and nutritional supplements, it is anticipated to play a significant role in the transition to personalized medical services, as shown in Table 14.2. It is anticipated that 3D printing will spread throughout pharmacies. Providing pharmacies with information medication formulations for drug manufacturing on demand could replace the current manufacturing and distribution practices utilized by pharmaceutical companies. The current medicine manufacturing and delivery procedures would undergo a considerable transition as a result, becoming more efficient. If maximum communal drugs are

Table 14.2 3D printing applications in customized medicine [26, 41, 42]

Area of usage	Definition	Use
Medical implants	Implants customized for each patient (e.g., hip, dental) Optimal fit, shorter surgical times, and better results	Optimum fit, shorter surgical times, and better results
Drug dosage forms	Customized doses and patterns of medication release	It is a customized medicine administration and the opportunity of increased patient compliance
Prosthetics	Prosthetic limbs or pieces manufactured to order	Increased patient comfort, more undertaking, and better fit
Bioprinted tissues/structures	Printed biomaterials and cells to promote tissue redevelopment	Probable remedies, customized tissue grafts, for the lack of organ donors
Personalized medical devices	Devices made to order (e.g., braces, orthotics)	Improved comfort and maximized functionality

completely obtainable in this way, consumers might be capable of reducing the number of pills they take each day to just one polypill; this would promote compliance from patients. The bioprinting process of intricate organs is anticipated to be the most technically advanced use case for three-dimensional printing. It is predicted that an entirely functioning printed heart will be available in less than 20 years. Despite the challenges associated with printing circulation networks, manufactured organs are still a long way off [5]. Nevertheless, the progress that has been made so far is impressive. It is anticipated that sophisticated heterogeneous tissue, like the kidneys and the liver, will be efficiently produced as technology advances. This allows for the creation of printed tissue and organ models for the purpose of finding new drugs, as well as functional living implants.

Additionally, it might be able to print a strip of a patient's tissue for usage in clinical trials to find the best course of treatment. One day, it may be possible to grow and build permanent replacement tissues and organs using stem cells derived from an infant's or a kid's tooth [20].

Another projected future breakthrough is the in situ printer technique, which produces implants or living organs inside the human body during operation. Following exact digital supervision, 3D bioprinting can be utilized to produce an architecture consisting of cells, growth factors, and biomaterials to repair a range of wound kinds and densities [22]. In situ biological printing techniques have been successfully used to mend external organs like the epidermis.

In the past 10 years, medical tissue engineering has seen a strong emergence of additive development, also recognized as 3D printing, which has ushered in a completely new era in health care technology. Bioprinting has also been among the most prominent applications of this integration. This technique does more than just create frameworks; it opens the way for complex arrangements that evenly distribute cells. The genius of bioprinting resides in its ability to precisely arrange many cell types inside its support structure, mimicking the complex structures of tissues composed of different kinds of cells or the points where two distinct tissues converge. Nonetheless, the resources utilized and the complexity of the scaffolding strategy have a direct impact on the bioprinting process' efficiency and effectiveness.

This is predominantly correct in light of its probable, mostly unexplored, straight in situ submissions [31]. A careful analysis shows there isn't a single bioprinting strategy that works for every application. Rather, a number of factors are taken into account, such as the required speed of manufacturing and solution, costs, and the special capacity to print in multiple orientations, including vertically.

These difficulties suggest that an alliance is in store for the next phase of bioprinting technology. The current research mindset is focused on combining multiple approaches so they can support one another. This cooperative method purposes to optimize the synthesis of assemblies that are functional and look like genuine tissues [41].

14.4 Conclusion

Digital creation with the use of progressive component adjustments and technical advancements, 3D printing, also known as additive manufacturing, turns geometrical plans into physical objects. This idea has become extremely common very rapidly, and it has applications in many other industries. The best examples of three-dimensional printing's versatility are its capacity to create freely available creates, mass customize products, and serve a variety of businesses, including medical treatment, agriculture, automotive, locomotives, and aviation. By depositing substance progressively, 3D printing produces objects based on a geometric pattern. The last few decades have seen a significant growth in this technique, signifying a significant turning point. In 1980, Charles Hull spearheaded the commercialization of 3D printing technologies. PGA rocket engines, an Amsterdam steel bridge, jewelry lines, 3D-printed corneas, artificial heart pumps, and a host of items for the food industry and aerospace sectors are just a few of the many uses for 3D printing that are currently underway. The three-dimensional printing technology is an innovative and flexible framework that builds three-dimensional objects layer by layer using computer-aided design (CAD) drawings.

There are many advantages to incorporating 3D printing technology into the health care sector, such as the capacity to personalize medications, tools, and medicinal supplies; financial advantages; heightened efficiency; democratized design and production procedures; and enhanced teamwork. The first uses of 3D production in the medicinal ground were to produce physiologically accurate orthopedic and therapeutic components tailored to each patient, including customized implants for teeth and operation schedules. This is particularly true in light of its relatively unexplored potential for direct in situ uses. A careful analysis shows there isn't a single bioprinting strategy that works for all purposes. Rather, a number of factors are taken into account, such as the required pace of production and conclusion, costs, and the special capacity to print in multiple beginnings, notably vertical.

All of these challenges suggest that a merger is in store for the development of biological printing. The present investigation approach is aimed at integrating many approaches and allowing them to complement one another. This collaborative technique aims to optimize the development of structures that imitate and operate like genuine tissues.

References

1. "3D printers for peace" contest—the results are in (n.d.).
2. Aimar A, Palermo A, Innocenti B. The role of 3D printing in medical applications: a state of the art. J Healthc Eng. 2019; https://doi.org/10.1155/2019/5340616.
3. Alzhrani RF, Alyahya MY, Algahtani MS, Fitaihi RA, Tawfik EA. Trend of pharmaceuticals 3D printing in the Middle East and North Africa (MENA) region: an overview, regulatory perspective and future outlook. Saudi Pharmaceutical Journal. 2024;32(6):7–8. https://doi.org/10.1016/j.jsps.2024.102098.
4. Awad A, Trenfield SJ, Gaisford S, Basit AW. 3D printed medicines: a new branch of digital healthcare. Int J Pharm. 2018;548(1):586–96. https://doi.org/10.1016/j.ijpharm.2018.07.024.
5. Banks J. Adding value in additive manufacturing: researchers in the United Kingdom and Europe look to 3D printing for customization. IEEE Pulse. 2013;4(6):22–6. https://doi.org/10.1109/MPUL.2013.2279617.
6. Beck RCR, Chaves PS, Goyanes A, Vukosavljevic B, Buanz A, Windbergs M, Basit AW, Gaisford S. 3D printed tablets loaded with polymeric nanocapsules: an innovative approach to produce customized drug delivery systems. Int J Pharm. 2017;528(1–2):268–79. https://doi.org/10.1016/j.ijpharm.2017.05.074.
7. Beer N, Hegger I, Kaae S, De Bruin ML, Genina N, Alves TL, Hoebert J, Kälvemark Sporrong S. Scenarios for 3D printing of personalized medicines – a case study. Exploratory Res Clin Social Pharm. 2021;4 https://doi.org/10.1016/j.rcsop.2021.100073.
8. Breitkreutz J, Boos J. Paediatric and geriatric drug delivery. Expert Opin Drug Deliv. 2007;4(1):37–45. https://doi.org/10.1517/17425247.4.1.37.
9. Brennan MD, Bokhari FF, Eddington DT. Open design 3D-printable adjustable micropipette that meets the ISO standard for accuracy. Micromachines. 2018;9(4):1–15. https://doi.org/10.3390/mi9040191.
10. Cailleaux S, Sanchez-Ballester NM, Gueche YA, Bataille B, Soulairol I. Fused Deposition Modeling (FDM), the new asset for the production of tailored medicines. J Control Release. 2021;330:821–41. https://doi.org/10.1016/j.jconrel.2020.10.056.
11. Calignano F, Manfredi D, Ambrosio EP, Biamino S, Lombardi M, Atzeni E, Salmi A, Minetola P, Iuliano L, Fino P. Overview on additive manufacturing technologies. Proc IEEE. 2017;105(4):593–612. https://doi.org/10.1109/JPROC.2016.2625098.
12. Chandekar A, Mishra DK, Sharma S, Saraogi GK, Gupta G. 3D printing technology: a new milestone in the development of pharmaceuticals. Curr Pharm Des. 2019;25(9):937–45.
13. Cooke MN, Fisher JP, Dean D, Rimnac C, Mikos AG. Use of stereolithography to manufacture critical-sized 3D biodegradable scaffolds for bone ingrowth. J Biomed Mater Res B Appl Biomater. 2003;64(2):65–9. https://doi.org/10.1002/jbm.b.10485.
14. Cui M, Pan H, Su Y, Fang D, Qiao S, Ding P, Pan W. Opportunities and challenges of three-dimensional printing technology in pharmaceutical formulation development. Acta Pharm Sin B. 2021;11(8):2488–504. https://doi.org/10.1016/j.apsb.2021.03.015.
15. Deshmukh K, Houkan MT, AlMaadeed MAA, Sadasivunid KK. Introduction to 3D and 4D printing technology: state of the art and recent trends. In: 3D and 4D printing of polymer nanocomposite materials: processes, applications, and challenges; 2019. p. 1–24. https://doi.org/10 1016/B978-0-12-816805-9.00001-6.

16. Fan D, Li Y, Wang X, Zhu T, Wang Q, Cai H, Li W, Tian Y, Liu Z. Progressive 3D printing technology and its application in medical materials. Front Pharmacol. 2020;11:24–5. https://doi.org/10.3389/fphar.2020.00122.
17. Food and Drug Administration. Technical considerations for additive manufactured medical devices: guidance for industry and food and drug administration staff document. In: Center for devices and radiological health; 2017.
18. Gomes C, Travitzky N, Greil P, Acchar W, Birolis H, De Oliveira APN, Hotza D. Laminated object manufacturing of LZSA glass-ceramics. Rapid Prototyp J. 2011;17(6):424–8. https://doi.org/10.1108/13552541111184152.
19. Goyanes A, Buanz ABM, Hatton GB, Gaisford S, Basit AW. 3D printing of modified-release aminosalicylate (4-ASA and 5-ASA) tablets. Eur J Pharm Biopharm. 2015;89:157–62.
20. Gross BC, Erkal JL, Lockwood SY, Chen C, Spence DM. Evaluation of 3D printing and its potential impact on biotechnology and the chemical sciences. Anal Chem. 2014;86(7):3240–53. https://doi.org/10.1021/ac403397r.
21. Hoffmann L, Breitkreutz J, Quodbach J. Fused Deposition Modeling (FDM) 3D printing of the thermo-sensitive peptidomimetic drug enalapril maleate. Pharmaceutics. 2022;14(11):1–14. https://doi.org/10.3390/pharmaceutics14112411.
22. Holzmann P, Breitenecker RJ, Soomro AA, Schwarz EJ. User entrepreneur business models in 3D printing. J Manuf Technol Manag. 2017;28(1):75–94. https://doi.org/10.1108/JMTM-12-2015-0115.
23. Hoy MB. 3D printing: making things at the library. Med Ref Serv Q. 2013;32(1):93–9. https://doi.org/10.1080/02763869.2013.749139.
24. Ibrahim AMS, Jose RR, Rabie AN, Gerstle TL, Lee BT, Lin SJ. Three-dimensional printing in developing countries. Plast Reconstr Surg Glob Open. 2015;3(7):1–17. https://doi.org/10.1097/GOX.0000000000000298.
25. Jakus AE. "An introduction to 3D printing—past, present, and future promise". In 3D printing in orthopaedic surgery. Am Ceram Soc Bull. 2019;98(4):1–15.
26. Joshua RJN, Raj SA, Hameed Sultan MT, Łukaszewicz A, Józwik J, Oksiuta Z, Dziedzic K, Tofil A, Shahar FS. Powder bed fusion 3D printing in precision manufacturing for biomedical applications: a comprehensive review. Materials. 2024;17(3):1–30. https://doi.org/10.3390/ma17030769.
27. Junker B. Discussing tomorrow' s regulatory risks today. PDA J Pharm Sci Technol. 2017;71:1–6.
28. Khorsandi D, Fahimipour A, Abasian P, Saber SS, Seyedi M, Ghanavati S, Ahmad A, De Stephanis AA, Taghavinezhaddilami F, Leonova A, Mohammadinejad R, Shabani M, Mazzolai B, Mattoli V, Tay FR, Makvandi P. 3D and 4D printing in dentistry and maxillofacial surgery: printing techniques, materials, and applications. Acta Biomater. 2021;122:26–49. https://doi.org/10.1016/j.actbio.2020.12.044.
29. Klein GT, Lu Y, Wang MY. 3D printing and neurosurgery-ready for prime time? World Neurosurg. 2013;80(3–4):233–5. https://doi.org/10.1016/j.wneu.2013.07.009.
30. Klingmann V, Spomer N, Lerch C, Stoltenberg I, Frömke C, Bosse HM, Breitkreutz J, Meissner T. Favorable acceptance of mini-tablets compared with syrup: a randomized controlled trial in infants and preschool children. J Pediatr. 2013;163(6):1–7. https://doi.org/10.1016/j.jpeds.2013.07.014.
31. Kollamaram G, Croker DM, Walker GM, Goyanes A, Basit AW, Gaisford S. Low temperature fused deposition modeling (FDM) 3D printing of thermolabile drugs. Int J Pharm. 2018;545(1–2):144–52. https://doi.org/10.1016/j.ijpharm.2018.04.055.
32. Krueger L, Miles JA. Clinical translation of 3D printed pharmaceuticals. 2024;1:5–9.
33. Lee Ventola C. Medical applications for 3D printing: current and projected uses. P and T. 2014;39(10):704–11.
34. Litman T. Personalized medicine—concepts, technologies, and applications in inflammatory skin diseases. APMIS. 2019;127(5):386–424. https://doi.org/10.1111/apm.12934.
35. Long J, Gholizadeh H, Lu J, Bunt C, Seyfoddin A. Application of fused deposition modelling (FDM) method of 3D printing in drug delivery. Curr Pharm Des. 2016;23(3):433–9. https://doi.org/10.2174/1381612822666161026162707.

36. McCracken H. How a TIME article led to the invention of a $100 3D-printed artificial limb I TIME.com. Time Mag. 2014:7–8. http://techland.time.com/2014/01/07/how-a-time-article-led-to-the-invention-of-a-100-3d-printed-artificial-limb/
37. Moreira M, Sarraguça M. How can oral paediatric formulations be improved? A challenge for the XXI century. Int J Pharm. 2020;590:1–8. https://doi.org/10.1016/j.ijpharm.2020.119905.
38. Mueller B, Kochan D. Laminated object manufacturing for rapid tooling and patternmaking in foundry industry. Comput Ind. 1999;39(1):47–53. https://doi.org/10.1016/S0166-3615(98)00127-4.
39. Norman J, Madurawe RD, Moore CMV, Khan MA, Khairuzzaman A. A new chapter in pharmaceutical manufacturing: 3D-printed drug products. Adv Drug Deliv Rev. 2017;108:39–50. https://doi.org/10.1016/j.addr.2016.03.001.
40. Özdemir V, Dove ES, Gürsoy UK, Şardaş S, Yıldırım A, Yılmaz ŞG, Ömer Barlas I, Güngör K, Mete A, Srivastava S. Personalized medicine beyond genomics: alternative futures in big data—proteomics, environtome and the social proteome. J Neural Transm. 2017;124(1):25–32. https://doi.org/10.1007/s00702-015-1489-y.
41. Pathak K, Saikia R, Das A, Das D, Islam MA, Pramanik P, Parasar A, Borthakur PP, Sarmah P, Saikia M, Borthakur B. 3D printing in biomedicine: advancing personalized care through additive manufacturing. Exploration of Medicine. 2023;4(6):1135–67. https://doi.org/10.37349/emed.2023.00200.
42. Pati F, Gantelius J, Svahn HA. 3D bioprinting of tissue/organ models. Angew Chem Int Ed. 2016;55(15):4650–65. https://doi.org/10.1002/anie.201505062.
43. Quodbach J, Bogdahn M, Breitkreutz J, Chamberlain R, Eggenreich K, Elia AG, Gottschalk N, Gunkel-Grabole G, Hoffmann L, Kapote D, Kipping T, Klinken S, Loose F, Marquetant T, Windolf H, Geißler S, Spitz T. Quality of FDM 3D printed medicines for pediatrics: considerations for formulation development, filament extrusion, printing process and printer design. Therapeutic Innovation and Regulatory Science. 2022;56(6):910–28. https://doi.org/10.1007/s43441-021-00354-0.
44. Robles-Martinez P, Xu X, Trenfield SJ, Awad A, Goyanes A, Telford R, Basit AW, Gaisford S. 3D printing of a multi-layered polypill containing six drugs using a novel stereolithographic method. Pharmaceutics. 2019;11(6) https://doi.org/10.3390/pharmaceutics11060274.
45. Schubert C, Van Langeveld MC, Donoso LA. Innovations in 3D printing: a 3D overview from optics to organs. Br J Ophthalmol. 2014;98(2):159–61. https://doi.org/10.1136/bjophthalmol-2013-304446.
46. Sodian R, Loebe M, Hein A, Martin DP, Hoerstrup SP, Potapov EV, Hausmann H, Lueth T, Hetzer R. Application of stereolithography for scaffold fabrication for tissue engineered heart valves. ASAIO J. 2002;48(1):12–6. https://doi.org/10.1097/00002480-200201000-00004.
47. Tabriz AG, Nandi U, Scoutaris N, Sanfo K, Alexander B, Gong Y, Hui HW, Kumar S, Douroumis D. Personalised paediatric chewable Ibuprofen tablets fabricated using 3D micro-extrusion printing technology. Int J Pharm. 2022;626 https://doi.org/10.1016/j.ijpharm.2022.122135.
48. Trenfield SJ, Awad A, Goyanes A, Gaisford S, Basit AW. 3D printing pharmaceuticals: drug development to frontline care. Trends Pharmacol Sci. 2018;39(5):440–51. https://doi.org/10.1016/j.tips.2018.02.006.
49. Wang S, Chen X, Han X, Hong X, Li X, Zhang H, Li M, Wang Z, Zheng A. A review of 3D printing technology in pharmaceutics: technology and applications, now and future. Pharmaceutics. 2023;15(2) https://doi.org/10.3390/pharmaceutics15020416.
50. Wickramasinghe S, Do T, Tran P. FDM-Based 3D printing of polymer and associated composite: a review on mechanical properties, defects and treatments. Polymers. 2020;12(7):1–42. https://doi.org/10.3390/polym12071529.
51. Zema L, Melocchi A, Maroni A, Gazzaniga A. Three-dimensional printing of medicinal products and the challenge of personalized therapy. J Pharm Sci. 2017;106(7):1697–705. https://doi.org/10.1016/j.xphs.2017.03.021.

Clinical Trials and Regulatory Approval of 3D-Printed Pharmaceuticals

15

Bannimath Gurupadayya, Meghraj Suryawanshi, Aparna Inamdar, Parashuram Bugadannavar, Arushi, Himanshu Sharma, Pranjal Gujarathi, and Kuldeep Vinchurkar

Abstract

This chapter explores the intersection of clinical trials and regulatory approval processes within the burgeoning field of 3D-printed pharmaceuticals (3D-PPs). As 3D-printing (3D-P) technology continues to evolve, its applications in pharmaceuticals offer promises of personalized medicine, enhanced drug delivery systems, and streamlined manufacturing processes. However, navigating the

B. Gurupadayya · A. Inamdar
Department of Pharmaceutical Chemistry, JSS College of Pharmacy, Mysuru, JSS Academy of Higher Education & Research, Mysuru, Karnataka, India
e-mail: bmgurupadayya@jssuni.edu.in

M. Suryawanshi
Department of Pharmaceutics and Pharmaceutical Technology, Krishna School of Pharmacy and Research, Drs. Kiran and Pallavi Patel Global University (KPGU), Varnama, Vadodara, India

P. Bugadannavar
KLE College of Pharmacy, KLE Academy of Higher Education and Research, Belagavi, Karnataka, India

Arushi
Shiva Institute of Pharmacy, Chandpur, Himachal Pradesh, India

H. Sharma
Teerthanker Mahaveer College of Pharmacy, Teerthanker Mahaveer University, Moradabad, (UP), India

P. Gujarathi
Department of Pharmacology, Vidhyadeep Institute of Pharmacy, Vidhyadeep University, Anita, Surat, Gujarat, India

K. Vinchurkar (✉)
Department of Pharmaceutics, Sandip Institute of Pharmaceutical Sciences (SIPS), Affiliated to Savitribai Phule Pune University (SPPU, Pune), Nashik, Maharashtra, India

K. Vinchurkar, S. Mane (eds.), *Innovations in Drug Manufacturing*,
https://doi.org/10.1007/978-981-96-9075-6_15

complex landscape of clinical trials and regulatory frameworks poses significant challenges. This chapter provides a comprehensive review of the status, challenges, and prospects of conducting clinical trials and obtaining regulatory approvals for 3D-PPs. It addresses key considerations such as regulatory requirements, quality control standards, patient safety, and efficacy assessment methodologies. Furthermore, it discusses emerging trends, regulatory updates, and potential strategies to facilitate the successful translation of 3D-PPs from bench to bedside.

Keywords

3D printed · Clinical trials · Regulatory agency · USFDA · MHRA

Abbreviations

3D-P	3D printing
3D-PPs	3D-printed pharmaceuticals
ADME	Absorption, distribution, metabolism, and excretion
ADRs	Adverse drug reactions
ANDA	Abbreviated new drug application
APIs	Active pharmaceutical ingredients
BIJ	Binder inkjet
BIMO	Bio-research monitoring program
CAD	Computer-aided design
CDRH	Center for Devices and Radiological Health
CJP	Continuous inkjet printing
CLIP	Continuous liquid interface production
DDD	Drug delivery devices
DOP	Drop-on-demand printing
DPE	Direct powder extrusion
EMA	European medicines agency
FDM	Fused deposition modeling
GCP	Good clinical practice
GLP	Good laboratory practice
HPMC	Hydroxypropyl methylcellulose
IND	Investigational new drug
INDA	Investigational new drug application
IVIVC	In-vitro and in-vivo correlation
MHRA	Medicines and Healthcare Products Regulatory Agency
PBF	Powder bed fusion
PD	Pharmacodynamics
PEG	Polyethylene glycol
PK	Pharmacokinetics

PLA	Polylactic acid
PVA	Polyvinyl alcohol
QA and QC	Quality assurance and control
RCTs	Randomized controlled trials
SLA	Stereolithography
SLS	Selective laser sintering
US FDA	United States Food and Drug Administration

15.1 Introduction

15.1.1 Overview of 3D Printing (3D-P) in Pharmaceuticals.

The advent of personalized medicine has led to a transformative shift in pharmaceutical manufacturing, emphasizing customized treatment approaches tailored to individual patient needs. Traditional pharmaceutical production methods, which have remained largely unchanged for over two centuries, rely on standardized dosage strengths designed for the average patient. However, such uniform dosing regimens often fail to account for interindividual variations in drug response. Studies indicate that up to 70% of patients in the UK do not achieve optimal therapeutic efficacy with conventional mass-manufactured medications, with only 30–50% of drugs proving effective in targeted populations and 7% of hospital admissions resulting from adverse drug reactions [42, 46].

A landmark moment in pharmaceutical manufacturing occurred in August 2015 when the United States Food and Drug Administration (US FDA) approved the first three-dimensional (3D) printed drug product, setting the stage for a new era in drug development and production [26]. Since the completion of the Human Genome Project, the pharmaceutical sector has increasingly explored personalized treatment approaches [5, 51, 72]. Conventional solid dosage forms, including tablets and capsules, are gradually being complemented by innovative drug delivery systems incorporating biomolecules such as DNA and proteins, offering targeted and optimized therapeutic benefits.

Despite its promise, the shift toward personalized medicine presents challenges for conventional bulk manufacturing systems. Traditional pharmaceutical production relies on high-speed machines capable of generating thousands of identical pills designed for extended stability and regulatory compliance. These products must remain chemically and physically stable over a prolonged shelf life, ensuring consistency in purity and quality. However, many promising drug candidates fail during development due to physicochemical instability, even after extensive formulation efforts to enhance their half-life. 3D printing (3D-P) offers an alternative, enabling on-demand drug fabrication with precise control over drug release profiles, impurity levels, and patient-specific needs. Although individualized compounding may seem a straightforward approach, ensuring precision in formulation design, regulatory compliance, and large-scale implementation remains complex.

The approval of the first 3D-printed pharmaceutical product has generated significant interest in personalized medicine, highlighting its potential for both large-scale and on-demand manufacturing. While 3D printing has already been widely adopted in medical device production and has received regulatory approvals through the Center for Devices and Radiological Health (CDRH) [23], its integration into pharmaceutical manufacturing is still in its early stages. Regulatory frameworks across different countries vary in their approaches to compounding, production, quality control, clinical studies, and distribution of 3D-printed pharmaceuticals [38]. Currently, the FDA has approved only one 3D-printed drug product, and regulatory bodies continue to develop guidelines addressing the technical and safety challenges associated with this emerging technology [47]. Before 3D-printed pharmaceutical products can become mainstream, several regulatory, technical, and clinical hurdles must be overcome to ensure their safety, efficacy, and widespread acceptance in global healthcare systems.

15.1.2 Importance and Potential Impact of 3D-Printed Pharmaceuticals (3D-PPs)

The novel 3D-PPs are the latest and most beneficial innovation in pharmaceutical science and the healthcare sector, as they design personalized treatment dosage regimens, varying geometries of dosage forms as per the patient's requirements, and cost-effective production. 3D-P technology permits the alterations in customized medicines as per individual specifications with adjusted doses and dosage forms. The 3D-P technology has many benefits in the healthcare profession because of its low economic burden and dosage forms that can be made available to each patient based on their need, but they still must overcome barriers of regulatory processes for on-demand tailored medication success. More research and constant refinements are essential in the 3D-P technology to meet the specifications of the regulatory bodies [55]. Spiratum, approved by the US FDA as the first 3D-P pharmaceutical drug used in the treatment of epilepsy in 2015, created a major milestone, prompting regulatory bodies to develop a set of guidelines for these emerging 3D-PPs [38]. 3D-P technology considers individual patient-related factors like genetic, physiological, and pathological conditions to design the medications as per the needs of the patients, helps to overcome the ADRs, and monitors the patient's good health in the healthcare profession. Also designs tailored medication dosages with controlled drug-releasing profiles and desired geometrical size and shape to improve therapeutic efficacy and reduce the systemic ADRs via target-specific drug delivery to the affected site. 3D-PPs can enhance the accuracy of the dosage regimen by increasing patient compliance in the pediatrics and geriatrics clinical sectors by complying with the regulatory guidelines [38, 58]. Overall, 3D-P technology contributes to the growth of the healthcare profession via patient-specific dosing with enhanced compliance with dosage forms. This technology helps to overcome the problems associated with the "one size fits all" paradigm by shifting it through personalized medications for individual patients [23, 58].

15.2 3D-P Technology in Pharmaceuticals

15.2.1 Basics of 3D-P Technology

3D-P technology is transforming the healthcare sector, making it possible to produce customized drugs according to the needs of patients and their pathological conditions. Advancements in the additive 3D-P techniques provide exact regulation of drug and excipient combinations, doses, and routes of administration, characteristics of customized medicines from the beginning till bulk manufacturing. Benefits of 3D-P technology include personalized treatments that can be designed via 3D-P technology, enabling the design of drug dosage forms with patient-specific characteristics, such as dose and drug combinations. This is particularly helpful for groups with specific needs, such as the elderly and pediatrics [8, 58]. The economic burden on patients can be decreased by reducing manufacturing expenses, labor costs, and time to market; the approach makes it possible to produce personalized medications in small quantities [13, 34]. Rapid prototype development can be achieved as 3D-P enables it to swiftly alter medication designs, allowing for more frequent modifications during the manufacturing process. 3D-P can be used to create multifunctional and complex drug delivery systems that enhance patient compliance and medical outcomes by combining many medications into a single dosage form [71]. Current application of 3D-P technology. A wide range of medicinal agents can be formulated via 3D-P technology, including capsules with both controlled and immediate effects, films that dissolve, patches of skin, tiny needles, personalized prosthetics, and inserts [71]. The techniques that are highly utilized in the 3D-P for the formulation of 3D-PPs are depicted in Fig. 15.1.

15.2.2 Types of 3D-P Techniques Used in Pharmaceuticals

15.2.2.1 Stereolithography (SLA)

Stereolithography (SLA) is a major 3D-P technique majorly utilized in the pharmaceutical stream due to its higher precision and capacity to develop intricately shaped 3D-PPs. It utilizes UV radiation in the formulation aspects for the layer-to-layer solidification of the liquid photopolymer resin on the active pharmaceutical ingredients (APIs) and excipient mixtures to enhance the binding between the particles. SLA has a wide range of applications in the field of pharmaceutical manufacturing, including personalized medication dosage administration to patients, where SLA can facilitate the creation of customized drug delivery systems that can be adapted to the unique requirements of various patients. The goal of the research is to develop multilevel polypills and pellets that can improve adherence among patients as well as efficacy by combining more APIs and excipients into one dosage form for the synergistic effect and enhanced therapeutic efficacy [20, 83]. Prototyping and rapid development of 3D-PPs by SLA due to their speed and accuracy make it an excellent choice for the accurate and timely development of novel medications. Experiments with various dimensions and discharge profiles allow scientists to

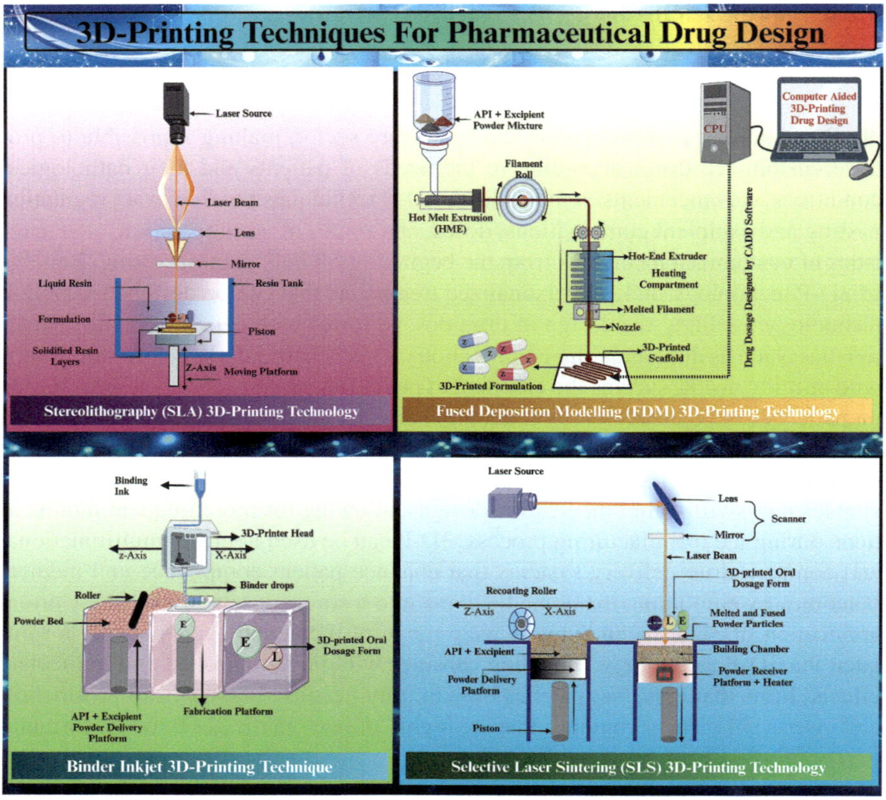

Fig. 15.1 3D-printing techniques in the formulation of 3D-pharmaceutical products

swiftly modify the designs to optimize the drug distribution patterns in the human body. During the early stages of drug discovery and development, these modifications can be quite beneficial, as adjustments can be made regularly to get achievable results with good therapeutic outcomes [41]. Oral dosage formulations where the printlets and pellets are major examples of oral dose forms that have been successfully manufactured using SLA. To manage treatment outcomes, medications can be prepared to achieve controlled drug release profiles, with regulated or immediate drug disintegration from the formulation. Various researchers reported that SLA can be successfully used to create systolic poly-printlets, underscoring the possibility of use in the fabrication of potent oral medicines [82].

15.2.2.2 Fused Deposition Modeling (FDM)

The FDM 3D-P technique works on the principle where the thermoplastic polymers are heated below their melting point temperature and then extruded through the nozzle in layers of API and excipients to construct the drug formulation. The movement between the printer head and the material deposition is controlled by using computer-aided design (CAD) technology. The built structure descends after every single layer has been printed to make vacant space for the unprinted subsequent layer, and this technique is repeated till the desired outcome is achieved [34, 58]. Applications of FDM include personalized medication regimens where the development of customized drugs is made possible by FDM. To enhance the patient's compliance and the effectiveness of the treatment regime, FDM was utilized, for example, to produce 3D-P pills that can administer several medications in a single treatment. Changing the concentration and amount of API and excipient fillings and shapes of the formulations enables customized release profiles that meet the needs of individual patients [31, 57]. 3D-PPs with controlled drug release profiles: here the formulations with a controlled release can be prepared with FDM technology and offer a regular release of medication throughout the shelf life of the product. This is accomplished through modifying a thermoplastic material composition that is utilized, in addition to printing parameters like speed of printing and nozzle diameter. These studies have demonstrated that the speed of release can be precisely adjusted to produce the intended therapeutic effects [78]. The development of thermolabile drug formulations is one of the major difficulties faced during the formulation of 3D-PPs of thermal-sensitive drugs, but it can be overcome with FDM technology, as it prevents the degradation of thermolabile medications by reducing their exposure to extremely high degrees of temperature while printing. Also, the research on FDM technology has shown that drug deterioration can be reduced by modifying printing parameters, such as utilizing a bigger nozzle size and modifying printing velocities. For instance, incorporating temperature-sensitive medications such as a maleate drug has been effectively formulated with FDM; however, the degree of drug integrity preservation has varied [31, 57].

15.2.2.3 Selective Laser Sintering [SLS]

SLS works by the principle of application of a thin layer of microscopic particle structure built on an API and excipient, and subsequently, the laser beam traverses the outermost layer, sintering the powder in specific areas by using an image as a guide. The platform moves down after applying one layer of powder, and the process is repeated until the intended 3D-P is achieved in the formulation. Application of SLS in the 3D-PPs includes the formulation of controlled-release drugs with fixed compositions, where the SLS is specifically useful in the production of drugs with regulated drug release in the human body upon their administration. Through the laser settings and film density adjustments, the formulation and development scientists can formulate a desired drug release profile, which can deliver the treatment medication agent at a consistent rate throughout the half-life of the drug. This ability is crucial for managing long-term conditions that need regular drug dosages. Similar and conventional formulations may not be beneficial for every patient, so the design of personalized medication plans for each patient via 3D-PPs through the SLS 3D-P technology has made it possible to create medications that are specifically tailored to each patient's needs. For example, SLS can create multi-drug printlets, which combine many APIs into a single dose form to enhance treatment strategies for patients with multiple health issues. The preparation of tablets that disintegrate upon oral administration as orally dispersing pills, which dissolve fast in the oral cavity to enhance compliance among patients, is satisfactorily prepared using SLS. These pills may have a rapid onset of action and pharmaceutical release of API that delivers instant therapeutic benefits [40].

15.2.2.4 Binder Inkjet (BIJ) 3D-P Technology

BIJ 3D-P technology is the most popular and highly preferred 3D-P technology in the pharmaceutical industry, as it develops multi-drug API and excipient mixtures in a precise manner. The following are the four primary uses of BIJ in 3D-P technology: customization of drug dosage forms. By using BIJ, the drug formulations can be made to meet the requirements of each patient. This includes the ability to incorporate many medications into a single dosage form, which enhances patient adherence and therapeutic efficacy. Furthermore, the BIJ-3D-P technology can handle many granular materials, which develops opportunities for various degrees of composition that are not achievable with traditional manufacturing methods [59]. The powder bed will be coated with the liquid binding agent in the powder BIJ 3D-P technique. In the process of enhancing the binding of the powder particles together, enabling the formation of solid drug structures. Its capacity to develop complicated geometries and rapidly soluble drugs without the requirement for high-temperature processing makes it more useful for pharmaceutical applications [63]. BIJ technology has been successfully applied to produce a tablet formulation that can disperse drugs rapidly due to their rapid dissolving nature orally, making it easier for patients, particularly the elderly and children, to stick to the prescriptions. Improving adherence by patients to treatment regimens requires this competence [32].

15.2.3 Material Used in 3D-P Pharmaceuticals

3D-P has enabled the development of novel pharmacological dosage forms by employing various materials. Some necessary elements for 3D-PPs are as follows:

Polymers: It has been demonstrated that polyvinyl alcohol [PVA] is used to create 3D-P caplets with controlled drug release characteristics. 3D-P tablets with extended-release and support structures use biodegradable polymers termed hydroxypropyl methylcellulose (HPMC) and methylcellulose [58]. Other polymers, such as polylactic acid (PLA) and polyethylene glycol (PEG), were also studied for use in 3D-printed drug delivery devices [70]. Active Pharmaceutical Ingredients: 3D-P dosage forms have been effectively infused with medications such as lidocaine, theophylline, isoniazid, and caffeine. Customized therapy can be achieved by carefully dosing APIs with limited therapeutic indices through 3D-P [8, 11, 33]. Excipients: Since the matrix of polymers and drugs are the two primary constituents in the 3D-PPs and the 3D-P permits the use of minimal excipients, which would decrease the potentially harmful consequences of the greater number of excipients and overcome these problems of the conventional drug dosage forms [11]. Bioinks: Cell structures and disease models are created using bioinks, which are composed of cells, biological elements, and biochemicals, for use in bioprinting applications. Collagen, fibrin, alginate, and gelatin protein hydrogels are the same materials used in 3D-P [33].

15.3 Clinical Trials for 3D-P Pharmaceuticals

3D-P novel technology in the field of pharmaceutical manufacturing leads to a paradigm shift in the pharmaceutical industry and clinical pharmacy practice, moving away from traditional mass manufacturing of pharmaceuticals and toward personalized, one-of-a-kind medicinal goods. The patients, healthcare professionals, chemists, the pharmaceutical industry, and healthcare sectors will gain a huge benefit from this 3D-P concept [33].

15.3.1 Overview of Clinical Trial Phases

Clinical studies might go so poorly that unanticipated adjustments to the population under study, the endpoints, or the analytic strategy are required. The number of patient therapies that are brought to market by researchers can be increased by better planning and executing clinical study protocols with the aid of an understanding of the fundamentals of the clinical trial process and its stages. Stages of the clinical trial phase are essential for one to follow for the successful development of formulation and its application in the market sector and healthcare sectors [33, 62]. Phase 0-IV are the major stages of the clinical trial investigation that need to be conducted by the researchers or the pharmaceutical industry to assess whether the medication under investigation will be beneficial or unfavorable to people. Pharmacokinetics (PK) and pharmacodynamics (PD) are recognized in Phase 0. In this phase, scientists confirm the behavior of the drugs in humans upon administration, whether in a way like the laboratory study reports or not [62]. Evaluating safety studies is involved in Phase I; Phase II involves evaluating efficacy; and Phase III involves confirming both safety and efficacy. Phase IV studies are post-marketing surveillance studies. Here, scientists also perform certain sets of studies to confirm the effectiveness of the formulation via community-based studies. While this may seem simple and uncomplicated, there is often ambiguity around the objectives and goals of the various stages, and studies conducted to evaluate whether a therapy administered to most patients may have complicated findings that are hard to analyze and come to proper findings [19]. The US FDA regulatory guidelines and the mandatory clinical trials for the 3D-PPs approval are depicted in Fig. 15.2.

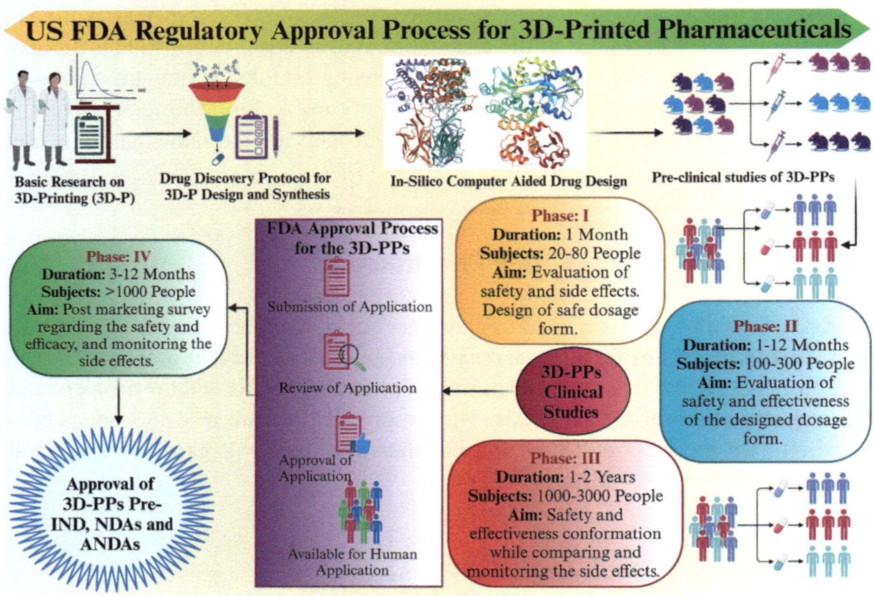

Fig. 15.2 US FDA regulatory guidelines and clinical trials for the 3D-PPs approval

15.3.2 Design and Conduct of Clinical Trials for 3D-P Drugs

The novel treatment drug under investigation may be superior to standard treatment already available in one of two scenarios: (1) It has shown a significant positive result (2). Equivalent to the standard treatment. Based on the preclinical review reports for safety and efficacy, the US FDA takes the responsibility for further assessment of the reports of the investigating drug in clinical studies. These researchers or the pharmaceutical industries are directed to follow good clinical practice (GCP) guidelines and are intended to address certain concerns regarding the behavioral nature and ADRs of the therapies under investigation. The trial's classification based on its goal or how the researchers plan to conduct clinical studies in their facilities (observational vs. interventional clinical trials) may reflect the differences and findings [45].

Randomized controlled trials (RCTs) are used to reveal information on side effects. RCTs are classified according to their research design (crossover, factorial, parallel-group, or equivalency) and their result obtained upon the conduct of these studies and the assessment of a hypothesis (superiority, non-inferiority, or equivalency) [35]. Random assignment is used to place participants in one of the several treatment groups under investigation. A randomized procedure reduces selection bias, minimizes allocation bias, and increases statistical power for optimal statistical analysis [14].

15.3.2.1 Preclinical Studies

The primary objectives of preclinical development, which begins before clinical trials, are to assess the safety and efficacy of the investigating drug. PK and PD investigations, ADME studies, and toxicity tests are involved. Both in-vitro and in-vivo correlation (IVIVC) testing are used for toxicity studies on mammalian reproduction and the long-term carcinogenic effects, and they also assess damages to the other targeted organs. The best animal model that correlates with human body physiology is selected to predict the investigating drug's behavior in the human body. For testing any medical device in preclinical research, one should use a higher number of animal species to assess the accurate results [81].

15.3.2.2 Phase I: Safety and Dosage

This stage evaluates the safety of medication or devices under investigation. This testing process is in the early stages of a clinical trial and takes up to a very few months to complete the study. Usually, 10–20 healthy individuals participate in this phase. The main aim of the phase I trial is to determine the drugs or device's PK and PD effects on humans, including their absorption, distribution, metabolism, and excretion (ADME) patterns. This stage also investigates ADRs observed by the tested dosage form in human subjects. Approximately 70% of experimental medications pass this stage of evaluation [64].

15.3.2.3 Phase II: Efficacy and Side Effects

This stage evaluates the effectiveness of the medications or devices under investigation. This is the testing phase II of clinical studies. It generally takes several months and up to one year for its completion, involving around 50–75 healthy subjects and patients. It is the RCT in which the drug under investigation is administered to one group of patients while a second "control" group is given a placebo or conventional care. Investigating drugs is often administered in a "blinded" fashion, meaning that neither the patients nor the researchers are aware of who has got it. Phase I and Phase II trials cover about one-third of investigational drug clinical trials [72].

15.3.2.4 Phase III: Efficacy and Monitoring of Adverse Reactions

This stage of the clinical study evaluates blind and RCT trials involving around 1000–3000 patients to assess both the safety and effectiveness of the investigating drug. This phase of clinical study may take up to 1–2 years for thorough testing. It provides complete information to researchers and the relevant regulatory body about the advantages, potential side effects, and efficacy of the medication or medical technology. Around 70% and 90% of medications that achieve success in this third phase of clinical trials will be utilized as successful and safe medications in further phase IV clinical trials. A pharmaceutical company can apply for FDA clearance for approval for the marketing of medicinal formulations upon completion of Phase III clinical studies.

15.3.2.5 Phase IV: Post-marketing Surveillance

Phase IV of clinical studies is referred to as post-marketing surveillance trials. In this phase, the pharmaceutical companies have multiple goals, like comparing the side effects of the investigating drug with the other medications that are administered to the same disease patients, and further risk-benefit analysis will be carried out to understand the safe therapeutic window of the medication agent. This also helps to gain further good market value for the medicinal agent by figuring out how cost-effective a drug therapy is in comparison to other existing and novel therapies [80].

15.3.3 Challenges and Considerations in Clinical Trials

15.3.3.1 Variability in 3D-P Drug Formulations

A specialized form of 3D-P called bioprinting is used to create biological organs and tissues. It can be used in tissue engineering applications, toxicity investigations, and pharmaceutical research for drug testing. Any variation in bioprinting due to the nozzle size and printer speed parameters changing would affect the viability of the cells, cause tissue damage, and differ in cell functioning, impacting the intended use of biologicals in the 3D-P [6]. Continuous liquid interface production (CLIP) is a very rapid 3D-P process that continually solidifies the liquid resin using oxygen-permeable optics. It makes it possible to produce precise dose forms and complex medication delivery systems. The alterations in the printing speed and UV/laser light exposure would affect the resolution of printing in 3D-P technologies [73]. Certain 3D printers can utilize several materials simultaneously, enabling the creation of intricate pharmaceutical designs over pharmaceutical formulations with many components, but there is a lack of compatibility between the resin materials chosen for printing that would reduce the mechanical strength of the printed objects due to biocompatibility issues [15]. The 3D-P blended technique utilizes the combinations of various techniques and resin materials to enhance the final product quality and strength. Any variation in these blending techniques leads to the altered mechanical strength of the formulation, different drug and excipient degradation times, and an unstable final product with irregular drug release properties [30].

15.3.3.2 Patient Recruitment and Data Collection

The ability to provide dosage flexibility based on patient demands is made possible via 3D-P technology. The pediatric population is one important group that requires dosage flexibility, where the child's age and body weight are considered when prescribing a therapeutic dosage. The above-mentioned parameters can be included, and pediatric dosage forms can be easily altered with 3D printers to provide patients with the optimal dose. Changing the geometry and forms of tablets is one of the best ways to achieve patient compliance with dosage forms. Low-dosage medications were made into immediate-release tablets, and it was reported by a few researchers that the preparation of thin tablets or enhancing the void volume between the particles in the formulated dosage forms would lead to improved drug-release properties or sometimes achieving complete drug release within a short period [53].

15.3.3.3 Ensuring Consistency and Quality

Quality assurance and control (QA and QC) techniques are essential considering the quickly expanding new in-hospital and pharmaceutical industrial technologies. There are very few reports on the QC of the entire 3D-P pharmaceutical process till today. Considering all the different QA and QC requirements for the success of the 3D-P technology, there are still various developed and validated analytical methods, as new research publications are essential to providing in-house 3D-P workflow for unsterilized anatomical models. Unexpected errors may occur at any point during the various stages of the 3D-PP formulation; they might be human or instrumental errors, such as miscommunication or the breakdown of other workflow-related components. Human error may be reduced or eliminated by process optimization and clear responsibility allotments; intrinsic error can only be observed and controlled for proper printing during the production of the 3D-PPs [28].

15.4 Regulatory Framework for 3D-P Pharmaceuticals

15.4.1 Overview of Regulatory Bodies

15.4.1.1 US FDA (US Food and Drug Administration)

It's a federal agency that governs the safety and efficacy of medicinal products marketed in the United States for safeguarding and advancing public health. This regulatory body, along with the regulation of the medicinal products intended for humans, also regulates the veterinary, medical devices, and other biological products' safety efficacy profiles before their marketing approval. The pharmaceutical industries and laboratories that research medicinal products to seek permission for marketing via Investigational New Drug Application (INDA) applications are audited by the FDA regularly. The FDA analyzes all the reports provided by the drug testing agencies, recognizes the flaws made during the conduct of the study, observes the honest findings in the report, and ranks them in Form 483. Every single observation is reported as per a standard set of guidelines made by the FDA that starts with the statement "rule or regulation" and ends with the circumstances that were seen and observed throughout the inspection period. The FDA bioresearch monitoring program (BIMO) monitors every aspect of the FDA-regulated research thoroughly via a set of data audits and visits for on-site inspections intended to keep an eye on every facet of conducting and disclosing research [47]. Some examples of medicinal formulations regulated by the USFDA are represented in Table 15.1.

15.4.1.2 EMA (European Medicines Agency)

The European Union (EU) organization in charge of assessing and overseeing pharmaceutical goods is the European Medicines Agency (EMA). More precisely, it

Table 15.1 Medical products approved by the FDA

FDA regulation	Product	Indication	Reference
I	Medical examination lamp powered by AC	Lens accessories to enhance magnified seeing	[9]
I	Backed thermal skin patch with adhesive	Momentary alleviation from joint and muscular pain brought on by sprains and arthritis	[7]
II	Angioscopy	To make bodily cavities, hollow organs, and canals accessible, illuminated, and manipulable	[18]
II	Test method for folic acid radioimmuneassay	Measurement of folic acid in plasma or serum for megaloblastic anemia diagnosis	[39]
III	Artificial heart	Prosthetic heart to replace the natural heart	[79]
III	Temporary blood pump for cardiac support	Brief circulatory support used for fewer than 6 hours after surgery, either with or without the need for an oxygenator	[25]

creates technical guidelines, offers sponsors scientific assistance, and coordinates the examination and monitoring of nationally recommended goods and centrally approved items [47].

15.4.1.3 Other International Regulatory Agencies

An FDA regulation that monitors, records, and archives lab research is known as good laboratory practice (GLP), and it governs the planning, execution, and other elements of a project. To provide reliable, accurate, and consistent results, the GLP requires the use of calibrated equipment and documentation methods that accurately reflect the original sequence of events and results. Every activity must be documented, and adhering to GLP documentation requirements will allow for an accurate reconstruction of the events as they occurred. Every laboratory procedure needs to be documented in standard operating procedures and followed by the laboratory; moreover, a functional quality assurance unit that is distinct from the analytical department needs to be in place [43]. It is unique in that it brings together regulatory authorities and the pharmaceutical sector to discuss the scientific and technical aspects of drug registration and approval processes. In Phase 5 of the ICH process, harmonized ICH recommendations are implemented by ICH Monitoring Members and Viewers in their respective countries or regions. The ICH guidelines are implemented while keeping in mind the stage at which each guideline is approved and by applicable national, local, and regional rules [61].

15.4.2 Regulatory Pathways for 3D-P Drugs

15.4.2.1 Investigational New Drug (IND) Application

According to current federal law, drugs cannot be transported or distributed over state boundaries unless they are covered by an approved selling request. Since it is likely to drive the distribution of the exploratory drug to experimental investigators in several circumstances, a guarantor requires appealing on exception following the legal duty. Through the IND, the patron receives this relief from the FDA and utilizes it during emergency circumstances; the FDA may authorize the use of an experimental drug in an emergency if there is insufficient time to get compliance. The IND is critical in getting permission for a novel drug based on the product's quality, safety, and efficacy. It acts as the impetus for clinical research in the United States. This often includes manufacturing data, preliminary product quality indicators, evidence from non-clinical testing, and published literature in marketplace. The first IND application is intended to provide the FDA with a broad investigative strategy and methods for particular human investigations, according to the FDA [74].

15.4.2.2 Abbreviated New Drug Application (ANDA) for Generics

An ANDA is a request for the licensing of a generic drug in the United States for a medicine that is already licensed or approved [12]. It includes information surrendered to the FDA intended for consideration and possible approval of a generic medication product [36].

15.4.3 Specific Guidelines for 3D-P Pharmaceuticals

Its basis is the concept of photo-polymerization, in which UV light and the photoinitiator interact to liberate free radicals. By permitting the UV laser beam to travel over the liquid resin's surface, the axis x and y baffles aid in accurately depicting the previously defined 3D model. Starting the procedure over again, add layers of liquid resin until the 3D object is formed layer by layer completely. Rugs, polymers, and other solid materials are combined in nozzle-based deposition techniques before 3D printing. Layer by layer, the mixture is created into a three-dimensional product by running it through a nozzle. There are two kinds of printing, depending on the material used [77]. It covers both continuous inkjet printing (CJP) and drop-on-demand (DOP) printing. In continuous inkjet printing, a high-pressure pump is utilized to direct the liquid or jet in droplets. A high-force pump is used in continuous inkjet printing to push the fluid link through an aperture that has a diameter of 50–80 μm, resulting in a continuous ink flow. A piezoelectric crystal causes the liquid to flow in a way that causes droplets of a certain size and speed to break off at regular intervals. An electrostatic field is created to control these factors. These methodologies must be followed by the pharmaceutical manufacturers during the formulation of the 3D-PPs [44].

15.4.3.1 Future Directions and Proposed Regulations

Personalized dosage forms and drug delivery devices (DDD) for every patient could be possibly manufactured by 3D-P technology as its major advantage is to create personalized medications. Pharmacological product customization is now possible due to the 3D-P technology, which has enabled the creation of patient-specific drug delivery device prototypes in a range of complicated levels of diseased states.

Technologies for printing might potentially enhance drug regimens for patients in the future. Several drugs and excipients, complex internal geometries, and solid dosage forms with different densities and diffusivities can be created with 3D-P technologies [54]. The release of several medications, peptides, potent drugs, and poorly water-soluble pharmaceuticals may all be handled by 3DP with considerable success. Extrusion, powder solidification, and stereolithography have all been used in the production of 3D-P drug product manufacturing. Most likely, the main barrier to their application in personalized medicine is related to the regulatory issues at play and the development of production models that could efficiently translate each patient's therapeutic requirements into modest amounts of appropriate pharmaceutical products that meet pre-defined quality standards. One of the biggest challenges to ensuring that 3D-printed medications are as stable, protective, and effective as those made by the traditional pharmaceutical sector. To ensure that 3D-P pharmaceuticals are used and ingested safely, the regulatory authorities must set standards, norms, and quality systems that meet the traditional demands of the pharmaceutical sector. Because of the availability of various computer designs, there are infinite methods to create suitable geometries with customized functionality and differing degrees of complexity to control the release characteristics of one or more pharmacological chemicals [24, 68].

15.5 Case Studies

The primary purpose of the case studies about 3D-P technology is to assess its viability and advantageous use in the pharmaceutical manufacturing industry. The primary use of 3D-P technology was the creation of efavirenz granulates, which were produced, transported, and processed at the 3D-P plant by Direct Powder Extrusion [DPE] to create 3D-P tablets [66]. The summary of 3D-P technologies and their reported case studies are represented in Table 15.2.

15.5.1 Approved 3D-P Pharmaceuticals

The US FDA approved Spiratum, the first 3D-P pharmaceutical product, in the year 2015 for the treatment of epilepsy. Spiratum is an API derived from levetiracetam. With the use of 3D-P technology, Spiratum can be formulated in oral dosage forms with a precise dose for each patient, having rapid disintegration properties in the aqueous media. These forms are especially useful for patients who have trouble swallowing pills [8, 78]. Spiratum is an advancement in the field of 3D-P, as it received FDA approval for clinical studies involving 3D-P tablets for rheumatoid arthritis treatment. The proposal from agencies like the Medicines and Healthcare Products Regulatory Agency [MHRA] in the UK to facilitate the development of personalized drugs through 3D-P technologies [78].

Table 15.2 Summary of reported case studies of 3D-P technologies

Case study	3D-P technology	Application	Key findings	References
Pediatric 3D-P mini tablets	Fused deposition modeling [FDM]	Pediatric treatment	Designed as mini tablets for children, customized dosage forms to enhance adherence to treatment regimen.	[17]
3D-P oral drug	Powder bed fusion [PBF]	Huge medication	Single dosage forms enable the production of multi-drug combinations, increasing simplification in the manufacturing process and enhancing patient compliance.	[22]
Polymer-based drug delivery system	Stereolithography [SLS]	Controlled drug release	The complex structure releases drugs in a controlled manner, enhancing therapeutic outcomes and minimizing side effects.	[37]
Custom implants for drug delivery	Fused deposition modeling [FDM]	Localized treatment	Specific implants for localized drug delivery by developed patients	[11]
Anticancer drug production via 3D-P	FDM	Anti-cancer treatment	This was achieved through the sustained release of anticancer medicine, enabling a prolonged reduction of dosing frequency by potential and therapeutic effect.	[10]
Personalized isoniazid drug	FDM	Medication and prevention of tuberculosis	It demonstrated the ability to create drug release profiles and customized dosing to individual patient requirements, enhancing therapeutic efficacy.	[50]
Smart pills with embedded sensors	FDM	Monitoring patient accumulation	It was an integrated sensor into 3D-P pills to provide real-time data to healthcare providers and monitor ingestion, enhancing patient management.	[2]
Decentralized manufacturing of efavirenz printouts	DPE	HIV treatment	By showcasing feasibility, over 80% of drugs are released within 60 minutes using real-time analytical techniques for QC in decentralized settings.	[1]

15.5.2 Spiratum [Levetiracetam]

Spiratum is a groundbreaking pharmaceutical that is the first 3D-P drug approved by the US FDA and manufactured by the Aprecia pharmaceutical industry. Levetiracetam is an API in tablet form that is primarily used for the treatment of epilepsy, using advanced zip dose technology from Aprecia, a high-dose medication that can be made soluble quickly in an aqueous media, making drug administration easy for patients while improving both drug absorption and therapeutic impacts [52]. For a better insight into oncology medicine, the formulation of the anti-cancer tablet involves combining more than two APIs customized to the patient's pathological conditions. This creates a synergistic anti-cancer dosage regimen for effective cancer treatment, enabled by 3D-P technology [48]. In another scenario, a pediatric medication in the form of a chewable tablet was developed utilizing 3D-P technology to ensure appropriate dosage forms for children. This innovative development, carried out at the University of Santiago de Compostela in Spain, aims to enhance the therapeutic efficacy of medications by offering easily administrable formulations that are tailored to the unique needs of pediatric patients [65].

15.5.3 Ongoing Clinical Trials and Research

Ongoing clinical trials and research studies use 3D-P technology in pharmaceuticals, including the M3DIMAKER GMP Printer for developing personalized drugs, particularly in cancer research. Personalized polypills: This study is centered on formulating customized polyfills utilizing 3D-P technology. Formulation and personalized dosing: In these trials, specific 3D-P dosage forms were developed by FabRx. This marks the first clinical trial used to treat a pediatric patient with rare metabolic disorders and urine diseases [27]. Triastek Inc. has received FDA approval to begin initial clinical studies of T21. T21 is a 3D-P drug designed to target specific segments in the colon. It is an isoleucine chewable tablet created using 3D-P technology [33]. Advanced drug delivery systems provide precise control over drug release rates, distribution, and dosages through technologies like inhalable formulations and microneedle patches that are formulated by 3D-P technology [16]. Early-phase trials and preclinical research 3D bioprinting speeds up early-stage human trials and drug development by creating tissue models that mimic human physiology, reducing the need for animal testing. 3D bio-printed drug products have been approved in China and the United States for human clinical trials [15, 49].

15.5.4 Lessons Learned from Case Studies

Case Study1: Implementing 3D-P for personalized drug dosages to enhance treatment efficacy in hospitals [58]. Case Study 2: The 3D-P of pharmaceutical products using semisolid extrusion necessitates precise material properties to ensure the production of high-quality pharmaceutical items [69]. Case Study 3 pertains to the use of fused filament 3D-P for drug items. In this context, the properties of drug release are influenced by the microstructure of 3D-printed caplets, underscoring the critical nature of judicious material selection [33]. Case Study 4: Development of customized dosage forms considering physiological and genetic differences among patients [58]. Case study 5 discusses using 3D-P to customize oral dosage forms for better patient compliance and bioavailability [11]. In their 2023 case study, "The Use of Fused Deposition Modeling," reported by Chakka LJ, et al., on the substantial influence of drug release properties on the microstructure of 3D-P tablets [8]. In a study by Huanbutta et al. [33], it was found that 3D-P technology can lower production costs for small batches [33].

15.6 Challenges and Future Perspective

15.6.1 Technical and Manufacturing Challenges

The implementation of 3D-P technology presents several technical and manufacturing challenges, each of which warrants careful consideration. Key challenges include certain technical challenges like mechanical properties: 3D-P technology often exhibits insufficient mechanical characteristics, such as high friability [8, 21]. Material limitation: The use of specific materials and excipients in 3D-P pharmaceuticals impacts the ability to produce a wide variety of doses [8, 67]. Regulatory framework: The regulatory landscape lacks clear definitions for 3D-P pharmaceuticals, posing unique challenges that require attention. Development of appropriate substances [26, 67]. Ensuring the development of stable, biocompatible materials during the printing process for drug encapsulation is crucial. The materials need to be both safe and effective [3].

A few manufacturing challenges that need to be addressed during the formulation of 3D-PPs are as follows: (1) Cost of Equipment Material: The significant initial investment required for large-scale production of 3D-P material and equipment can be a barrier for many pharmaceutical companies [76] (2) Quality Control and Regulatory Compliance: 3D-P pharmaceuticals are vital for meeting regulatory requirements and ensuring safety and efficacy [96] (3) Scale-Up Issues: The transition from small-scale to large-scale production presents considerable logistical and technical challenges [72] (4) Expertise and Training: Specialized skills and expertise are essential for operating advanced 3D-P equipment and developing complex drug formulations [51].

15.6.2 Regulatory and Compliance Challenges

The pharmaceutical industry faces challenges in adhering to laws and regulations, particularly with 3D-P technology. Some key issues include regulatory and intellectual property considerations, lack of clear regulatory guidelines, quality control, quality assurances, verification and validation, and post-market longevity. It's important to ensure patient safety and efficacy by assessing the impact of the printing process on drug stability, bioavailability, and therapeutic effectiveness [35].

15.6.3 Future Trends and Innovations

In future developments and trends in 3D pharmaceutical technology, we can expect the incorporation of nanotechnology to improve therapeutic results and drug delivery. Sustainable manufacturing practices will reduce waste and energy usage, and advanced materials will be utilized. Point-of-care manufacturing and regenerative medicine will improve patient outcomes. Digital health integration will enable real-time monitoring and personalized treatment adjustments. Additionally, bioprinting and personalized medicine will offer customized drug formulations and dosages. Lastly, sophisticated drug distribution systems will allow focused and monitored drug release [35, 51, 72, 76].

15.6.4 Potential Impact on Personalized Medicines

This 3D-P technology has a significant influence on personalized medicine in the pharmaceutical sector and presents several innovative applications. The following significant findings are the result of a recent study: Polypills & drug combinations of many prescriptions into a single tablet—this technology simplifies life for individuals who must take multiple medications daily. Here, taking all drugs as prescribed not only enhances treatment efficacy but also promotes adherence. The medication's shape is now personalized to make it easier for patients to take it, especially for younger individuals who might prefer various flavors or forms. On-demand manufacturing, particularly for vaccinations, makes it possible to fabricate medications at the site of treatment using 3D printing. During pandemics or in isolated areas, the capacity to swiftly and locally create vaccinations might revolutionize the distribution of serum [75]. Improved drug delivery systems suggest targeted therapeutic delivery, such as 3D-printed microrobots. These systems may deliver drugs at precise times and locations because of their enhanced capacity to move through the body, which enhances therapeutic efficacy and minimizes adverse effects [40]. The future trends and the present applications of 3D-P pharmaceutical dosage forms are represented in Fig. 15.3.

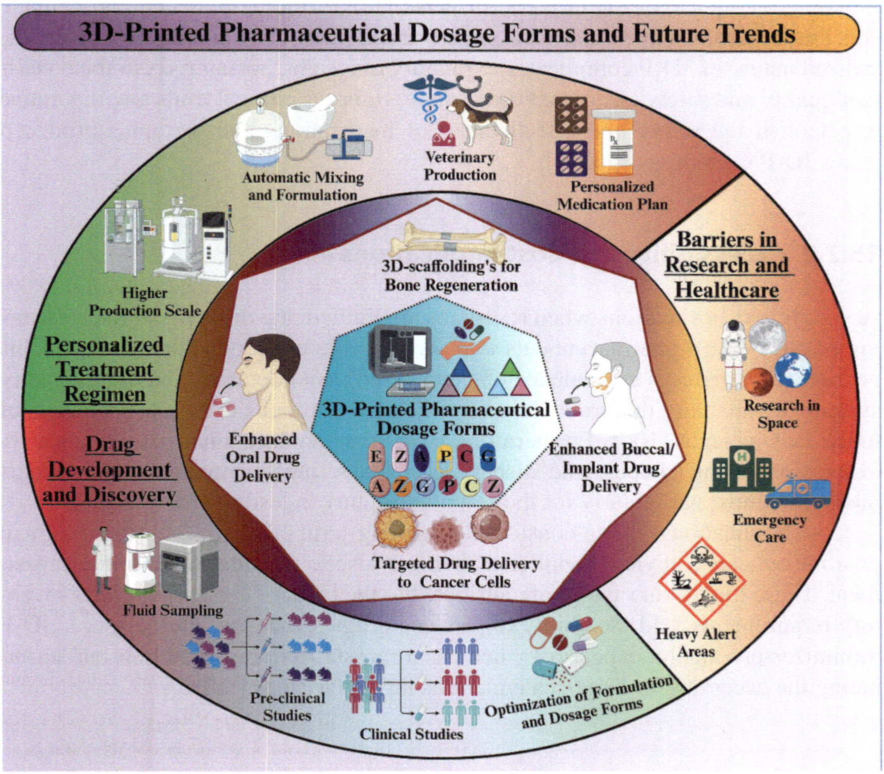

Fig. 15.3 The future trends and the present applications of 3D-P pharmaceutical dosage forms

15.7 Ethical and Social Considerations

15.7.1 Patient Safety and Ethical Concerns

Ensuring patient safety in 3D-P is a major criterion to be considered due to the elimination of hazardous gases, especially when utilizing materials like PLA and ABS. Implementing effective ventilation and filtration techniques is essential to minimize exposure. Furthermore, product liability risks arise when pharmaceutical companies grant production licenses, potentially leading to intricate liability issues involving various parties. Addressing these challenges is imperative to safeguard patient safety and maintain industry integrity [4, 75].

The growing use of 3D printers for personalized drug treatments raises ethical concerns regarding equity and access to advanced medical technologies. The decentralized nature of 3D-P complicates regulatory oversight, posing risks to the consistent quality and safety of drugs. Furthermore, rigorous clinical trials are imperative to establish the safety and effectiveness of medications and therapies produced using 3D-P technology [56, 60].

15.7.2 Accessibility and Cost Implications

Accessibility: In situations when resources are limited, the on-demand manufacturing of customized pharmaceuticals is made possible using 3D-P technology. This novel method reduces dependence on centralized manufacturing and drug delivery systems by enabling the production of customized dosages that meet the needs of individual patients [104]. Furthermore, 3D-P can produce pharmaceuticals with exact dimensions, shapes, and dispersion profiles, meeting patient requirements most efficiently, particularly for those with difficulty ingesting pills [12, 29].

Cost Implications: When considering the long-term effects, 3D-P technology in pharmaceuticals can yield significant savings, despite the substantial initial investment. These long-term savings are attributed to the reduction of waste, lower inventory requirements, and the ability to produce drugs as needed. Furthermore, 3D-P minimizes production expenses by decreasing waste from raw materials and eliminating the necessity for large-scale manufacturing facilities [38].

15.8 Conclusion

The advent of 3D-P medications has revolutionized pharmaceutical manufacturing by allowing the production of personalized doses and controlled drug release patterns. However, the clinical research and regulatory approval processes for these medications present significant challenges. Like traditional pharmaceuticals, clinical trials for 3D-P medications must confirm their quality, safety, and effectiveness. The customized nature of these medications introduces complexities, requiring precise designs for tailored doses to ensure consistent therapeutic outcomes. Trials must also evaluate the stability and bioavailability of the printed form compared to conventional medications. Validation of these customized treatments requires real-world evidence and adaptive trial designs. Additionally, the development of regulatory frameworks for 3D-printed medications is an ongoing effort, with organizations such as the FDA creating oversight structures for these innovations. Approval for 3D-P medications necessitates well-documented processes covering material requirements, printer calibration, and QC procedures. Regulatory bodies need evidence that the integrity, potency, and purity of the drugs remain unchanged during the printing process. The FDA's approval of Spritam, a 3D-P tablet for epilepsy treatment, highlights the importance of a comprehensive assessment of additive manufacturing technology. In conclusion, despite the significant potential of 3D-printed medications for personalized healthcare, establishing robust and adaptable frameworks for their clinical and regulatory processes is imperative.

Acknowledgments The authors would like to acknowledge the management of colleges and universities of all authors for overall support in carrying out the review work.

References

1. Aguilar-de-Leyva Á, Casas M, Ferrero C, Linares V, Caraballo I. 3D printing direct powder extrusion in the production of drug delivery systems: state of the art and future perspectives. Pharmaceutics. 2024;16(4):437. https://doi.org/10.3390/pharmaceutics16040437.
2. Ahn S, Montero M, Odell D, Roundy S, Wright PK. Anisotropic material properties of fused deposition modeling ABS. Rapid Prototyp J. 2002;8(4):248–57. https://doi.org/10.1108/13552540210441166.
3. Alhnan MA, Okwuosa TC, Sadia M, Wan K-W, Ahmed W, Arafat B. Emergence of 3D printed dosage forms: opportunities and challenges. Pharm Res. 2016;33(8):1817–32. https://doi.org/10.1007/s11095-016-1933-1.
4. Alzoubi L, Aljabali AAA, Tambuwala MM. Empowering precision medicine: the impact of 3D printing on personalized therapeutic. AAPS PharmSciTech. 2023;24(8):228. https://doi.org/10.1208/s12249-023-02682-w.
5. Awad A, Trenfield SJ, Goyanes A, Gaisford S, Basit AW. Reshaping drug development using 3D printing. Drug Discov Today. 2018;23(8):1547–55. https://doi.org/10.1016/j.drudis.2018.05.025.
6. Babbar A, et al. 3D bioprinting in pharmaceuticals, medicine, and tissue engineering applications. Adv Manuf Process Technol CRC Press. 2020:147–61.
7. Banerjee S, Chattopadhyay P, Ghosh A, Datta P, Veer V. Aspect of adhesives in transdermal drug delivery systems. Int J Adhes Adhes. 2014;50:70–84. https://doi.org/10.1016/j.ijadhadh.2014.01.001.
8. Basit AWTS. 3D printing of pharmaceuticals and the role of pharmacy. Pharm J. 2022;308:7959. https://doi.org/10.1211/PJ.2022.1.135581.
9. Baura G. Medical device technologies: a systems based overview using engineering standards. Elsevier; 2021. eBook ISBN: 9780128119853. https://shop.elsevier.com/books/medical-device-technologies/baura/978-0-12-811984-6
10. Cailleaux S, Sanchez-Ballester NM, Gueche YA, Bataille B, Soulairol I. Fused deposition modeling (FDM), the new asset for the production of tailored medicines. J Control Release. 2021;330:821–41. https://doi.org/10.1016/j.jconrel.2020.10.056.
11. Chakka LRJ, Chede S. 3D printing of pharmaceuticals for disease treatment. Front Med Technol. 2023;4:1040052. https://doi.org/10.3389/fmedt.2022.1040052.
12. Chandrakar B. 3D printing in pharmaceutical and medical applications recent achievements and challenges. Int J Health Sci (Qassim). 2022:8109–21. https://doi.org/10.53730/ijhs.v6nS3.7939.
13. Charoo NA, Barakh Ali SF, Mohamed EM, Kuttolamadom MA, Ozkan T, Khan MA, Rahman Z. Selective laser sintering 3D printing—an overview of the technology and pharmaceutical applications. Drug Dev Ind Pharm. 2020;46(6):869–77. https://doi.org/10.1080/03639045.2020.1764027.
14. Chen C, Cai L, Zheng W, Wang J, Guo X, Chen H. The efficacy of using 3D printing models in the treatment of fractures: a randomised clinical trial. BMC Musculoskelet Disord. 2019;20(1):65. https://doi.org/10.1186/s12891-019-2448-9.
15. Chen G, Xu Y, Chi Lip Kwok P, Kang L. Pharmaceutical applications of 3D Printing. Addit Manuf. 2020;34:101209. https://doi.org/10.1016/j.addma.2020.101209.

16. Cheng S, Tracy TS, Li X. 3D Printing pharmaceuticals: current status and future opportunities. Pharm Front. 2024;06(02):e192–4. https://doi.org/10.1055/s-0044-1782512.
17. Chennakesava P, Shivraj Narayan Y. Fused deposition modeling-insights. In: In Proceedings of the international conference on advances in design and manufacturing ICAD&M. 2014. 1345.
18. Cortis BS, Harris DM, Principe J. From angiography to angioscopy: informal discussion. Texas Hear Inst J. 1986;13(3):281–9.
19. Desai PB, Karve AS, Zawit M, Arora P, Dave N, Awosika J, Li N, Fuhrman B, Medvedovic M, Sallans L, Kendler A, DasGupta B, Plas D, Curry R, Zuccarello M, Chaudhary R, Sengupta S, Wise-Draper TM. A phase 0/I pharmacokinetic and pharmacodynamics and safety and tolerability study of Letrozole in combination with standard therapy in recurrent high-grade Gliomas. Clin Cancer Res. 2024;30(10):2068–77. https://doi.org/10.1158/1078-0432.CCR-23-3341.
20. Deshmane S, Kendre P, Mahajan H, Jain S. Stereolithography 3D printing technology in pharmaceuticals: a review. Drug Dev Ind Pharm. 2021;47(9):1362–72. https://doi.org/10.1080/03639045.2021.1994990.
21. Desu PK, Maddiboyina B, Vanitha K, Rao Gudhanti SNK, Anusha R, Jhawat V. 3D printing technology in pharmaceutical dosage forms: advantages and challenges. Curr Drug Targets. 2021;22(16):1901–14. https://doi.org/10.2174/1389450122666210120142416.
22. Dev Singh D, Mahender T, Raji Reddy A. Powder bed fusion process: a brief review. Mater Today Proc. 2021;46:350–5. https://doi.org/10.1016/j.matpr.2020.08.415.
23. Di Prima M, Coburn J, Hwang D, Kelly J, Khairuzzaman A, Ricles L. Additively manufactured medical products—the FDA perspective. 3D Print Med. 2016;2(1):1. https://doi.org/10.1186/s41205-016-0005-9.
24. Elhadad AA, Rosa-Sainz A, Cañete R, Peralta E, Begines B, Balbuena M, Alcudia A, Torres Y. Applications and multidisciplinary perspective on 3D printing techniques: recent developments and future trends. Mater Sci Eng R Rep. 2023;156:100760. https://doi.org/10.1016/j.mser.2023.100760.
25. Franko L, D'Alessandro D. Durable mechanical circulatory support. In: Cardiac surgery clerkship: a guide for senior medical students. Cham: Springer International Publishing; 2024. p. 337–44.
26. Bhusnure OG, Gholve SV, Sugave BK, Dongre RC, Gore SA, Giram PS. 3D printing & pharmaceutical manufacturing: opportunities and challenges. Int J Bioassays. 2016;5(01):4723. https://doi.org/10.21746/ijbio.2016.01.006.
27. Gioumouxouzis CI, Karavasili C, Fatouros DG. Recent advances in pharmaceutical dosage forms and devices using additive manufacturing technologies. Drug Discov Today. 2019;24(2):636–43. https://doi.org/10.1016/j.drudis.2018.11.019.
28. Goyanes A, Scarpa M, Kamlow M, Gaisford S, Basit AW, Orlu M. Patient acceptability of 3D printed medicines. Int J Pharm. 2017;530(1–2):71–8. https://doi.org/10.1016/j.ijpharm.2017.07.064.
29. Halagali P, Inamdar A, Singh J, Anand A, Sadhu P, Pathak R, Sharma H, Biswas D. Phytochemicals, herbal extracts, and dietary supplements for metabolic disease management. Endocr Metab Immune Disord Drug Targets. 2024;24 https://doi.org/10.2174/0118715303287911240409055710.
30. Hirschberg C, Boetker JP, Rantanen J, Pein-Hackelbusch M. Using 3D printing for rapid prototyping of characterization tools for investigating powder blend behavior. AAPS PharmSciTech. 2018;19(2):941–50. https://doi.org/10.1208/s12249-017-0904-0.
31. Hoffmann L, Breitkreutz J, Quodbach J. Fused deposition modeling (FDM) 3D printing of the thermo-sensitive peptidomimetic drug enalapril maleate. Pharmaceutics. 2022;14(11):2411. https://doi.org/10.3390/pharmaceutics14112411.
32. Hong X, Han X, Li X, Li J, Wang Z, Zheng A. Binder jet 3D printing of compound LEV-PN dispersible tablets: an innovative approach for fabricating drug systems with multicompartmental structures. Pharmaceutics. 2021;13(11):1780. https://doi.org/10.3390/pharmaceutics13111780.

33. Huanbutta K, Burapapadh K, Sriamornsak P, Sangnim T. Practical application of 3D printing for pharmaceuticals in hospitals and pharmacies. Pharmaceutics. 2023;15(7):1877. https://doi.org/10.3390/pharmaceutics15071877.
34. Islam RSP. An insight of 3d printing technology in pharmaceutical development and application: an updated review. Curr Trends Pharm Res. 2020;7:56–80.
35. Jamróz W, Szafraniec J, Kurek M, Jachowicz R. 3D printing in pharmaceutical and medical applications—recent achievements and challenges. Pharm Res. 2018;35(9):176. https://doi.org/10.1007/s11095-018-2454-x.
36. Jun SY, Sanz-Izquierdo B, Parker EA, Bird D, McClelland A. Manufacturing considerations in the 3-D printing of fractal antennas. IEEE Trans Components, Packag Manuf Technol. 2017;7(11):1891–8. https://doi.org/10.1109/TCPMT.2017.2730366.
37. Kafle A, Luis E, Silwal R, Pan HM, Shrestha PL, Bastola AK. 3D/4D printing of polymers: fused deposition modelling (FDM), selective laser sintering (SLS), and stereolithography (SLA). Polymers (Basel). 2021;13(18):3101. https://doi.org/10.3390/polym13183101.
38. Khairuzzaman A. Regulatory Perspectives on 3D Printing in Pharmaceuticals. In: 3D-Printing of Pharmaceuticals. Cham: Springer International Publishing. 2018;215–236.
39. Kim J, Nguyen T and Eydelman MB. "The FDA's Role in the Regulation of New Diagnostic and Surgical Devices." In: Chandler and Grant's Glaucoma. CRC Press., 2024;751–56.
40. Kruth J, Mercelis P, Van Vaerenbergh J, Froyen L, Rombouts M. Binding mechanisms in selective laser sintering and selective laser melting. Rapid Prototyp J. 2005;11(1):26–36. https://doi.org/10.1108/13552540510573365.
41. Lakkala P, Munnangi SR, Bandari S, Repka M. Additive manufacturing technologies with emphasis on stereolithography 3D printing in pharmaceutical and medical applications: a review. Int J Pharm X. 2023;5:100159. https://doi.org/10.1016/j.ijpx.2023.100159.
42. Lancet T. Personalised medicine in the UK. Lancet. 2018;391 https://doi.org/10.3892/br.2017.922.
43. Lu A, Williams RO, Maniruzzaman M. 3D printing of biologics—what has been accomplished to date? Drug Discov Today. 2024;29(1):103823. https://doi.org/10.1016/j.drudis.2023.103823.
44. Lynn AQ, Pflibsen LR, Smith AA, Rebecca AM, Teven CM. Three-dimensional printing in plastic surgery: current applications, future directions, and ethical implications. Plast Reconstr Surg Glob Open. 2021;9(3):e3465. https://doi.org/10.1097/GOX.0000000000003465.
45. Mahan VL. Clinical trial phases. Int J Clin Med. 2014;05(21):1374–83. https://doi.org/10.4236/ijcm.2014.521175.
46. Mathur S, Sutton J. Personalized medicine could transform healthcare. Biomed Reports. 2017;7(1):3–5. https://doi.org/10.3892/br.2017.922.
47. Mirza MA, Iqbal Z. 3D printing in pharmaceuticals: regulatory perspective. Curr Pharm Des. 2019;24(42):5081–3. https://doi.org/10.2174/1381612825666181130163027.
48. Morris G, O'Brien D, Henshall DC. Opportunities and challenges for microRNA-targeting therapeutics for epilepsy. Trends Pharmacol Sci. 2021;42(7):605–16. https://doi.org/10.1016/j.tips.2021.04.007.
49. Muhindo D, Elkanayati R, Srinivasan P, Repka MA, Ashour EA. Recent advances in the applications of additive manufacturing (3D printing) in drug delivery: a comprehensive review. AAPS PharmSciTech. 2023;24(2):57. https://doi.org/10.1208/s12249-023-02524-9.
50. Mwema FM, Akinlabi ET. Basics of Fused Deposition Modelling (FDM). In: Fused deposition modeling: strategies for quality enhancement. Cham: Springer International Publishing., 2020;1–15
51. Norman J, Madurawe RD, Moore CMV, Khan MA, Khairuzzaman A. A new chapter in pharmaceutical manufacturing: 3D-printed drug products. Adv Drug Deliv Rev. 2017;108:39–50. https://doi.org/10.1016/j.addr.2016.03.001.
52. Northrup L, Christopher MA, Sullivan BP, Berkland C. Combining antigen and immunomodulators: emerging trends in antigen-specific immunotherapy for autoimmunity. Adv Drug Deliv Rev. 2016;98:86–98. https://doi.org/10.1016/j.addr.2015.10.020.

53. Parhi R. A review of three-dimensional printing for pharmaceutical applications: quality control, risk assessment and future perspectives. J Drug Deliv Sci Technol. 2021;64:102571. https://doi.org/10.1016/j.jddst.2021.102571.
54. Parikh N, Sharma P. Three-dimensional printing in urology: history, current applications, and future directions. Urology. 2018;121:3–10. https://doi.org/10.1016/j.urology.2018.08.004.
55. Park BJ, Choi HJ, Moon SJ, Kim SJ, Bajracharya R, Min JY, Han H-K. Pharmaceutical applications of 3D printing technology: current understanding and future perspectives. J Pharm Investig. 2018:1–11. https://doi.org/10.1007/s40005-018-00414-y.
56. Park BJ, Choi HJ, Moon SJ, Kim SJ, Bajracharya R, Min JY, Han H-K. Pharmaceutical applications of 3D printing technology: current understanding and future perspectives. J Pharm Investig. 2018;49:575–85. https://doi.org/10.1007/s40005-018-00414-y.
57. Parulski C, Jennotte O, Lechanteur A, Evrard B. Challenges of fused deposition modeling 3D printing in pharmaceutical applications: where are we now? Adv Drug Deliv Rev. 2021;175:113810. https://doi.org/10.1016/j.addr.2021.05.020.
58. Pawar R, Pawar A. 3D printing of pharmaceuticals: approach from bench scale to commercial development. Futur J Pharm Sci. 2022;8(1):48. https://doi.org/10.1186/s43094-022-00439-z.
59. Pereira BC, Isreb A, Forbes RT, Dores F, Habashy R, Petit J-B, Alhnan MA, Oga EF. 'Temporary Plasticiser': a novel solution to fabricate 3D printed patient-centred cardiovascular 'Polypill' architectures. Eur J Pharm Biopharm. 2019;135:94–103. https://doi.org/10.1016/j.ejpb.2018.12.009.
60. Rogers H, Baricz N, Pawar KS. 3D printing services: classification, supply chain implications and research agenda. Int J Phys Distrib Logist Manag. 2016;46(10):886–907. https://doi.org/10.1108/IJPDLM-07-2016-0210.
61. Sanicola HW, Stewart CE, Mueller M, Ahmadi F, Wang D, Powell SK, Sarkar K, Cutbush K, Woodruff MA, Brafman DA. Guidelines for establishing a 3-D printing biofabrication laboratory. Biotechnol Adv. 2020;45:107652. https://doi.org/10.1016/j.biotechadv.2020.107652.
62. Schreiber K, Graversgaard C, Hunt BJ, Wason JMS, Costedoat-Chalumeau N, Aguilera S, Guerra MM, Salmon JE. Challenges of designing and conducting cohort studies and clinical trials in populations of pregnant people. Lancet Rheumatol. 2024;6(8):e560–72. https://doi.org/10.1016/S2665-9913(24)00118-8.
63. Sen K, Mehta T, Sansare S, Sharifi L, Ma AWK, Chaudhuri B. Pharmaceutical applications of powder-based binder jet 3D printing process—a review. Adv Drug Deliv Rev. 2021;177:113943. https://doi.org/10.1016/j.addr.2021.113943.
64. Seoane-Viaño I, Otero-Espinar FJ, Goyanes Á. 3D printing of pharmaceutical products. In: Additive Manufacturing. Elsevier. 2021a;569–597.
65. Seoane-Viaño I, Trenfield SJ, Basit AW, Goyanes A. Translating 3D printed pharmaceuticals: from hype to real-world clinical applications. Adv Drug Deliv Rev. 2021;174:553–75. https://doi.org/10.1016/j.addr.2021.05.003.
66. Seoane-Viaño I, Xu X, Ong JJ, Teyeb A, Gaisford S, Campos-Álvarez A, Stulz A, Marcuta C, Kraschew L, Mohr W, Basit AW, Goyanes A. A case study on decentralized manufacturing of 3D printed medicines. Int J Pharm X. 2023;5:100184. https://doi.org/10.1016/j.ijpx.2023.100184.
67. Shahrubudin N, Koshy P, Alipal J, Kadir MHA, Lee TC. Challenges of 3D printing technology for manufacturing biomedical products: a case study of Malaysian manufacturing firms. Heliyon. 2020;6(4):e03734. https://doi.org/10.1016/j.heliyon.2020.e03734.
68. Sharma H, Anand A, Halagali P, Inamdar A, Pathak R, Taghizadeh-Hesary FAS. Advancement of Nanoengineered Flavonoids for Chronic Metabolic Diseases. In: Role of Flavonoids in Chronic Metabolic Diseases. Wiley Publishers. 2024;459–510.
69. Sun W, Rantanen J, Genina N. Lessons to learn for 3D printing of drug products by semisolid extrusion (SSE). J Pharm Sci. 2024; https://doi.org/10.1016/j.xphs.2024.05.032.
70. Tappa K, Jammalamadaka U. Novel biomaterials used in medical 3D printing techniques. J Funct Biomater. 2018;9(1):17. https://doi.org/10.3390/jfb9010017.

71. Tasneem I, Ariz A, Bharti D, Haleem A, Javaid M, Bahl S. 3D printing technology and its significant applications in the context of healthcare education. J Ind Integr Manag. 2023;08(01):113–30. https://doi.org/10.1142/S2424862221500159.
72. Trenfield SJ, Awad A, Goyanes A, Gaisford S, Basit AW. 3D printing pharmaceuticals: drug development to frontline Care. Trends Pharmacol Sci. 2018;39(5):440–51. https://doi.org/10.1016/j.tips.2018.02.006.
73. Tumbleston JR, Shirvanyants D, Ermoshkin N, Janusziewicz R, Johnson AR, Kelly D, Chen K, Pinschmidt R, Rolland JP, Ermoshkin A, Samulski ET, DeSimone JM. Continuous liquid interface production of 3D objects. Science. 2015;347((6228)):1349–52. https://doi.org/10.1126/science.aaa2397.
74. Utela B. Development and application of new material systems for three dimensional printing (3DP). In: University of Washington ProQuest Dissertations & Theses; 2008. p. 3345611.
75. Vaz VM. Kumar L. 3D printing as a promising tool in personalized medicine. AAPS PharmSciTech. 2021;22(1):49. https://doi.org/10.1208/s12249-020-01905-8.
76. Ventola CL. Medical applications for 3D printing: current and projected uses. P T. 2014;39(10):704–11.
77. Vinogradov P. 3D printing in medicine: Current challenges and potential applications. In: 3D Printing Technology in Nanomedicine. Elsevier Inc. 2019;1.
78. Wang S, Chen X, Han X, Hong X, Li X, Zhang H, Li M, Wang Z, Zheng A. A review of 3D printing technology in pharmaceutics: technology and applications, now and future. Pharmaceutics. 2023;15(2):416. https://doi.org/10.3390/pharmaceutics15020416.
79. Warraich HJ, Califf RM. The FDA and the cardiovascular community. J Am Coll Cardiol. 2024;84(1):124–9. https://doi.org/10.1016/j.jacc.2024.05.013.
80. Witowski J, Sitkowski M, Zuzak T, Coles-Black J, Chuen J, Major P, Pdziwiatr M. From ideas to long-term studies: 3D printing clinical trials review. Int J Comput Assist Radiol Surg. 2018;13(9):1473–8. https://doi.org/10.1007/s11548-018-1793-8.
81. Wong RMY, et al. 3D printing in orthopaedic surgery: a scoping review of randomized controlled trials. Bone Joint Res. 2021;10(12):807–19.
82. Xu X, Goyanes A, Trenfield SJ, Diaz-Gomez L, Alvarez-Lorenzo C, Gaisford S, Basit AW. Stereolithography (SLA) 3D printing of a bladder device for intravesical drug delivery. Mater Sci Eng C. 2021;120:111773. https://doi.org/10.1016/j.msec.2020.111773.
83. Xu X, Robles-Martinez P, Madla CM, Joubert F, Goyanes A, Basit AW, Gaisford S. Stereolithography (SLA) 3D printing of an antihypertensive polyprintlet: case study of an unexpected photopolymer-drug reaction. Addit Manuf. 2020;33:101071. https://doi.org/10.1016/j.addma.2020.101071.

New Horizons: Investigations of Natural Polymers and Fibers in Personalized Drug Delivery Systems

16

Ushasi Das, Meghraj Suryawanshi, Hardik Rana, Pranjal Gujarathi, and Kuldeep Vinchurkar

Abstract

This book chapter presents an exploration of the innovative utilization of natural polymers and fibers in personalized drug delivery systems. Natural polymers and fibers, sourced from renewable biopolymers such as cellulose, chitosan, alginate, and silk, offer unique properties that make them promising candidates for personalized medicine applications. Their biocompatibility, biodegradability, and tunable physicochemical properties enable the design of tailored drug delivery systems to meet individual patient needs. This chapter provides an in-depth analysis of the characteristics, formulation approaches, and applications of natural polymers and fibers in personalized drug delivery. It discusses the mechanisms of drug release, stability considerations, and regulatory aspects associated with incorporating these biomaterials into pharmaceutical formulations. Furthermore, it highlights recent advancements, challenges, and future prospects in harnessing the potential of natural polymers and fibers for personalized drug delivery.

U. Das
Department of Pharmaceutical Technology, Jadavpur University, Kolkata, West Bengal, India

M. Suryawanshi (✉) · K. Vinchurkar
Department of Pharmaceutics, Sandip Institute of Pharmaceutical Sciences (SIPS), Affiliated to Savitribai Phule Pune University (SPPU, Pune), Nashik, Maharashtra, India

H. Rana
Department of Pharmaceutics, Anand Pharmacy College, Anand, Gujarat, India

P. Gujarathi
Department of Pharmacology, Vidhyadeep Institute of Pharmacy, Vidhyadeep University, Anita, Surat, Gujarat, India

K. Vinchurkar, S. Mane (eds.), *Innovations in Drug Manufacturing*,
https://doi.org/10.1007/978-981-96-9075-6_16

Keywords

Natural polymers · Fibers · Polymer-based drug delivery systems · Personalized drug delivery

16.1 Introduction to Natural Polymers and Fibers in Drug Delivery

Natural or organic polymers provide an alternative to petroleum-based polymers because of their varied mechanical, physical, chemical, and biological attributes. Organic polymers are obtained from naturally renewable resources such as plant-based materials, animal sources, microbes, or algae [8]. These polymers have minimal toxicity, biocompatibility, durability, and renewable resources. When subjected to anaerobic, aerobic, or microbiological processes, biodegradable polymers degrade due to a variety of parameters, including dimension, diameter, and content. Examples of these include polysaccharides, proteins, fibers, and secondary metabolites [9, 20]. Organic polymers with particular interactions, controlled degeneration, and biological compatibility, such as silk fibroin, cellulose, chitosan, alginate, and hyaluronic acid, make them useful for drug delivery applications. These systems, which may hold different payloads, including proteins, DNA, and tiny molecules, are utilized in tissue engineering, wound healing, and anticancer treatment. Advances in drug delivery techniques are being driven by the fabrication of derivatives and modifications, which hold promise for more sophisticated and versatile carriers [24, 85]. pH-sensitive hydrogels based on Salecan are a promising option for the administration of protein/peptide drugs since they facilitate regulated release rates as well as dose and spatiotemporal customization [68]. Natural fibers are inexpensive, lightweight, sustainable, biodegradable, and ecologically beneficial substitutes for manufactured fibers like carbon fiber and glass [4]. The biodegradable property of plant-based natural fiber composites renders them a possible substitute for synthetic fiber augmented polymer matrix composite materials. Regarding tensile strength, impact strength, interlaminar shear strength, thermal qualities, water absorption, and tribological qualities, they provide qualities that are equivalent to those of synthetic fibers. However, a number of variables affect their characteristics, including the kind of resin, the fiber's origin, the type of reinforcement, the fiber's orientation, the manufacturing process, the crystallinity index, the size of the crystallites, the chemical functional groups, the volume and weight fraction of the fiber, and the fiber's state [75]. The intriguing ability of polymeric nanofibers to overcome the drawbacks of traditional pharmaceutical formulations and provide a way to regulate the site, rate, and timing of drug release to accomplish targeted therapeutic effects has drawn curiosity regarding them. These solid fibers, which have a diameter of less than 1 μm, are potential universal drug delivery approaches because of their intrinsic nanoscale features and distinctive functionality, which include high surface area-to-volume ratio, significant mass transfer, large surface areas, and linked nanoporosity [30, 36]. They can be made with proven technology to provide a broad range of drug release kinetics and perhaps shield medications from breaking down in the body prior to approaching their intended destination. Formulations for oral, ophthalmic, topical, transmucosal, and transdermal routes have been developed using nanofibers [22].

Polysaccharides such as guar gum, pectin, and starch are utilized in pharmaceutical dosage variations, such as diltiazem and isoniazid regulated release formulations. Because of guar gum's capacity to form films, breath films, cough strips, and sore throat strips have been created. Borax-guar gum and xyloglucan have impacted colon-specific medication delivery formulations. Xanthan gum is a highly branched glucamannan that is isolated from microorganisms and employed in culinary, medicinal, and cosmetic products because of its consistency over a broad pH range. It can be found in nitazoxanide tablets and cefdinir oral suspension [31, 39, 40]. Treatments for cancer, hepatitis, diabetes, rheumatoid arthritis, and leukemia all depend on proteins and peptides. However, problems with pharmaceuticals and biopharmaceuticals restrict their therapeutic application. Parenteral administration is the usual mode of administration for therapeutic proteins and peptides; however, because of their short half-life in vivo, many injections are required. Carriers such as liposomes, solid lipid nanoparticles, polymeric nanoparticles, and microparticles can be employed to address this. Because polymeric nanoparticles are smaller than microspheres, parenteral administration is an appropriate application for them. All living things produce natural biodegradable polymers, which are being researched as oral protein and peptide delivery systems. It is simple to break down, digest, and process these naturally occurring polymers without causing any residue [33, 96].

Systems for delivering drugs are essential to individualized therapy. These systems facilitate increased patient compliance, fewer side effects, and better treatment results by customizing medication delivery to each patient's unique features [66]. The focus of personalized medicine is on an individual's distinct genetic composition, way of life, and medical background. By delivering designed nanoparticles that react to certain stimuli, innovative drug delivery systems—which fuse cutting-edge technology with drug delivery—have completely changed the treatment of cancer and other chronic diseases. This improves treatment outcomes for neoplasia and chronic diseases by enabling accurate, customized therapy catered to the needs of specific patients [34, 66]. This chapter scrutinizes the possibilities of natural fibers and polymers in pharmaceutical formulations as well as their stability, regulatory considerations, and release mechanisms for customized drug administration.

16.2 Characteristics and Properties of Natural Polymers and Fibers

The chemical structure of natural polymers determines their special qualities, which include mechanical strength, elasticity, thermal stability, and biodegradability. Chain length, branching, and cross-linking are among the elements that affect these features and their potential use in regulated drug delivery as well as their function in organisms [24].

16.2.1 Biodegradability

Crystallinity, hydrophobicity, and rising macromolecule molecular weights are general criteria for assessing biodegradability improvement. The biodegradability of polymers, including both hydrophobic and hydrophilic segments, is greater than that of polymers containing only one of these characteristics, such as shape, processing conditions, unexpected units, configuration structures, sterilization process, distribution, molecular-weight distribution, annealing, hydrolysis mechanism, surface area, hydrophilic and hydrophobic character, chemical structure, glass transition temperature, melting point, elasticity, and crystal structure. In general, side-chained polymers degrade less quickly than those without them. The biodegradability of a polymer is also significantly influenced by its molecular weight. When the molecular weight rises, the rate of degradation declines. The degree of biodegradation of a polymer is also greatly influenced by its shape. Biodegradability is significantly influenced by the degree of crystallinity since amorphous parts are often attacked by enzymes. Because of its tighter packing, the crystalline portion of the polymer is more resilient to deterioration. An important factor influencing a polymer's enzymatic breakdown is its melting temperature (Tm). The enthalpy change and entropy change during melting are what define the melting point (Tm) [63, 73].

16.2.2 Biocompatibility

Natural polymers, or biopolymers, have a critical role in medicine as imaging agents, scaffolds for tissue growth, medication delivery systems, and medical devices. For undesirable reactions and difficulties, such as immunological responses and inflammation, to be avoided, they must be biocompatible. To guarantee the safety of biomaterials for use in pharmaceuticals, thorough testing—including both in vitro and in vivo evaluations—is required. Comprehending these interactions is essential to the design of biomaterials that harmoniously live with biological settings, hence averting problems and implant malfunction [41]. In order to minimize the possibility of unfavorable responses, biomaterials are generated using molecules and structures that the human system can identify or digest. Surface characteristics like functionalization or coatings can have a direct impact on how a biomaterial communicates with its physiological surroundings. The physical attributes that affect biocompatibility include mechanical strength, flexibility, and rate of degradation. These qualities have to be compatible with the particular use of the biomaterial. The fabrication of smart biomaterials that adapt proactively to the biological milieu to improve biocompatibility is the result of advances in the field of biomaterial research. In order to lessen the possibility of negative responses and enhance patient outcomes, these materials can release medications, grow with tissues, or modify their characteristics to account for changes in the body [86]. In order to generate biomaterials that effortlessly interact with the human body and, ultimately, advance medicine and improve patient care, biocompatibility is an essential and mandatory aspect of biomaterial design and development. Biocompatibility testing and careful consideration of physical, surface, and chemical properties are essential.

16.3 Formulation Approaches for Personalized Drug Delivery Systems

Nanoparticle-Based Delivery Systems

In pharmaceutical applications, biopolymers are essential considering that they perform as precise drug delivery systems with a variety of structures to meet different physiological and medical requirements [12, 13, 47]. Chitosan [19, 62], silk fibroin [17], starch [80], shellac [84], gelatin [59], lignin [18], cellulose [97], alginate [65], and collagen [26] are examples of well-known naturally derived polymers that are utilized in drug administration using suspensions and techniques such as microemulsion, electrospraying, freeze-drying, and supercritical fluid extraction. Biopolymer composites are becoming more and more popular because of their lower toxicity, biodegradability, durability, and renewable nature. Polymeric drug delivery systems are the main emphasis, with approaches such as albumin microspheres and elastin-like polypeptides (ELPs) being investigated [25, 70]. Table 16.1 depicts some of the most important naturally derived polymers and their nanoparticle-based delivery.

Chitosan

Chitosan, a biopolymer derived from chitin found in crustacean shells, is gaining attention for drug delivery due to its biocompatibility, biodegradability, non-toxicity, and ability to interact with biomolecules. Chitosan-based drug delivery systems have shown promising results in improving bioavailability and targeted delivery of drugs, including anticancer agents, vaccines, proteins, and genes. Chitosan can form nanoparticles and microparticles through methods like ionic gelation, emulsion cross-linking, and coacervation, which can be used for sustained release, controlled release, and targeted delivery. However, its low solubility in neutral or high pH mediums limits its applications in biology. By functionalizing its backbone, chitosan can be transformed into hydrogels, nanoparticles, micro- or nano-spheres, and micelles, which are used in cancer treatment [10].

Alginate

Sodium alginate is a linear anionic polysaccharide found in brown algae like Sargassum and giant algae and is a key component in seaweed cell stroma and cell walls. It forms a viscous colloidal liquid when dissolved in water, increasing its viscosity with molecular weight and concentration. The molecule consists of homopolymerization regions (GG, MM, GM) of L-guluronic acid residues, D-mannuronic acid residues, and two types of uronic acid residues connected by β-1,4 and α-1,4 glycosidic bonds. The region ratio of sodium alginate varies among organisms, and the content of M and G significantly impacts its performance. High G content results

Table 16.1 Some of the most important naturally derived polymers and their nanoparticle-based delivery

Polymers	Nanoparticle-based delivery	Drug used	Application	Reference
Chitosan	Thermosensitive liposome	DOX	Triple-negative breast cancer	[58]
	Silver nanoparticles	–	Human hepatocellular carcinoma	[88]
	Glycyrrhetinic acid-modified nanoparticles	5-fluorouracil	Liver cancer	[16]
	Thermoresponsive hydrogels	Umbilical cord mesenchymal stem cells	Acute myocardial infarction	[37]
Alginate	Core-shell nanoparticle	Naringenin	Diabetes	[51]
	Microspheres	Nystatin	Oral candidiasis	[53]
	Hydrocolloid films	Vicenin-2 (VCN-2)	Chronic wound healing	[82]
	Chitosan/alginate/hyaluronic acid sponges	Genipin	Wound healing	[55]
Silk fibroin	Nanospheres	Fluoxetine	Anticancer	[98]
	Coated liposomes	Emodin	Breast cancer	[15]
	Microcomposite tablet	Theophylline	Controlled drug delivery	[72]
	Nanoparticles	Doxorubicin	Lysosomotropic anticancer	[89]
	Microparticle scaffolds	Bone Morphogenic Protein-2	Osteochondral tissue engineering	[91]
	Hydrogel	Benfotiamine	Diabetic neuropathy	[27]
Lignin	Electrospun PVA/PVP nanofiber	Paclitaxel	Cervical cancer	[42]
	Folic acid-PEG-alkaline LNPs	Hydroxycamptothecin	Anticancer	[46]
	Fe_3O_4-infused nanoparticles	Sorafenib	Anticancer	[23]
	Nanoparticles	Curcumin	Anticancer	[6]
	Hydrogel	Mesenchymal stem cells	Wound healing	[71]
Starch	CMC/starch/cu-CQDs	Quercetin	Anticancer	[57]
	Modified nanoparticles	Paclitaxel	Anticancer	[67]
	Nanospheres	Ginkgo biloba extracts	Oral drug delivery	[90]
	Self-assembled nanoparticles	Flavonoid morin	Hyperuricemia therapy	[43]
	Nanoparticles	Irbesartan	Hypertension	[11]
Gelatin	Hydrogel	Anti-TGF-β antibody	Glaucoma	[49]

in a hard and fragile hydrogel, while high M content provides good elasticity but poor adhesion and immune stimulation [2, 64, 95]. Alginate-based drug delivery systems target specific body tissues or organs, providing controlled drug release over time. Alginate hydrogels are used for wound healing, tissue engineering, and drug delivery. Alginate nanoparticles and microspheres are used for targeted drug delivery to cancer cells or diseased tissues. Alginate thin films can be applied to medical devices for sustained drug release to prevent infection or inflammation [1].

Silk Fibroin

Silks are ideal for DDS due to their biocompatibility, biodegradability, and non-antigenic properties. Silk fibroin (SF), a natural protein from the cocoons of Bombyx mori, is particularly biocompatible and has potential applications in biomedicals, photonics, electronics, and optoelectronics. Researchers are exploring the development of a delivery system based on SF for drug release and loading. Silk fibroin-designed nanoparticles have been utilized as drug delivery systems, wound dressings, tissue engineering scaffolds, and cosmetic formulations [28, 100].

Lignin

Lignin, containing phenylpropane units and phenolic and aliphatic hydroxyl groups, has been used in drug delivery and controlled release studies due to its ability to respond to stimuli or be modified [35]. The potential application of lignin nanocarriers in chemotherapeutic drugs has drawn attention. According to studies, lignin contains anticancer and antioxidant properties that may work in concert with cancer treatment. Cancer progression is linked to reactive oxygen species (ROS), as seen by elevated levels of oxidative stress indicators in cancer patients. Antioxidant levels, however, drastically drop, indicating that they may have anti-cancer properties. Because of its phenolic hydroxyl group moiety, lignin, a potential natural antioxidant, scavenges free radical species [7, 14].

Starch

A naturally occurring polymer and carbohydrate, starch is predominantly composed of corn, cassava, wheat, and potatoes. Depending on the source, the quantities of the two macromolecules—amylose and amylopectin—in this combination vary. The functional characteristics of starch, such as gel stability, viscosity, and gelatinization, are influenced by the ratio of amylose to amylopectin concentration. Because starch is inexpensive and readily available, it is utilized extensively in the food sector as well as various pharmaceuticals, drug delivery, and composites [52, 81, 92].

Gelatin

Gelatin is a biodegradable polymer that is becoming more and more popular because of its environmentally beneficial qualities and its uses in the food, pharmaceutical, and bioengineering industries. It is mostly derived from the partial hydrolysis of collagen in animal tissues such as bones, hide, and pigskin. There are two varieties of gelatin: anionic Type B and cationic Type A. Gelatin is likewise approved by the FDA as a safe polymer [5, 48, 83].

Hydrogels and Scaffolds

Biocompatibility, biodegradability, and sustainability characteristics of natural polymers such as alginate, starch, cellulose, chitosan, gelatin, collagen, and hyaluronic acid are ideal for hydrogel fabrication. Hydrogels are three-dimensional networks made of hydrophilic polymers through chemical or physical cross-linking; they explode in water while preserving shape despite absorbing water, and they have garnered attention since they were originally discovered in the 1960s. These hydrogels have a wide range of uses in the medical field, including drug delivery, wound dressings, cell culture substrates, and scaffolds for tissue regeneration [38, 99]. Additionally, the cost-effective synthesis of hydrogels and nanogels, which may have uses in the treatment of cancer, wound healing, and tissue regeneration, is made possible by the abundance of naturally occurring biopolymers [94].

Scaffolding for bone tissue engineering uses natural polymer-based nanomaterials because of their capacity for regeneration and biodegradation. Polysaccharides, polynucleotides, and proteins are examples of these scaffolds. Since they resemble extracellular matrix components, they have improved biocompatibility, cell adhesion, and growth promotion. In bone tissue engineering, natural polymers such as collagen/gelatin, hyaluronic acid, alginate, silk fibroin, chitosan, and peptides are frequently used [76, 79].

16.4 Mechanisms of Drug Release and Controlled Delivery

Drug delivery systems are being explored more and more due to their low cost and good quality. DDSs are perfect for administering medications through the body cavity since they enable the delivery of the drug in its active state or stabilized by carrier functionalization. Because of their effectiveness and affordability, they also provide superior treatments. Various drug delivery methods are employed, such as quick release via tablets, capsules, and injections; however, these methods have restricted pharmacokinetic profiles and are not appropriate for all types of treatments. Implantable devices—which are frequently used in cancer treatments and contraception—achieve longevity release. Because of their enhanced effectiveness, increased patient compliance, and decreased toxicity, controlled release systems utilizing biopolymers or other biomolecules are recommended [3, 87]. The study of a drug's physicochemical properties is crucial for optimizing the delivery system. Key properties include drug solubility, molecular weight, chemical stability, and surface tension. The right carrier is chosen for a drug, and the drug is loaded into it. The ideal loading strategies involve compatibility between the drug, carrier, and excipients, while also considering the release environment. Covalent bond-based systems are used to improve drug solubility and biocompatibility, but not all bonds can be used due to potential external stimulations [60, 74].

Swelling is a crucial mechanism for drug delivery in polymers, causing a material to increase in size and volume due to absorption phenomena. This process affects the physical properties of materials like biopolymers, such as permeability, strength, and flexibility, leading to drug release. Hydrogels, in particular, are affected by this mechanism, as they can absorb multiple times their weight in water. The forces of osmotic, electrostatic, and entropy-favored dissolving drive the process of water intake and swelling. Swelling is coupled with diffusion in hydrophilic polymers, stabilizing a drug release rate that would otherwise be controlled by dissolution. Swelling behavior has been extensively studied for both biopolymers and hybrid-enhanced biopolymers, leading to numerous publications. Osmosis is another important mechanism, transferring a solvent through a membrane to equalize concentrations of the non-permeable solute [29, 60].

Erosion and degradation are crucial for sustained drug delivery, as they can delay the distribution velocity and increase the active role of the polymer. These processes can be caused by chemical reactions or external stimulation, such as pH, T, or mechanical stress. These systems are useful for implantable or injectable therapies, as they allow for less discomfort for patients. Research is ongoing to understand the impacts of degradation and erosion on drug delivery, and the use of complementary materials in drug release systems may increase bioavailability. External stimulation, such as ultrasounds, magnetic fields, lights, and electrochemical devices, can also stimulate drug release. However, controlling internal stimuli like pH, temperature, and enzymatic and redox activities is challenging. The choice of external stimulus depends on the carrier's chemical and physical structure [22, 24, 33, 60].

16.5 Regulatory Perspectives on Natural Polymers and Fibers in Pharmaceutical Formulations

Regulatory bodies defend consumers by advancing and defending human health. In the realm of regenerative medicine and medication delivery, biomaterials like polysaccharides are often governed as medical devices. Because the safety and efficacy of these biomaterials should be beyond dispute, medical devices provide significant issues for regulators, necessitating the development of appropriate regulatory structures. The physicochemical qualities, agglomeration, and size distribution of nanomaterials are evaluated by the FDA based on attributes such as stability, porosity, shape, solubility, density, and contaminants. The FDA offers health and safety guidelines, as well as identification criteria and possible safety hazards, for the use of nanomaterials and nanotechnological techniques in cosmetic products. Drugs and skincare items need pre-market approval, and producers need to make sure everything is safe before going on sale. The FDA stresses that misbranding or adulteration of skin-biocompatible products or their ingredients is prohibited. The toxicological consequences of nanomaterials, with their physicochemical characteristics such as stiffness and surface qualities, have been investigated. Their tendency for aggregation, which may result in immunological responses, is one of the primary characteristics and factors influencing these investigations. The absorption and interaction of nanomaterials with the cell membrane can be influenced by surface functionalization, which can have a positive or negative effect on subsequent biological reactions. Nevertheless, because of their phagocytic activity, macrophages can trigger mild to severe inflammatory responses [54, 56].

16.6 Case Studies and Examples of Natural Polymer-Based Drug Delivery Systems

1. Case Study Phenol functionalized polymer induced in-situ microfiber formation for 3D printing of marine-based hydrogel [32]

Description The paper describes a method for 3D printing marine-based hydrogels with enhanced mechanical properties using synergistic complexation of phenol-functionalized polymers. The design of 3D printable bio-based hydrogels with enhanced mechanical properties and minimal chemical modification can open new opportunities in the field of biomedical applications

Main Findings (1) The authors developed a tough and self-healable chitosan-based hydrogel via a green and sustainable approach by taking advantage of the chitosan's inherent cationic nature, enabling chitosan to form a dynamic reversible electrostatic interaction with an anionic polymer (alginate) (2) The hydrogel exhibited enhanced mechanical properties, toughness, flexibility, and self-healing capability due to the synergistic effect of the phenolated polyelectrolyte complex (PHEC) formation between phenolated chitosan and alginate (3) The PHEC hydrogel was 3D printable due to the reversible nature of the weak physical interactions, which allowed the formed network to be broken and reformed when the shear caused by the injection through the needle was removed.

Limitations (1) Schiff-base linkages can be hydrolyzed under acidic conditions, limiting their applicability (2) Previous methods using synthetic polymers and extensive chemical modifications are not green and hinder biomedical applications (3) More green approaches are needed to develop chitosan-based hydrogels for 3D printing without using toxic chemicals, solvents, and extensive modifications.

2. Case Study 3D Printing of Cytocompatible Gelatin-Cellulose-Alginate Blend Hydrogels [21].

Description This paper presents the development of a natural polymer-based hydrogel ink composed of gelatin, alginate, and cellulose for 3D printing of cytocompatible scaffolds.

Main Findings (1) The study developed a 3D printable hydrogel ink composed of natural polymers—gelatin, alginate, and cellulose (2) The study examined the physicochemical interactions between the components of the gelatin-cellulose-alginate hydrogel by varying the copolymer ratios (3) The study successfully 3D printed multilayer cylindrical hydrogel structures and confirmed their porous structure using SEM and BET analysis (4) The study confirmed the cytocompatibility of the hydrogel scaffolds using fibroblast cells.

Limitations (1) The mechanical properties of natural hydrogels alone may be insufficient for 3D printing, necessitating the development of composite hydrogels (2) The optimal crosslinking strategy (using glutaraldehyde or $CaCl_2$) is still an open question (3) While the developed material has promising properties, further research and development may still be needed to fully realize its potential for biomedical applications.

3. Case Study 3D Printing of Photocurable Cellulose Nanocrystal Composite [61].

Description This paper demonstrates the 3D printing of cellulose nanocrystal-filled biomaterial with improved mechanical and surface properties for potential tissue engineering applications.

Main Findings (1) The study successfully 3D printed a cellulose nanocrystal (CNC)-filled biomaterial that had significantly improved mechanical and surface properties compared to previous polymers used in 3D printing (2) The findings from this work could lead to innovative and cost-effective patient-specific solutions in the medical industry (3) This is the first successful demonstration of 3D printing a CNC nanocomposite hydrogel using stereolithography, resulting in complex architectures with enhanced material properties suitable for tissue engineering applications.

Limitations (1) Challenges in developing suitable materials for 3D printing in industry applications (2) Weak mechanical properties of polymers used in biomedical applications (3) Limitations of current options for patient-specific solutions in the medical industry.

4. Case Study Development of PLA-HAp-CS-based biocompatible functional prototype [69].

Description This case study outlines the development of a biocompatible PLA-HAp-CS composite feedstock filament for 3D printing.

Main Findings (1) The study found the optimal settings for the twin-screw extruder (TSE) used to prepare the feedstock filament, including a barrel temperature of 190 °C, screw speed of 140 r/min, and dead weight of 12 kg (2) The study also found the optimal settings for the fused deposition modeling (FDM) 3D printer used to print the biocompatible composite-based prototype, including a layer thickness of 0.2 mm, deposition angle of 30/45°, and infill density of 100% (3) The results were supported by scanning electron microscopic analysis.

Limitations (1) The study only optimized the process for tensile and flexural samples and did not explore other potential applications or properties of the material (2) The study only used SEM analysis and did not explore other characterization techniques that could provide additional insights (3) The study only explored a limited range of parameters for the TSE and FDM processes and did not investigate the effects of other parameters that could potentially impact the final properties of the material.

16.7 Emerging Trends and Novel Applications

Recent advances in 3D printing technology have sparked significant interest in using natural biopolymers for tissue engineering and biomedical applications. These eco-friendly materials, derived from sources such as lignocellulose, starch, algae, and chitosan, offer customizable biochemical and mechanical properties [45]. Natural polysaccharide-based bioinks, including those of terrestrial and marine origin, have shown promise in reproducing complex tissue microarchitectures and providing biomimetic environments for cell growth [50]. The combination of 3D printing technology with biopolymers has led to the development of numerous research programs exploring material systems for tissue engineering [44]. These natural biopolymer-based bioinks have been applied in various medical fields, including cancer treatment, dental care, biosensors, cardiovascular disease, and muscle restoration [78].

Biobased polymers are the most used materials for 3D printing due to their ability to improve ink flow behavior and mechanical strength of printed structures. Modifying the rheological properties of biopolymeric-based inks can improve the resolution, precision, and geometry of 3D-printed constructs [77]. Combining biopolymers with other biomacromolecules and nanoparticles can enhance the multifunctionality of 3D-printed structures. Despite their potential, challenges remain in customizing these polymers for specific printing requirements and functional needs in different biomedical applications [93].

16.8 Conclusion

This chapter offers a comprehensive overview of natural polymers and fibers used in biomedical applications. Natural polymers are widely used in drug delivery, tissue engineering, wound healing, and regenerative medicine. They have properties like bioactivity, biocompatibility, antigenicity, and structural resemblance. However, they face challenges like microbial contamination, decreased tunability, immunogenic reactions, uncontrollable degradation rate, and poor mechanical strength. Polymers and fibers are essential resources with numerous benefits. Future research in biomedical applications will focus on synthesis and research on multifunctional nanocarriers, including micelles, nanogels, and polymerzomes.

References

1. Abasalizadeh F, Moghaddam SV, Alizadeh E, Akbari E, Kashani E, Fazljou SMB, Torbati M, Akbarzadeh A. Alginate-based hydrogels as drug delivery vehicles in cancer treatment and their applications in wound dressing and 3D bioprinting. J Biol Eng. 2020;14(1):8. https://doi.org/10.1186/s13036-020-0227-7.
2. Abu-Rabeah K, Polyak B, Ionescu RE, Cosnier S, Marks RS. Synthesis and characterization of a pyrrole–alginate conjugate and its application in a biosensor construction. Biomacromolecules. 2005;6(6):3313–8. https://doi.org/10.1021/bm050339j.
3. Adepu S, Ramakrishna S. Controlled drug delivery systems: current status and future directions. Molecules. 2021;26(19):5905. https://doi.org/10.3390/molecules26195905.
4. Akter M, Uddin MH, Tania IS. Biocomposites based on natural fibers and polymers: a review on properties and potential applications. J Reinfor Plast Composit. 2022;41(17–18):705–42. https://doi.org/10.1177/07316844211070609.
5. Alipal J, Mohd Pu'ad NAS, Lee TC, Nayan NHM, Sahari N, Basri H, Idris MI, Abdullah HZ. A review of gelatin: properties, sources, process, applications, and commercialisation. Mater Today Proc. 2021;42:240–50. https://doi.org/10.1016/j.matpr.2020.12.922.
6. Alqahtani MS, Alqahtani A, Al-Thabit A, Roni M, Syed R. Novel lignin nanoparticles for oral drug delivery. J Mater Chem B. 2019;7(28):4461–73. https://doi.org/10.1039/C9TB00594C.
7. Alqahtani MS, Kazi M, Ahmad MZ, Syed R, Alsenaidy MA, Albraiki SA. Lignin nanoparticles as a promising vaccine adjuvant and delivery system for ovalbumin. Int J Biol Macromol. 2020;163:1314–22. https://doi.org/10.1016/j.ijbiomac.2020.07.026.
8. Arif ZU. The role of polysaccharide-based biodegradable soft polymers in the healthcare sector. Adv Ind Eng Polym Res. 2024. S2542504824000241; https://doi.org/10.1016/j.aiepr.2024.05.001.
9. Arif ZU, Khalid MY, Sheikh MF, Zolfagharian A, Bodaghi M. Biopolymeric sustainable materials and their emerging applications. J Environ Chem Eng. 2022;10(4):108159. https://doi.org/10.1016/j.jece.2022.108159.
10. Baharlouei P, Rahman A. Chitin and chitosan: prospective biomedical applications in drug delivery, cancer treatment, and wound healing. Mar Drugs. 2022;20(7):460. https://doi.org/10.3390/md20070460.
11. Bashir Pathan I, Subhashrao Misal N, Bairagi S, Mallikarjuna Setty C. Palmitic acid grafted maize starch (PAgMS) nanoparticles as potential drug carrier for irbesarten: in vitro and in vivo evaluation. Curr Nanomed. 2016;6(2):156–64. https://doi.org/10.2174/2468187306666160622082419.
12. Bejenaru C, Radu A, Segneanu A-E, Biţă A, Ciocîlteu MV, Mogoşanu GD, Bradu IA, Vlase T, Vlase G, Bejenaru LE. Pharmaceutical applications of biomass polymers: review of current research and perspectives. Polymers. 2024;16(9):1182. https://doi.org/10.3390/polym16091182.
13. Chandakavathe BN, Kulkarni RG, Dhadde SB. Grafting of natural polymers and gums for drug delivery applications: a perspective review. Crit Rev™ Ther Drug Carrier Syst. 2022;39(6):45–83. https://doi.org/10.1615/CritRevTherDrugCarrierSyst.2022035905.
14. Chaudhary M, Sinha VR. Lignin-based carriers for drug delivery applications: from an industrial waste to a pharmaceutical aid. Eur Polym J. 2023;195:112206. https://doi.org/10.1016/j.eurpolymj.2023.112206.
15. Cheema SK, Gobin AS, Rhea R, Lopez-Berestein G, Newman RA, Mathur AB. Silk fibroin mediated delivery of liposomal emodin to breast cancer cells. Int J Pharm. 2007;341(1–2):221–9. https://doi.org/10.1016/j.ijpharm.2007.03.043.

16. Cheng M, Gao X, Wang Y, Chen H, He B, Xu H, Li Y, Han J, Zhang Z. Synthesis of glycyrrhetinic acid-modified chitosan 5-fluorouracil nanoparticles and its inhibition of liver cancer characteristics in vitro and in vivo. Mar Drugs. 2013;11(9):3517–36. https://doi.org/10.3390/md11093517.
17. Crivelli B, Bari E, Perteghella S, Catenacci L, Sorrenti M, Mocchi M, Faragò S, Tripodo G, Prina-Mello A, Torre ML. Silk fibroin nanoparticles for celecoxib and curcumin delivery: ROS-scavenging and anti-inflammatory activities in an in vitro model of osteoarthritis. Eur J Pharm Biopharm. 2019;137:37–45. https://doi.org/10.1016/j.ejpb.2019.02.008.
18. Dai L, Liu R, Hu L-Q, Zou Z-F, Si C-L. Lignin nanoparticle as a novel green carrier for the efficient delivery of resveratrol. ACS Sustain Chem Eng. 2017;5(9):8241–9. https://doi.org/10.1021/acssuschemeng.7b01903.
19. Das U, Kapoor DU, Singh S, Prajapati BG. Unveiling the potential of chitosan-coated lipid nanoparticles in drug delivery for management of critical illness: a review. Zeitschrift Für Naturforschung C. 2024;79(5–6):107–24. https://doi.org/10.1515/znc-2023-0181.
20. Dirauf M, Muljajew I, Weber C, Schubert US. Recent advances in degradable synthetic polymers for biomedical applications – beyond polyesters. Prog Polym Sci. 2022;129:101547. https://doi.org/10.1016/j.progpolymsci.2022.101547.
21. Erkoc P, Uvak I, Nazeer MA, Batool SR, Odeh YN, Akdogan O, Kizilel S. 3D Printing of cytocompatible gelatin-cellulose-alginate blend hydrogels. Macromol Biosci. 2020;20(10):2000106. https://doi.org/10.1002/mabi.202000106.
22. Farhaj S, Conway BR, Ghori MU. Nanofibres in drug delivery applications. Fibers. 2023;11(2):21. https://doi.org/10.3390/fib11020021.
23. Figueiredo P, Lintinen K, Kiriazis A, Hynninen V, Liu Z, Bauleth-Ramos T, Rahikkala A, Correia A, Kohout T, Sarmento B, Yli-Kauhaluoma J, Hirvonen J, Ikkala O, Kostiainen MA, Santos HA. In vitro evaluation of biodegradable lignin-based nanoparticles for drug delivery and enhanced antiproliferation effect in cancer cells. Biomaterials. 2017;121:97–108. https://doi.org/10.1016/j.biomaterials.2016.12.034.
24. Gaikwad D, Sutar R, Patil D. Polysaccharide mediated nanodrug delivery: a review. Int J Biol Macromol. 2024;261:129547. https://doi.org/10.1016/j.ijbiomac.2024.129547.
25. Geng Z, Laakko T, Hokkanen A, Södergård C, Maasilta I, Mohammadi P. Material engineering and application of hybrid biomimetic-de novo designed elastin-like polypeptides. Commun Mater. 2024;5(1):152. https://doi.org/10.1038/s43246-024-00597-y.
26. Hall Barrientos IJ, Paladino E, Szabó P, Brozio S, Hall PJ, Oseghale CI, Passarelli MK, Moug SJ, Black RA, Wilson CG, Zelkó R, Lamprou DA. Electrospun collagen-based nanofibres: a sustainable material for improved antibiotic utilisation in tissue engineering applications. Int J Pharm. 2017;531(1):67–79. https://doi.org/10.1016/j.ijpharm.2017.08.071.
27. Hanawa T, Watanabe A, Tsuchiya T, Ikoma R, Hidaka M, Sugihara M. New oral dosage form for elderly patients. II. Release behavior of benfotiamine from silk fibroin gel. Chem Pharm Bull. 1995;43(5):872–6. https://doi.org/10.1248/cpb.43.872.
28. Harishchandra Yadav R, Kenchegowda M, Angolkar M, Meghana TS, Osmani RAM, Palaksha S, Veerabhadrappa Gangadharappa H. A review of silk fibroin-based drug delivery systems and their applications. Eur Polym J. 2024;216:113286. https://doi.org/10.1016/j.eurpolymj.2024.113286.
29. Harting R, Johnston K, Petersen S. Correlating *in vitro* degradation and drug release kinetics of biopolymer-based drug delivery systems. Int J Biobased Plast. 2019;1(1):8–21. https://doi.org/10.1080/24759651.2018.1563358.
30. Hrib J, Sirc J, Hobzova R, Hampejsova Z, Bosakova Z, Munzarova M, Michalek J. Nanofibers for drug delivery—incorporation and release of model molecules, influence of molecular weight and polymer structure. Beilstein J Nanotechnol. 2015;6:1939–45. https://doi.org/10.3762/bjnano.6.198.
31. Idrees H, Zaidi SZJ, Sabir A, Khan RU, Zhang X, Hassan S. A review of biodegradable natural polymer-based nanoparticles for drug delivery applications. Nanomaterials. 2020;10(10):1970. https://doi.org/10.3390/nano10101970.

32. Jafari H, Delporte C, Bernaerts KV, Alimoradi H, Nie L, Podstawczyk D, Tam KC, Shavandi A. Synergistic complexation of phenol functionalized polymer induced *in situ* microfiber formation for 3D printing of marine-based hydrogels. Green Chem. 2022;24(6):2409–22. https://doi.org/10.1039/D1GC04347A.
33. Jain S, Jain A, Jain R, Chauhan NS. Potential of natural polymeric materials in pharmaceutics. Pharmacol ResNat Prod. 2024;2:100014. https://doi.org/10.1016/j.prenap.2024.100014.
34. Jian J, He D, Gao S, Tao X, Dong X. Pharmacokinetics in pharmacometabolomics: towards personalized medication. Pharmaceuticals. 2023;16(11):1568. https://doi.org/10.3390/ph16111568.
35. Kai D, Tan MJ, Chee PL, Chua YK, Yap YL, Loh XJ. Towards lignin-based functional materials in a sustainable world. Green Chem. 2016;18(5):1175–200. https://doi.org/10.1039/C5GC02616D.
36. Kajdič S, Planinšek O, Gašperlin M, Kocbek P. Electrospun nanofibers for customized drug-delivery systems. Jl Drug Deliv Sci Technol. 2019;51:672–81. https://doi.org/10.1016/j.jddst.2019.03.038.
37. Ke X, Li M, Wang X, Liang J, Wang X, Wu S, Long M, Hu C. An injectable chitosan/dextran/β-glycerophosphate hydrogel as cell delivery carrier for therapy of myocardial infarction. Carbohydr Polym. 2020;229:115516. https://doi.org/10.1016/j.carbpol.2019.115516.
38. Klein M, Poverenov E. Natural biopolymer-based hydrogels for use in food and agriculture. J Sci Food Agric. 2020;100(6):2337–47. https://doi.org/10.1002/jsfa.10274.
39. Krishnaiah YSR, Satyanarayana V, Dinesh Kumar B, Karthikeyan RS. In vitro drug release studies on guar gum-based colon targeted oral drug delivery systems of 5-fluorouracil. Eur J Pharm Sci. 2002;16(3):185–92. https://doi.org/10.1016/S0928-0987(02)00081-7.
40. Kumar A, Gulati M, Singh SK, Gowthamarajan K, Prashar R, Mankotia D, Gupta JP, Banerjee M, Sinha S, Awasthi A, Corrie L, Kumar R, Patni P, Kumar B, Pandey NK, Sadotra M, Kumar P, Kumar R, Wadhwa S, Khursheed R. Effect of co-administration of probiotics with guar gum, pectin and eudragit S100 based colon targeted mini tablets containing 5-Fluorouracil for site specific release. J Drug Deliv Sci Technol. 2020;60:102004. https://doi.org/10.1016/j.jddst.2020.102004.
41. Langer R, Peppas NA. Advances in biomaterials, drug delivery, and bionanotechnology. AIChE Journal. 2003;49(12):2990–3006. https://doi.org/10.1002/aic.690491202.
42. Li B, Xia X, Chen J, Xia D, Xu R, Zou X, Wang H, Liang C. Paclitaxel-loaded lignin particle encapsulated into electrospun PVA/PVP composite nanofiber for effective cervical cancer cell inhibition. Nanotechnology. 2021;32(1):015101. https://doi.org/10.1088/1361-6528/abb55a.
43. Li J, Yang Y, Lu L, Ma Q, Zhang J. Preparation, characterization and systemic application of self-assembled hydroxyethyl starch nanoparticles-loaded flavonoid Morin for hyperuricemia therapy. Int J Nanomedicine. 2018;13:2129–41. https://doi.org/10.2147/IJN.S158585.
44. Li X, Cui R, Sun L, Aifantis KE, Fan Y, Feng Q, Cui F, Watari F. 3D-printed biopolymers for tissue engineering application. Int J Polym Sci. 2014;2014:1–13. https://doi.org/10.1155/2014/829145.
45. Liu J, Sun L, Xu W, Wang Q, Yu S, Sun J. Current advances and future perspectives of 3D printing natural-derived biopolymers. Carbohydr Polym. 2019;207:297–316. https://doi.org/10.1016/j.carbpol.2018.11.077.
46. Liu K, Zheng D, Lei H, Liu J, Lei J, Wang L, Ma X. Development of novel lignin-based targeted polymeric nanoparticle platform for efficient delivery of anticancer drugs. ACS Biomater Sci Eng. 2018; https://doi.org/10.1021/acsbiomaterials.8b00260.
47. Lohani A, Singh G, Bhattacharya SS, Verma A. Interpenetrating polymer networks as innovative drug delivery systems. J Drug Deliv. 2014;2014:1–11. https://doi.org/10.1155/2014/583612.
48. Madkhali OA. Drug delivery of gelatin nanoparticles as a biodegradable polymer for the treatment of infectious diseases: perspectives and challenges. Polymers. 2023;15(21):4327. https://doi.org/10.3390/polym15214327.
49. Maeda M, Kojima S, Sugiyama T, Jin D, Takai S, Oku H, Kohmoto R, Ueki M, Ikeda T. Effects of gelatin hydrogel containing anti-transforming growth factor-β antibody in a canine filtration surgery model. Int J Mol Sci. 2017;18(5):985. https://doi.org/10.3390/ijms18050985.

50. Mahendiran B, Muthusamy S, Sampath S, Jaisankar SN, Popat KC, Selvakumar R, Krishnakumar GS. Recent trends in natural polysaccharide based bioinks for multiscale 3D printing in tissue regeneration: a review. Int J Biol Macromol. 2021;183:564–88. https://doi.org/10.1016/j.ijbiomac.2021.04.179.
51. Maity S, Mukhopadhyay P, Kundu PP, Chakraborti AS. Alginate coated chitosan core-shell nanoparticles for efficient oral delivery of naringenin in diabetic animals—an in vitro and in vivo approach. Carbohydr Polym. 2017;170:124–32. https://doi.org/10.1016/j.carbpol.2017.04.066.
52. Marta H, Rizki DI, Mardawati E, Djali M, Mohammad M, Cahyana Y. Starch nanoparticles: preparation, properties and applications. Polymers. 2023;15(5):1167. https://doi.org/10.3390/polym15051167.
53. Martín MJ, Calpena AC, Fernández F, Mallandrich M, Gálvez P, Clares B. Development of alginate microspheres as nystatin carriers for oral mucosa drug delivery. Carbohydr Polym. 2015;117:140–9. https://doi.org/10.1016/j.carbpol.2014.09.032.
54. Meftahi A, Samyn P, Geravand SA, Khajavi R, Alibkhshi S, Bechelany M, Barhoum A. Nanocelluloses as skin biocompatible materials for skincare, cosmetics, and healthcare: formulations, regulations, and emerging applications. Carbohydr Polym. 2022;278:118956. https://doi.org/10.1016/j.carbpol.2021.118956.
55. Meng X, Lu Y, Gao Y, Cheng S, Tian F, Xiao Y, Li F. Chitosan/alginate/hyaluronic acid polyelectrolyte composite sponges crosslinked with genipin for wound dressing application. Int J Biol Macromol. 2021;182:512–23. https://doi.org/10.1016/j.ijbiomac.2021.04.044.
56. Morgan SE, Havelka KO. In: Lochhead RY, editor. Cosmetic nanotechnology: polymers and colloids in cosmetics, vol. 961. American Chemical Society; 2007. https://doi.org/10.1021/bk-2007-0961.
57. Najafi M, Pourmadadi M, Abdous M, Rahdar A, Pandey S. Formulation of double nanoemulsions based on pH-sensitive carboxymethyl cellulose/Starch copper doped carbon quantum dots for quercetin controlled release. J Mol Liq. 2024;400:124543. https://doi.org/10.1016/j.molliq.2024.124543.
58. Niu S, Williams GR, Wu J, Wu J, Zhang X, Chen X, Li S, Jiao J, Zhu L-M. A chitosan-based cascade-responsive drug delivery system for triple-negative breast cancer therapy. J Nanobiotechnol. 2019;17(1):95. https://doi.org/10.1186/s12951-019-0529-4.
59. Nouri-Felekori M, Khakbiz M, Nezafati N, Mohammadi J, Eslaminejad MB. Comparative analysis and properties evaluation of gelatin microspheres crosslinked with glutaraldehyde and 3-glycidoxypropyltrimethoxysilane as drug delivery systems for the antibiotic vancomycin. Int J Pharm. 2019;557:208–20. https://doi.org/10.1016/j.ijpharm.2018.12.054.
60. Opriş O, Mormile C, Lung I, Stegarescu A, Soran M-L, Soran A. An overview of biopolymers for drug delivery applications. Appl Sci. 2024;14(4):1383. https://doi.org/10.3390/app14041383.
61. Palaganas NB, Mangadlao JD, De Leon ACC, Palaganas JO, Pangilinan KD, Lee YJ, Advincula RC. 3D printing of photocurable cellulose nanocrystal composite for fabrication of complex architectures via stereolithography. ACS Appl Mater Interfaces. 2017;9(39):34314–24. https://doi.org/10.1021/acsami.7b09223.
62. Pathak K, Misra SK, Sehgal A, Singh S, Bungau S, Najda A, Gruszecki R, Behl T. Biomedical applications of quaternized chitosan. Polymers. 2021;13(15):2514. https://doi.org/10.3390/polym13152514.
63. Patwary MAS, Surid SM, Gafur MA. Properties and applications of biodegradable polymers. J Res Updat Polym Sci. 2020;9:32–41. https://doi.org/10.6000/1929-5995.2020.09.03.
64. Pawar SN, Edgar KJ. Alginate derivatization: a review of chemistry, properties and applications. Biomaterials. 2012;33(11):3279–305. https://doi.org/10.1016/j.biomaterials.2012.01.007.
65. Petchsomrit A, Sermkaew N, Wiwattanapatapee R. Alginate-based composite sponges as gastroretentive carriers for curcumin-loaded self-microemulsifying drug delivery systems. Sci Pharm. 2017;85(1):11. https://doi.org/10.3390/scipharm85010011.

66. Puccetti M, Pariano M, Schoubben A, Giovagnoli S, Ricci M. Biologics, theranostics, and personalized medicine in drug delivery systems. Pharmacol Res. 2024;201:107086. https://doi.org/10.1016/j.phrs.2024.107086.
67. Putro JN, Ismadji S, Gunarto C, Soetaredjo FE, Ju YH. A study of anionic, cationic, and nonionic surfactants modified starch nanoparticles for hydrophobic drug loading and release. J Mol Liq. 2020;298:112034. https://doi.org/10.1016/j.molliq.2019.112034.
68. Qi X, Wei W, Li J, Zuo G, Pan X, Su T, Zhang J, Dong W. Salecan-based pH-sensitive hydrogels for insulin delivery. Mol Pharm. 2017;14(2):431–40. https://doi.org/10.1021/acs.molpharmaceut.6b00875.
69. Ranjan N, Singh R, Ahuja I. Development of PLA-HAp-CS-based biocompatible functional prototype: a case study. J Thermoplast Compos Mater. 2020;33(3):305–23. https://doi.org/10.1177/0892705718805531.
70. Rathod S, Deshpande S. Albumin microspheres as an ocular delivery system for pilocarpine nitrate. Indian J Pharm Sci. 2008;70(2):193. https://doi.org/10.4103/0250-474X.41454.
71. Ravishankar K, Venkatesan M, Desingh RP, Mahalingam A, Sadhasivam B, Subramaniyam R, Dhamodharan R. Biocompatible hydrogels of chitosan-alkali lignin for potential wound healing applications. Mater Sci Eng C. 2019;102:447–57. https://doi.org/10.1016/j.msec.2019.04.038.
72. Rodrigues M, Peiriço N, Matos H, Gomes De Azevedo E, Lobato MR, Almeida AJ. Microcomposites theophylline/hydrogenated palm oil from a PGSS process for controlled drug delivery systems. J Supercrit Fluids. 2004;29(1–2):175–84. https://doi.org/10.1016/S0896-8446(03)00034-2.
73. Saini RD. New age biodegradable and compostable plastics. Asian J Res Chem. 2018;11(1):179. https://doi.org/10.5958/0974-4150.2018.00037.8.
74. Salamanca CH, Yarce CJ, Moreno RA, Prieto V, Recalde J. Natural gum-type biopolymers as potential modified nonpolar drug release systems. Carbohydr Polym. 2018;189:31–8. https://doi.org/10.1016/j.carbpol.2018.02.011.
75. Sanjay MR, Madhu P, Jawaid M, Senthamaraikannan P, Senthil S, Pradeep S. Characterization and properties of natural fiber polymer composites: a comprehensive review. J Clean Prod. 2018;172:566–81. https://doi.org/10.1016/j.jclepro.2017.10.101.
76. Saurav S, Sharma P, Kumar A, Tabassum Z, Girdhar M, Mamidi N, Mohan A. Harnessing natural polymers for nano-scaffolds in bone tissue engineering: a comprehensive overview of bone disease treatment. Curr Issues Mol Biol. 2024;46(1):585–611. https://doi.org/10.3390/cimb46010038.
77. Shahbazi M, Jäger H. Current status in the utilization of biobased polymers for 3D printing process: a systematic review of the materials, processes, and challenges. ACS Appl Bio Mater. 2021;4(1):325–69. https://doi.org/10.1021/acsabm.0c01379.
78. Shaji SS, Kamalasanan K, Harika S, Tiwari A, Raj B. Natural biopolymer for 3D printing. J Polym Sci Eng. 2023;6(1):3016. https://doi.org/10.24294/jpse.v6i1.3016
79. Sivakumar PM, Yetisgin AA, Sahin SB, Demir E, Cetinel S. Bone tissue engineering: anionic polysaccharides as promising scaffolds. Carbohydr Polym. 2022;283:119142. https://doi.org/10.1016/j.carbpol.2022.119142.
80. Sousa ACC, Romo AIB, Almeida RR, Silva ACC, Fechine LMU, Brito DHA, Freire RM, Pinheiro DP, Silva LMR, Pessoa ODL, Denardin JC, Pessoa C, Ricardo NMPS. Starch-based magnetic nanocomposite for targeted delivery of hydrophilic bioactives as anticancer strategy. Carbohydr Polym. 2021;264:118017. https://doi.org/10.1016/j.carbpol.2021.118017.
81. Tagliapietra BL, De Melo BG, Sanches EA, Plata-Oviedo M, Campelo PH, Clerici MTPS. From micro to nanoscale: a critical review on the concept, production, characterization, and application of starch nanostructure. Starch – Stärke. 2021;73(11–12):2100079. https://doi.org/10.1002/star.202100079.
82. Tan WS, Arulselvan P, Ng S-F, Taib CNM, Sarian MN, Fakurazi S. Healing effect of vicenin-2 (VCN-2) on human dermal fibroblast (HDF) and development VCN-2 hydrocolloid film based on alginate as potential wound dressing. Biomed Res Int. 2020;2020:1–15. https://doi.org/10.1155/2020/4730858.

83. Tan Y, Zi Y, Peng J, Shi C, Zheng Y, Zhong J. Gelatin as a bioactive nanodelivery system for functional food applications. Food Chem. 2023;423:136265. https://doi.org/10.1016/j.foodchem.2023.136265.
84. Thombare N, Kumar S, Kumari U, Sakare P, Yogi RK, Prasad N, Sharma KK. Shellac as a multifunctional biopolymer: a review on properties, applications and future potential. Int J Biol Macromol. 2022;215:203–23. https://doi.org/10.1016/j.ijbiomac.2022.06.090.
85. Tong X, Pan W, Su T, Zhang M, Dong W, Qi X. Recent advances in natural polymer-based drug delivery systems. React Funct Polym. 2020;148:104501. https://doi.org/10.1016/j.reactfunctpolym.2020.104501.
86. Trucillo P. Biomaterials for drug delivery and human applications. Materials. 2024;17(2):456. https://doi.org/10.3390/ma17020456.
87. Uhrich KE, Cannizzaro SM, Langer RS, Shakesheff KM. Polymeric systems for controlled drug release. Chem Rev. 1999;99(11):3181–98. https://doi.org/10.1021/cr940351u.
88. Vijayakumar M, Priya K, Ilavenil S, Janani B, Vedarethinam V, Ramesh T, Arasu MV, Al-Dhabi NA, Kim Y-O, Kim H-J. Shrimp shells extracted chitin in silver nanoparticle synthesis: expanding its prophecy towards anticancer activity in human hepatocellular carcinoma HepG2 cells. Int J Biol Macromol. 2020;165:1402–9. https://doi.org/10.1016/j.ijbiomac.2020.10.032.
89. Wang S, Xu T, Yang Y, Shao Z. Colloidal stability of silk fibroin nanoparticles coated with cationic polymer for effective drug delivery. ACS Appl Mater Interfaces. 2015;7(38):21254–62. https://doi.org/10.1021/acsami.5b05335.
90. Wang T, Wu C, Fan G, Li T, Gong H, Cao F. Ginkgo biloba extracts-loaded starch nanospheres: Preparation, characterization, and in vitro release kinetics. Int J Biol Macromol. 2018;106:148–57. https://doi.org/10.1016/j.ijbiomac.2017.08.012.
91. Wang X, Wenk E, Zhang X, Meinel L, Vunjak-Novakovic G, Kaplan DL. Growth factor gradients via microsphere delivery in biopolymer scaffolds for osteochondral tissue engineering. J Control Release. 2009;134(2):81–90. https://doi.org/10.1016/j.jconrel.2008.10.021.
92. Waterschoot J, Gomand SV, Fierens E, Delcour JA. Production, structure, physicochemical and functional properties of maize, cassava, wheat, potato and rice starches. Starch – Stärke. 2015;67(1–2):14–29. https://doi.org/10.1002/star.201300238.
93. Xu W, Wang X, Sandler N, Willför S, Xu C. Three-dimensional printing of wood-derived biopolymers: a review focused on biomedical applications. ACS Sustain Chem Eng. 2018;6(5):5663–80. https://doi.org/10.1021/acssuschemeng.7b03924.
94. Yang G, Xiao Z, Ren X, Long H, Qian H, Ma K, Guo Y. Enzymatically crosslinked gelatin hydrogel promotes the proliferation of adipose tissue-derived stromal cells. Peer J. 2016;4:e2497. https://doi.org/10.7717/peerj.2497.
95. Yang J-S, Xie Y-J, He W. Research progress on chemical modification of alginate: a review. Carbohydr Polym. 2011;84(1):33–9. https://doi.org/10.1016/j.carbpol.2010.11.048.
96. Yu D-G, Zhao P. The key elements for biomolecules to biomaterials and to bioapplications. Biomolecules. 2022;12(9):1234. https://doi.org/10.3390/biom12091234.
97. Yu H-Y, Zhang H, Song M-L, Zhou Y, Yao J, Ni Q-Q. From cellulose nanospheres, nanorods to nanofibers: various aspect ratio induced nucleation/reinforcing effects on polylactic acid for robust-barrier food packaging. ACS Appl Mater Interfaces. 2017;9(50):43920–38. https://doi.org/10.1021/acsami.7b09102.
98. Yu S, Yang W, Chen S, Chen M, Liu Y, Shao Z, Chen X. Floxuridine-loaded silk fibroin nanospheres. RSC Adv. 2014;4(35):18171–7. https://doi.org/10.1039/C4RA02113D.
99. Zhao L, Zhou Y, Zhang J, Liang H, Chen X, Tan H. Natural polymer-based hydrogels: from polymer to biomedical applications. Pharmaceutics. 2023;15(10):2514. https://doi.org/10.3390/pharmaceutics15102514.
100. Zhao Z, Li Y, Xie M-B. Silk fibroin-based nanoparticles for drug delivery. Int J Mol Sci. 2015;16(3):4880–903. https://doi.org/10.3390/ijms16034880.

4D Bioprinting Using Biomaterials: A Future of 3D Printing

17

Akanksha Dwivedi, Shivangi Sharma, Disha Sharma, Anuradha Derashri, and Kuldeep Vinchurkar

Abstract

With 4D bioprinting, the creation of biological structures may incorporate time, a transformational factor, which is a substantial advancement above typical 3D printing. This development, which makes printed constructions capable of dynamically changing and responding to a variety of stimuli, including temperature, pH, and biochemical signals, has the potential to completely transform tissue engineering and regenerative medicine. Smart biomaterials, which may change their composition, structure, or function after creation to more accurately resemble the adaptive behaviors of real tissues, are at the heart of this breakthrough.

This chapter explores the state of 4D bioprinting technology today and provides a thorough synopsis of the fundamental ideas in this area. Important ideas are carefully considered, such as the notion of 4D bioprinting and the mechanics of dynamic metamorphosis. Many kinds of smart biomaterials are discussed with their distinct characteristics, behaviors, and synthesis and characterization techniques. 4D bioprinting has several potential uses, including customized medicine, medication delivery, tissue engineering, and regenerative medicine. A

A. Dwivedi (✉)
Acropolis Institute of Pharmaceutical Education and Research, Indore, MP, India

S. Sharma
Amity Institute of Pharmacy, Amity University, Gwalior, MP, India

D. Sharma · A. Derashri
LSHGCT's Gahlot Institute of Pharmacy, Navi Mumbai, Maharashtra, India

K. Vinchurkar
Department of Pharmaceutics, Sandip Institute of Pharmaceutical Sciences (SIPS), Affiliated To Savitribai Phule Pune University (SPPU, Pune), Nashik, Maharashtra, India

K. Vinchurkar, S. Mane (eds.), *Innovations in Drug Manufacturing*,
https://doi.org/10.1007/978-981-96-9075-6_17

comparison with 3D bioprinting is presented through case studies and recent research, highlighting noteworthy experiments and results that highlight the improved capabilities of 4D bioprinting. In addition to discussing potential issues and offering solutions, the chapter looks forward, spotting new developments and trends. Critical analysis is used to address ethical and regulatory issues, defining the frameworks and rules required to negotiate the complexity of this quickly developing technology.

Keywords

4D bioprinting · Tissue engineering · Regenerative medicine · Customized medicine · Ethical · Regulatory

17.1 Introduction

17.1.1 Evolution from 3D to 4D Bioprinting

Science and the globe are advancing at a breakneck pace. New technologies that will enhance quality of life are being introduced on a daily basis. 3D printing, often known as additive manufacturing, is one of them. This technique, which can be improved by the addition of intelligent materials such as smart polymers as feed, fills the gap left by the present production processes. The product that follows is capable of adjusting to various situations, including variations in temperature and tension. These reactions led to the development of 4D printing, a sophisticated 3D printing technique. Applications for 3D and 4D printing technologies have been discovered across all sectors and sizes of businesses, from small scale to enormous scale. Biological chemicals, biomaterials, and live cells are combined in the additive manufacturing process known as "bioprinting" to create physiologically useful structures [36]. Compared to two-dimensional cell culture, three-dimensional (3D) bioprinting is a more realistic approximation of in vivo settings and is a frequently used in vitro modelling method. While 3D bioprinting has been applied in a number of tissue engineering and therapeutic contexts, it only considers the scaffold or item in its initial condition. In order to include the extra dimension of time inside the printed 3D scaffolds, a new technique known as four-dimensional (4D) bioprinting has arisen recently. The printed construct is subjected to an external stimulus throughout the 4D bioprinting process, which eventually modifies its form or functioning [62].

As the next-generation biological tissue engineering solution, four-dimensional (4D) bioprinting—where time is combined with three-dimensional (3D) bioprinting as the fourth dimension—has recently come to light because it has the potential to create intricate, functional components. By using materials that respond to stimuli, 4D bioprinting may be utilized to create dynamic, three-dimensional biological constructions that will change shape in response to different stimuli. One further aspect of 4D bioprinting is the functional transition and maturation of printed cell-laden constructions over time, which offers the previously unheard-of possibility of bone tissue creation. The ability of printed structures to retain their shape allows for the customized repair of connective tissue defects, while the processes involved in functional maturation encourage stem cells to differentiate into osteoblasts [7].

The utilization of alginate-gelatin hydrogels in the bioprinting process allowed for the creation of a complex and diverse aortic valve. This breakthrough demonstrated the potential of 3D bioprinting to produce anatomically intricate and heterogeneously enclosed hydrogel conduits for aortic valves. The full potential of hydrogels in bioprinting became evident when methacrylated gelatine (GelMA) gained popularity. GelMA exhibits increased stiffness and swelling properties when exposed to ultraviolet light, making it suitable for bioprinting due to its desired mechanical properties. A recent development in the field of bionic tissue and organ creation involves the successful replication of a human ear. This was achieved by using 3D-printing technology to create a matrix made of hydrogel that was seeded with cells. Additionally, an inductive coil antenna was incorporated into the matrix, enabling the ear to receive radiofrequency signals [56]. In 2014, the advancement of vascular pathways within printed structures made it possible to sustain the viability of cells in thicker tissues. This breakthrough allowed the cells to keep growing and maturing even after being printed. In addition, tumor reconstructions were conducted for research purposes. As an illustration, HeLa cells were fabricated using 3D printing technology to generate an artificial representation of a cervical tumor in a controlled laboratory environment. It was shown that the morphology and force exerted by the needle employed in the bioprinting process could potentially influence the viability of the cells. In addition, bioinks made from decellularized extracellular matrix have been created to enhance tissue specificity due to the intricate composition and vital role of the extracellular matrix in cellular development and maintenance [34].

17.1.2 Advancement of 4-Dimensional (4D) Bioprinting

In 2015, researchers demonstrated the development of a tissue construct made of soft hydrogels and high-porosity microfiber networks. This construct exhibited mechanical and biological compatibility, with stiffness and elasticity comparable to that of cartilage in articulation tissue. In addition, due to the high conductivity of graphene, the formulation of a bioink containing it was modified to manipulate various aspects such as adhesion, viability, proliferation, and differentiation of mesenchymal cells into neurological tissue [25]. The development of bioprinting materials for bone regeneration and the investigation of potential hydrogel combinations and printing settings in order to achieve optimal outcomes persisted in 2018. In order to as closely as possible replicate this kind of tissue utilizing bioprinting technologies and provide more accurate and realistic tests to fight the illness, research into the tumor microenvironment and its function in cell communication in the development of cancer has proceeded [26].

Biological chemicals, biomaterials, and live cells are combined in the additive manufacturing process known as "bioprinting" to create physiologically useful structures. Compared to two-dimensional cell culture, three-dimensional (3D) bioprinting is a more realistic approximation of in vivo settings and is a frequently used in vitro modelling method. While 3D bioprinting has been applied in a number of tissue engineering and therapeutic contexts, it only considers the scaffold or item in its initial condition. In order to include the extra dimension of time inside the printed 3D scaffolds, a new technique known as four-dimensional (4D) bioprinting has arisen recently [43]. The printed construct is subjected to an external stimulus throughout the 4D bioprinting process, which eventually modifies its form or functioning.

Through examining the responses of the attached cells and structures to different stimuli, researchers can get a more profound comprehension of the functions of natural tissues. Furthermore, to illustrate possible insights for new 4D bioprinting applications, the usage of smart biomaterials and 4D printing methods for tissue engineering applications are presented. In conclusion, we will discuss future approaches, including the integration of self-assembling nanomaterials and biological scaffolds in bioprinted tissue structures to overcome the present problems with this technology [21, 32].

17.1.3 Significance and Potential Impact

Smart materials are utilized in 4D printing, which is an advanced form of additive manufacturing. This enables the integration of 3D printing principles with the capability to alter the structure, characteristics, or functionality of materials over time in response to external stimuli. The term "4D" emphasizes the dynamic characteristics of these printed structures by associating time with a fourth dimension. 4D printing technology revolutionizes biomedical applications by facilitating the creation of dynamic structures that can seamlessly adjust to their environment through the integration of stimuli-responsive materials such as hydrogels, shape-memory polymers, and bio-inks. The transformative capabilities of 4D printing in the domains of medication delivery, medical devices, tissue engineering, diagnostics, and medical devices themselves render it a highly consequential technology in the realm of biomedical engineering. The ability to create more complex and adaptable devices that can replicate the intricate behavior of biological systems is made possible by the dynamic nature of 4D-printed materials [66]. This can eventually improve therapeutic outcomes and enable patient-specific therapies. For example, 4D printing may be used in tissue engineering and regenerative medicine to produce constructs that, upon implantation, change into the appropriate shape or structure, allowing for better integration with the surrounding tissue and encouraging cell proliferation and differentiation. Similarly, the use of 4D printing might facilitate the creation of adaptive drug delivery systems, which can administer drugs more precisely by releasing their payload when exposed to certain physiologic cues like pH and temperature changes. 4D-printed sensors and other technologies might be used in diagnostics to detect infections, biomarkers, and other analyses more precisely and consistently by adapting to different physiological situations [29].

The development of smart implants and prosthetics has advanced significantly with the advent of 4D printing technology. 4D-printed objects may self-transform or adjust in response to certain stimuli, such as light, moisture, magnetic fields, or temperature, by including time as an additional dimension. Biomedical engineering has seen a substantial transformation as a result of this special quality, especially in the area of prostheses and implant design and manufacture. The need for intrusive operations and modifications may decrease with the use of 4D-printed smart implants and prostheses. Patients may experience physical and psychological strain when undergoing repeated surgical procedures for the installation, replacement, or alterations of traditional implantation and prostheses [23].

The impact of 4D bioprinting is tremendous in the biomedical field and is depicted in Fig. 17.1. The applications of 4D printing technology in tissue engineering and regenerative medicine have shown great potential. Through the use of bio-inks infused with living cells and the special powers of 4D printing, scientists have created structures that have the ability to grow and change over time to become functioning tissue. This innovative method can revolutionize donor organ transplantation and encourage quicker tissue repair. Bio-inks, biocompatible polymers infused with living cells, are an essential part of tissue engineering 4D printing. By combining bio-inks with the dynamic properties of 4D printing, scientists can create complex, multi-layered structures that closely mimic the natural composition of human tissues [61]. As an illustration, cartilage material can be produced using a 4D printing technique that utilizes a hydrogel capable of expanding in response to the quantity of human mesenchymal stromal cells present in the bio-ink.

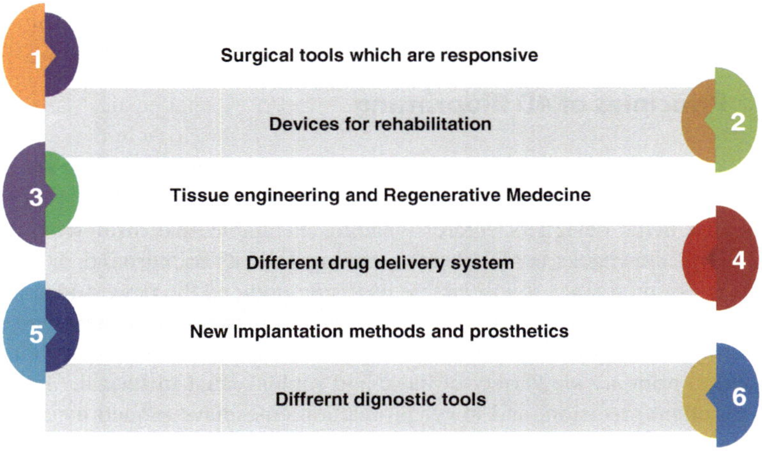

Fig. 17.1 Potential Impact of 4D printing in the biomedical field

With the use of 4D printing techniques, surgeons will be able to perform intricate surgeries with better control and accuracy thanks to the creation of surgical instruments that are responsive to changes in their surroundings. These cutting-edge instruments may modify their stiffness and form under certain stimuli by using the special qualities of 4D-printed materials, which enhances surgical results and shortens recovery periods for patients [22].

The capacity of responsive surgical instruments to alter in shape and stiffness is essential because it minimizes the possibility of tissue injury by enabling the instruments to fit to various surgical settings and anatomical features.

The development of sophisticated diagnostic instruments that have the potential to completely transform the medical diagnostics industry has been made possible by 4D printing technology. Scientists can enhance the accuracy, sensitivity, and individualized nature of diagnostic tools by leveraging the unique properties of 4D-printed materials, which can change their shape or properties in response to specific stimuli. This will ultimately improve the quality of patient care and outcome [65]. An instance of a portable smart sensor made with thermoplastic polyurethane (TPU) printed on cloth is a 4D-printed diagnostic instrument. Using the stimuli-responsive qualities of the TPU material, this sensor can measure vital indicators, including blood pressure, body temperature, and heart rate.

The subject of biomedical rehabilitation has seen a paradigm change with the introduction of 4D printing technology, which has opened up new avenues for the development of responsive, adaptable, and intelligent devices. With this innovative method, biomedical rehabilitation devices might be designed, manufactured, and used in a completely new way that is more efficient, patient-centered, and individualized [35].

The production of dynamic braces and splints for the treatment of musculoskeletal disorders is one instance of 4D printing in rehabilitation. By adjusting their form or stiffness in response to muscle activation or joint position, these smart devices can minimize the risk of stiffness in the joint or muscle degeneration while providing customized encouragement and facilitating recovery [16].

17.2 Principles of 4D Bioprinting

It is discovered that 4DP represents the most notable advancement over the current 3DP process and serves as a model for additive manufacturing (AM). Another clever concept that helps designers create dynamic, adaptable structures while getting around 3DP's drawbacks is 4DP. Understanding 3DP, its background, and printing methods is essential since it will enable us to comprehend the newest idea in smart 4DP and its discovery more fully. Recent years have seen the widespread use of computer-aided design (CAD) with the 3DP technology, which is controlled by a computer, to print a wide variety of basic and sophisticated materials. 3DP's rapid speed, excellent precision, and lower production costs have piqued the interest of businesses and research institutions. 3DP is a multidisciplinary technique that brings together many scientific disciplines such as the study of materials, mechanical engineering, engineering science, and data processing [47]. 3DP is a novel approach for designing complicated structures that are not viable using standard techniques. Significant discoveries have been made in the fields of remotely actuated robots, bio-inspired designs, microbial environments and tissues, and medication delivery systems. 3DP has shown to be a creative and clever technology in the biomedical and other industrial sectors. While 4DP is still in its earliest days, it has a chance to alter the production sector in the years to come [18].

The foundational concepts were formulated at the Massachusetts Institute of Technology (MIT), with the inclusion of time as the fourth dimension. 4D bioprinting implies that in the future, it will be possible to incorporate live cells into biocompatible materials that are 3D printed using bioinks. Subsequently, a series of step-by-step methods were employed to advance the concept of 4D bioprinting based on identified stimuli that are relevant to particular biological uses. The initial method of 4D printing closely resembled the MIT concept, where the printed material (such as a smart biopolymer or responsive hydrogel) folds into a predetermined 3D shape when triggered, and the tissues or cells attach to the folded surface to create the desired form [31]. As the tissue or organ grows stronger, the scaffold progressively dissolves, ideally in a controlled manner, and is absorbed by the body. Tissue growth might be seen as a primary stimulus in this method. However, due to their biodegradability, 3D-printed scaffolds are extremely divisive.

17.3 Mechanisms of Stimulation Response

17.3.1 Pathways for 4D Bioprinting

Self-adaptability, self-sensing, shape memory, responsiveness, multifunctionality, and self-repair are the primary characteristics of smart materials. These traits leverage a number of interesting applications by determining their after-printing behaviors in response to external stimuli. Even though certain reviews of stimuli-responsive materials have already been published in other domains, it is still important to determine whether or not they are appropriate for use in biomedical applications. In fact, the stimulus provided and the material selection—which is based on the intended application—have a significant impact on how a 4D bio construct functions [42, 44].

When temperature, light, electric, mechanical, magnetic, and surface stimuli are applied to polymer compounds, which are stimuli-responsive, the polymers' size, shape, permeability, mechanical, surface, optical, and electrical properties fluctuate. Stimulus-responsive hydrogels are considered smart materials because, as was previously said, they can react to different variables in the environment. In reaction to outside influences, adaptive hydrogels can alter their permeability, or the tension strength, network topology, and swelling behavior. It's noteworthy to note that a large number of stimuli-responsive hydrogels exhibit completely reversible changes, making them highly desirable for biological applications [33].

17.4 Smart Biomaterials in 4D Bioprinting

17.4.1 Types of Smart Biomaterials

Smart hydrogels have two main advantages over conventional substances: they have a high water content that closely resembles the environment found in biological tissues, and they facilitate more effective mass movement. Sol-gel transition, shape memory, and self-healing are some of the special properties of smart hydrogels that make them very useful for bioprinting devices in medicine. The following characteristics are necessary for a successful bioprinted hydrogel construct:

- Printing capability, which is determined by the appropriate viscosity, quick response, transition time, and a suitable sol-gel transition stimulus;
- Biocompatibility, which encompasses biodegradability, the ability to withstand cell-cell and cell-matrix interactions, and absence of toxicity;
- Mechanical properties, which should match those of the tissue being studied in terms of stiffness, elasticity, and durability; and
- Shape and framework, as the printed structure should exhibit high structural characteristics similar to the natural tissue [37].

17.4.2 Materials That Respond to Humidity

Humidity-sensitive polymers are gaining a lot of attention for numerous commercial and technological uses, as well as for applications related to personal comfort and health, because water is ubiquitous in nature. The feature in the TE field that describes the various degrees of temporal/spatial swelling deformation that can be caused in a scaffold is called humidity-responsiveness. Nonetheless, the prolonged response times and intricate control actuation of these materials pose practical obstacles to their widespread application, mostly stemming from the sluggish kinetics of water diffusion. Owing to its carcinogenic qualities, one contentious substance is based on poly(ethylene glycol) (PEG) and is created by mixing agarose (AG) with azobenzene derivative (PCAD) to create PCAD@AG. In any case, scientists have been examining its characteristics since PCAD and agarose, which has a low desorption rate but a quick absorption of water rate, can be combined to create a moisture-responsive system that increases adsorption while decreasing absorption rate. The PCAD@AG film rapidly absorbs wetness, swells, and folds up when it comes into interaction with moisture. A humidity differential can be used to direct this folding; PCAD@AG folds or coils in accordance with the expansion caused by absorption of water on the surface of the contact side [67]. On the other hand, a membrane will quickly coil and unwind in successively reverse directions if it is placed on wet filter paper, causing it to move quickly across the paper. Emphasis has been given to polymers whose water-induced shape memory is relevant.

Due to their biocompatibility and biodegradability, PCL and PEG are both appropriate candidates for use as biomaterials in medical applications. This has been noted in the literature and recognized by the US Food and Drug Administration.

Due to its new use in biomedical applications, little is known about CNC biocompatibility. Nevertheless, cytotoxicity testing has demonstrated the outstanding cytocompatibility of nanocomposites, indicating their potential use in medical applications including drug administration, smart sutures, vascular and esophageal stents, and scaffolds for tissue creation. Additionally responsive to water stimulation, PEG and PEG-diacrylate hydrogel have found uses as sensors and actuators, as well as in the development of soft robots, artificial muscles, energy generators, programmable origami, and scaffolding for TE technologies. The three films' bending curvatures grew as the relative humidity (ΔRH) variance increased. In addition to increasing the polymer networks' crosslinking density, a longer exposure duration resulted in a reduced bending curvature for the film at the same ΔRH [39]. Self-acting structures that can fold and unfurl are called active origami. Origami can offer appropriate solutions for minimally invasive surgery by creating structures that fold up and fit into tiny openings. Actuators that are sensitive to moisture can also be built on a liquid-crystalline (LC) polymer network. These can produce complex anisotropic deformations including helicoids, spiral ribbons, conic, and anticonic shapes.

Generally, the alignment and molecular order of the LC units, in all three dimensions that comprise the polymeric network, determine the management of the targeted deformations. Similarly, similar networks that have been turned on by an alkaline solution can be employed in intelligent fabrics as humidity-responsive actuators. Recent proposals for new biomaterials include elastomeric, soft, water-swelling, shape-memory liquid-crystalline anisotropic hydrogels [63].

17.4.3 Materials That Respond to Magnetism

Reactive polymers can be free strands in solution, framed on surfaces, cross-linked inside polymer networks, or reactive to magnetic fields either way. A nonuniform magnetic attraction causes the materials to instantly change in size and shape, which makes the procedure reversible. Typically, inorganic magnetic particles known as "nanos" are covalently immobilized on 3D lattices. The electrical stimulation of the polymers in this instance produces a magnetic vulnerability, which has sparked interest in these materials for applications as drug delivery systems, separated media, mechanical muscles, soft biomimetic actuators, sensors, and cancer therapeutic agents. A magnetic field is used to regulate the orientation of printed anisotropic particles with stiff magnetized plates throughout the printing procedure. By controlling the chemical makeup of supplies, biomaterials can be created with a single two-component unit or with multiple materials forming a single geometry [64]. This adds another dimension to the space of design that can be used to create functional constructs that can eventually resemble complex biological structures found in nature.

Combining hydrogel systems with magnetic nanoparticles (MNP) results in magnetic hydrogels. In response to magnetic stimuli, MNPs such as cobalt ferrite, iron platinum (FePt), iron (III) oxide (Fe_2O_3), and iron (II, III) oxide (Fe_3O_4) cause hydrogel deformation [45]. A magnetic field is used to regulate the orientation of printed anisotropic particles with stiff magnetized plates throughout the printing procedure. By controlling the chemical makeup of supplies, biomaterials can be created with a single two-component unit or with multiple materials forming a single geometry [19]. This adds another dimension to the space of design that can be used to create functional constructs that can eventually resemble complex biological structures found in nature.

The latest study using human liver cancer cells and PAA shows that they exhibit the intended cytotoxic action. Hydrophilic, biocompatible, and non-immunogenic is the polymer itself, PHPMAm. Toxicological testing should always be done; the purity of the polymer affects the outcome as well. Tests using PNIPAAm on various cell kinds showed that the cell sensitivity varies according to cell type. One key characteristic of light-sensitive polymers is that they can be stimulated by radiation in an extremely easy and non-invasive way, which results in a responsive behavior. UV light exposure can easily cause cell-containing polymers to crosslink. Radicals that are free are produced by photoinitiators throughout the curing phase, which starts with the polymerization procedure. Free radicals are produced by photoinitiators during the curing phase, which starts the polymerization process. It is important to monitor and evaluate the time spent exposed, duration, light intensity, and suitable photoinitiator to make certain the cells won't sustain any damage.

Reversible optical storage, polymer viscosity control, transduction and photomechanical performance, the administration of drugs, interchange for protein biological activity, and TE are a few potential uses for photoresponsive polymers [1]. In order to create micelles for chemotherapy for cancer, light-responsive polymers such as poly(1-pyrenylmethyl methacrylate) (PEO-PPyMA), poly(2-nitrobenzylmethyl methacrylate) (PEO-b-PNBMA), and PEO-b-P(MA-DEACM) have been utilized.

17.4.4 pH-Adaptive Substances

Both normal physiological conditions (such as in the digestive system or vagina) and abnormal pathological conditions (such as bone fractures, inflammation, tumors, certain cardiovascular abnormalities, and infected wounds) can lead to a substantial fluctuation in the body's pH levels. The gastrointestinal tract exemplifies this phenomenon, as the pH gradually increases from 1 in the stomach to 8 in the intestine. Drug delivery could significantly benefit from the use of responsive biomaterials that can effectively interact with pH fluctuations. Specifically, hydrogels that are sensitive to changes in pH in their immediate surroundings exhibit either expansion or contraction of their volume, commonly referred to as swelling or deswelling. The ionization of pendant groups, such as amine and carboxylic acid groups, is the primary cause of this phenomenon [13]. Proteins (such as gelatin and albumin) and polysaccharides (such as alginate and chitosan) have the ability to create hydrogels that respond to changes in pH. Poly(N-isopropyl acrylamide-co-butyl methacrylate-co-acrylic acid) and star-branched poly(ε-caprolactone)-b-poly(2-(dimethylamino)ethyl methacrylate) (HPs-star-PCL-b-PDMAEMA) are polymers that are sensitive to changes in pH and temperature. These polymers are used for applications involving controlled drug delivery. Several of these polymers have been utilized for 4D bioprinting, where pH acts as a designated stimulus [24].

17.4.5 Other Materials That Respond to Stimuli

This section reports on other stimulus-responsive materials, in addition to the previously mentioned types, that are activated by chemical, mechanical, and glucose-based stimuli.

Mechanically or shear-responsive hydrogels exhibit a reaction to external mechanical disturbances. They can change their inherent viscoelastic properties and display either shear-thinning or shear-thickening behaviors, depending on the applied shear stress. Indeed, the viscosity of shear-thickening hydrogel increases in response to an external force, while the viscosity of shear-thinning hydrogel decreases. Self-assembled polymeric structures exhibit a reversible phenomenon known as shear-thinning. Producing injectable biomaterials has the potential to be highly practical. Shear-thickening, on the other hand, only occurs in specific shear ranges and deals with colloidal suspensions [13]. One such is a hydrogel with a cysteine and elastin-like structure.

Proteins (such as gelatin and albumin) and polysaccharides (such as alginate and chitosan) have the ability to create hydrogels that respond to changes in pH. Poly(N-isopropyl acrylamide-co-butyl methacrylate-co-acrylic acid) and star-branched poly(ε-caprolactone)-b-poly(2-(dimethylamino)ethyl methacrylate) (HPs-star-PCL-b-PDMAEMA) are polymers that are sensitive to changes in pH and temperature. These polymers are used in controlled drug delivery applications. Several of these polymers have been utilized for 4D bioprinting, with pH acting as a designated stimulus. Table 17.1 shows different types of material used in the progression of 4D printing and what their individual applications are [45].

Table 17.1 Types of materials used in 4D bioprinting

Material	Application
Materials that respond to humidity	
PEG–PCAD@AG	For situations that involve contactless actuation in response to the day-night cycle of humidity in the atmosphere
PEG–PCL–CNC	Therapeutic uses include smart stitches, vascular stents and esophagus stents, tissue-engineered scaffolds, and delivery of drugs
Liquid–crystalline (LC) polymer networks activated with an alkaline solution	Humidity-responsive actuators for use in smart fabrics
Polyethylene glycol	Tissue engineering
Cellulose stearoyl esters (CSEs)	Sensors, actuators, or the development of soft robots

(continued)

Table 17.1 (continued)

Material	Application
Hydrogel composite ink composed of stiff cellulose fibrils embedded in a soft acrylamide matrix	Biomedical devices, tissue engineering, soft robotics
Materials that respond to magnetism	
Cobalt ferrite ($CoFe_2O_4$)	Controlled drug release
Iron (III) oxide (Fe_2O_3)	Application in drug delivery
CoPt	Application in drug delivery
(Fe_3O_4) with PNIPAM, PVA, poly(acrylamide), alginate	Acts as a semiconductor, actively supports drug on-demand and cell delivery
Iron nanoparticles/[11-(2-bromo-2-methyl)-propionyloxy] undecyltrichlorosilane (Fenp-PS gel)	Cancer treatment, sensors, switches, different separations, membranes, and drug delivery systems
pH-adaptive substance	
Poly(acrylic acid) (PAA)	Peroral-controlled medication delivery, taste-masking of bitter pharmaceuticals, and intravenous drug release with elevated blood pH in specific cardiac defects
Poly(acrylic acid) (PAA):PEO	Application in drug delivery
Based on gelatin (G) and acrylic acid (AAc)	Oral drug delivery (colon-specific)
Poly(acrylamide/maleic acid) (P(AAm/MA))	Application in drug delivery
Polyacrylamide and chitosan (PAAm)	Agriculture and biomedical field
Sulfonamide/polyethyleneimine (PEI)	Gene delivery (tumor-specific)
Alginate	Application in drug delivery
Other materials that respond to stimuli (chemistry, mechanical force, stress, and thermomechanical)	
Glucose-responsive hydrogels	Monitoring of diabetes
Cysteine-containing hydrogel	Biomaterials that are injectable
Barium titanate ($BaTiO_3$, BTO) nanoparticles into a polyethylene glycol diacrylate (PEGDA) matrix	Medical devices that are implantable
$BaTiO_3$ (BTO) filler in a poly(vinylidene) fluoride (PVDF)	Pressure sensor
$BaTiO_3$ powder and photocurable resin SI500	Ultrasonic sensing and energy concentrating
Shape memory polymer	Origami in active form
Multiwall carbon nanotubes (MWCNTs)/PVDF/$BaTiO_3$ nanoparticles	Sensor

17.5 Technological Advances

17.5.1 Printing Techniques and Equipment

Typically, standard 3D printing materials like acrylonitrile styrene (ABS) or PLA are tailor-made for pre-established printing settings in 3D printers. Current 3D printers may encounter challenges with smart materials that have specific functions and multi-components, as they have the potential to clump together and create obstacles during the printing process. Consequently, several technologies have been adopted for 4D printers. In order to maintain the proper heat circulation while printing, the printer additionally features a heated bed [17].

A method like this one was used to create a manufacturing technology for building 2D and 3D solid structures with built-in electrical circuitry. The process involves designing the parts, planning the process, carrying out integrated manufacturing (including multiple starts and stops for both SL and DP, as well as various intermediate processes), and then doing postprocessing. The SL developed the substrate/mechanical structure, and conductive inks were directly printed onto the connections. Examples of simple practical use were performed using 2D and 3D circuit designs [5, 52, 58, 68].

Espalin et al. recommended using professional-grade ME systems for discrete multi-material production [20]. A system incorporating multiple materials and technologies was developed and put into operation to facilitate the production of components utilizing various materials or process adjustments. Two obsolete manufacturing systems underwent upgrades and were consolidated into a single production unit, enabling precise, spatially controlled deposition of thermoplastic materials using multiple extrusion nozzles within the same manufacturing process. This methodical approach was made possible through the integration of a build platform connected to a pneumatic slide for transferring the platform between the two manufacturing systems, a comprehensive control system, a central PC, a custom application (FD Motion), and a user-friendly graphical interface.

17.5.2 Stimuli-Responsive Mechanisms

The emergence of intelligent platforms in biomedical applications is a product of the new material age. These platforms react to external stimuli, enabling precise medicine and tailored treatment. The materials used in the 4D bioprint should have good printing and form-making capabilities, meaning that external triggers will need to regulate the final shape. These can be classified into physical, chemical, and biological stimuli. Physical stimulations include magnetic fields, temperature, sound, electric fields, and light, pH, solvents, humidity, and chemical triggers, and biological stimulations, including proteins, enzymes, glucose, as well as cell attraction forces, which can be used to control the structure and function of receptive materials. The platform for construction was linked to a pneumatic slide, which enabled the platform to move between two ME systems. It was also connected to a central PC, an overall control system, a custom program (FD Motion), and a graphical user interface. This systematic approach was made possible by these connections [8, 9, 51, 53, 60].

17.5.2.1 Physical Stimuli

Light

Light-responsive materials can alter physically or chemically by catching light using chromophores in the polymer chain. Due to the presence of various chromophores, such as azobenzene, sulfuric acid, and fluorides, light radiation results in chemical structure, load, water affinity, and polymer polarity changes that transfer to the final properties of 4D printing materials. Biomaterials that react to light can be stimulated remotely by ultraviolet radiation (UV), infrared radiation (IR), and near-IR radiation (NIR), allowing exact adjustment of intensity and wavelength. Light stimuli provide several benefits, including the ability to be employed quickly, readily switched, and targeted with great accuracy in time and place utilizing non-invasive/minimally invasive procedures.

The sorts of photochemical functional groups employed in SMP play an important role in the production of light-responsive 4D materials. Light-induced substances can be transformed reversibly or irreversibly, depending on the properties of photosensitive molecules and the kind of polymer material. Light-responsive polymers include liquid crystal elastomers, composites, hydrogels, and SMPs.

An intriguing study looked into the synthesis of a functional oligomer of cholesteric liquid crystals (azo-ChLC) using azobenzene. This oligomer yields a photoisomerizable elastomer and allows for the production of various nematic alignments using the same color ink in a single continuous direct ink writing process (DIW) without the need to alter print parameters.

The retention of deformation, NIR-sensitive structures, and the biocompatibility of hydrogel-based ink render these methods appealing for the 4D bioprinting of artificial tissues and organs.

Temperature

Temperature is one of the most common external stimuli used in 4D printing, allowing you to regulate and apply it simply, allowing you to produce deformations of forms and geometric arrangements of responsive materials in an efficient manner. When polymers are heated at high temperatures, the original shape is restored. The original form is restored when the polymer is heated at a high temperature. When healing and recovering from bone abnormalities, this capacity to regain its shape after the stimulus is administered might be quite helpful. Only polymers with a Tg of less than or equal to body temperature can use this technique.

For instance, self-adapting tissue engineering implants may be made using 3D-printed porous scaffolds made of hydroxyapatite (HA) and polylactide (PLA), which may regain their form following cycles of compression, heating, and compression.

Electric Field

Many biological applications, such as medication delivery, tissue engineering, and regenerative medicine, are intriguing for electroactive biomaterials. In this regard, the 4D printing paradigm has also been used to study electrically conductive materials. 4D electroactive devices were created by the combined deposit method of printing composites of PLAs and CNTs. Excellent electroactive responses were also displayed by the most conductive printed 2D and 3D structures, with 90% form restitution upon voltage application. The study demonstrates how 4D technology may be used to produce new, multipurpose, adaptable gadgets.

Magnetic Field

Magnetic fields may also be used to operate 4D printing remotely and safely from a distance. Magnetization-responsive materials are created by adding ferromagnetic or paramagnetic compounds into polymer architectures that may be triggered by magnetic field triggers. Magnetic nanoparticles, metal alloys, and metal oxides are the three most often used magnetic additives. By adding the electromagnetic reaction components, a 4D printed material can change shape directly by magnetic, thermodynamic, or electrodynamic means. To develop a 4D-printed magnetic active material, its shape change and mechanical ability can be controlled, and a 3D magnetic active material based on microparticles such as butyl phthalate, polydimethylsiloxane (PDMS), NdFeB, and blown silicon was printed.

Studies conducted recently have outlined the creation of 4D-printed shape-memory materials that are sensitive to magnets. This was achieved by blending thermoplastic PU (TPU) with PLA particles and either Fe_3O_4 or NdFeB with PPR. Intelligent printed structures exhibit excellent tensile strength and rapid responsiveness to external magnetic fields. These findings serve as the foundation for future research into magneto-active structures developed via 4D printing.

17.5.2.2 Chemical Stimuli

pH

Fluctuations in pH levels can lead to interesting changes in the shape of 3D-printed materials, making pH-responsive materials commonly used in biomedical applications. These materials are used in therapies for conditions such as cancer and inflammation, as they can adapt to different pH environments. Natural pH-responsive biopolymers like gelatin, alginate, keratin, hyaluronic acid, collagen, and chitosan, as well as synthetic polymers made from acetate, acrylic acid, and L-glutamic acid monomers, are used to create pH-sensitive 3D printing materials. These materials are categorized into basic and acid polymers and have also been used to create pH-responsive tablets using semi-solid extrusion 3D printing, with the aim of enhancing the bioavailability of oral medications. They produce novel polypropylenes by mixing varying ratios of sodium alginate, carboxymethyl chitosan, and PEG diacrylate (PEGDA) that regulate the placement and sustained release of acid-sensitive medicines in the stomach and intestines. In this situation, a secondary cross-link between Ca^{2+} and the substance gives an active reaction over the tablet's pH range. The human body experiences a variety of pH levels, making it possible to create a new pH-sensitive device for biomedical applications.

Humidity

Humidity-sensitive materials can alter their size, function, and form in addition to scaffolds that respond to pH variations. Humidity-resistant materials are appealing for 4D printing because they may swell or contract depending on whether liquids are present or not. Even if these qualities are intriguing for biological applications, the process of swelling to rupture should be carefully managed to preserve the printed material's integrity. A palette of different stiffness and hygro-responsive filaments filled with cellulose was 3D printed to produce hygro-morphic structures using fused filament manufacturing technology. All of the prototypes demonstrated completely reversible cyclic opening and closure under various relative humidity settings because of the high hygroscopicity of cellulose.

These characteristics open up new possibilities for the development of intelligent materials that can adjust on their own to changes in relative humidity. Another use of moisture-responsive polymers in 4D printing is the creation of a soft robot resembling a seed. The development of an artificial seed involved the combination of coaxial electrospinning of hygroscopic fibers crafted from PEO and cellulose nanocrystals with the fused deposition modeling of hygroscopic PCL. This type of hygroscopic actuator could potentially function as a sustainable energy source for small robots.

17.5.2.3 Biological Stimuli

Materials with biological activity utilize biological stimulants like proteins, glucose, enzymes, and other biological macromolecules. Alongside chemical and physical stimuli, the goal of 4D printing technology is to manufacture materials that demonstrate responsive behavior in the presence of biological stimuli.

Enzymes

Enzymes are molecules that are highly selective and specialized, and they are involved in many different biological processes. Given that the body contains a large number of enzymes, interest in using printed enzyme-responsive materials for biological purposes has increased over time. For example, enzymes may be included in 3D-printed materials to facilitate tissue regeneration, which can be used to customize devices that are comfortable for patients or to accelerate implant degradation in preparation for eventual natural removal.

A recent study utilized a thermal paste printing method to produce PCL composites with lipases, leading to the creation of a novel biomaterial that could be naturally inserted and broken down in the body. The ability of lipases to degrade biodegradable polymers was demonstrated, and 3D-printed PCL-lipase composites were broken down in a water-based environment at 37 °C within a reasonable timeframe. These 4D-printed materials could be utilized as a biomedical implant, with a portion of the structure being absorbed into the body before introducing another component.

The use of 3D-printed structures to immobilize enzymes shows promise in controlling calcification processes and providing an alternative approach to bone regeneration. In addition to tissue engineering, the immobilization of enzymes through printing introduces a new category of 3D-printed biocatalysts for various applications in industrial biotechnology, including organic synthesis, drug screening, industrial processes, biosensing, and environmental uses.

Biomolecules

These days, routinely checking blood sugar and urine levels is a straightforward process for identifying renal disease early on and diabetes early on, respectively. A lot of work has gone into creating more straightforward and precise biosensors over time in an attempt to enhance the detection of glucose and urea. When it comes to producing biomolecule-responsive materials for the quantitative detection of urea and glucose in complicated biological samples, 4D printing has proven to be an effective technique in all the fabrication processes.

A digital light processing (DLP) 3D-printing technology was used to develop an all-in-one needle panel meter for measuring glucose and urea. This meter utilized photocurable polymers with or without 2-carboxyethyl acrylate. Reusability, suitability for usage in intricate biological matrices, ease of use, affordability, and independence from analytical conditions (temperature, buffer, pH) are some of this innovative device's benefits.

17.6 Application of 4D Bioprinting

17.6.1 Tissue Engineering and Regenerative Medicine

4D printing has the potential to be used in biomanufacturing for tissue engineering and regenerative medicine. This technology has three primary uses: converting planar printed structures into anatomically appropriate curved shapes, replicating the dynamics of native tissue, and adjusting printed designs for less invasive use in surgeries.

Tube-like channels, with diameters ranging from micrometers to centimeters, are vital components of various organ systems such as the neurological, pulmonary, gastrointestinal, and genitourinary systems. These structures act as essential conduits, enabling the passive circulation of fluids and, in certain instances, altering fluid composition.

While the mechanisms behind natural tissue development and tube formation are not fully understood, the numerous factors influencing tube morphogenesis can be used as a basis for innovative 4D printing technologies. The formation of tubular structures involves various processes, such as wrapping, budding, cavitation, cord hollowing, and cell hollowing, each contributing to the creation of tubular shapes through individual and collective cell behaviors. A comprehensive study by Lubarsky and Krasnow delves into the mechanics governing tube morphogenesis. Conventional 3D printing technologies encounter challenges when stacking circular layers, especially during extended print durations corresponding to the tubular structure's length. Additionally, initiating cell growth on planar surfaces and transforming them into irregular or curved arrangements leads to more successful uniform or planned cell dispersion. The early versions of self-folding tube constructs created through 4D printing were relatively straightforward in theory, but they faced challenges due to complex mesh-like vascular networks and issues with the strength and tightness of the connections. Nonetheless, recent developments have made it possible to 4D print intricate, branching vascular junctions, including T- and Y-shaped bifurcations. Ongoing advancements are expected to match or even surpass the progress made in 3D printing technology, especially when it comes to creating intricate, multi-vascular networks similar to those found in organs like the lungs [41].

Achieving optimal therapeutic results depends on the least disruptive placement and seamless incorporation of tissue scaffolds into defect voids. Tissue scaffolds should be designed as temporary, small structures in 4D to facilitate less invasive deployment.

17.6.2 Drug Delivery Systems

Design considerations for drug delivery systems (DDS) include the precise temporal and geographical release of encapsulated medicinal compounds. An innovative approach to address these crucial aspects involves integrating 4D printing principles with DDSs, allowing for personalized drug administration to specific tissues and sites with unique physiological conditions.

New cage-like microstructures have been created to capture or release microparticles on demand, taking advantage of differences in pore widths when the cage is expanded or contracted. This development has intriguing implications for medication delivery.

When exposed to near-infrared (NIR) light, nanoscale shape changes in liquid metal-based particles with a GQD shell, which have been endocytosed, can effectively disrupt cellular structures by rupturing the endosomal membrane, leading to rapid drug release. The potential of this is tremendous, especially when it comes to delivering personalized medicine to tumor cells. The microscale form-morphing is especially intriguing because the shape of the microparticle determines whether it can be phagocytosed, which has extensive implications for biomedicine [3, 41, 48, 49, 70]. These are represented in Fig. 17.2:

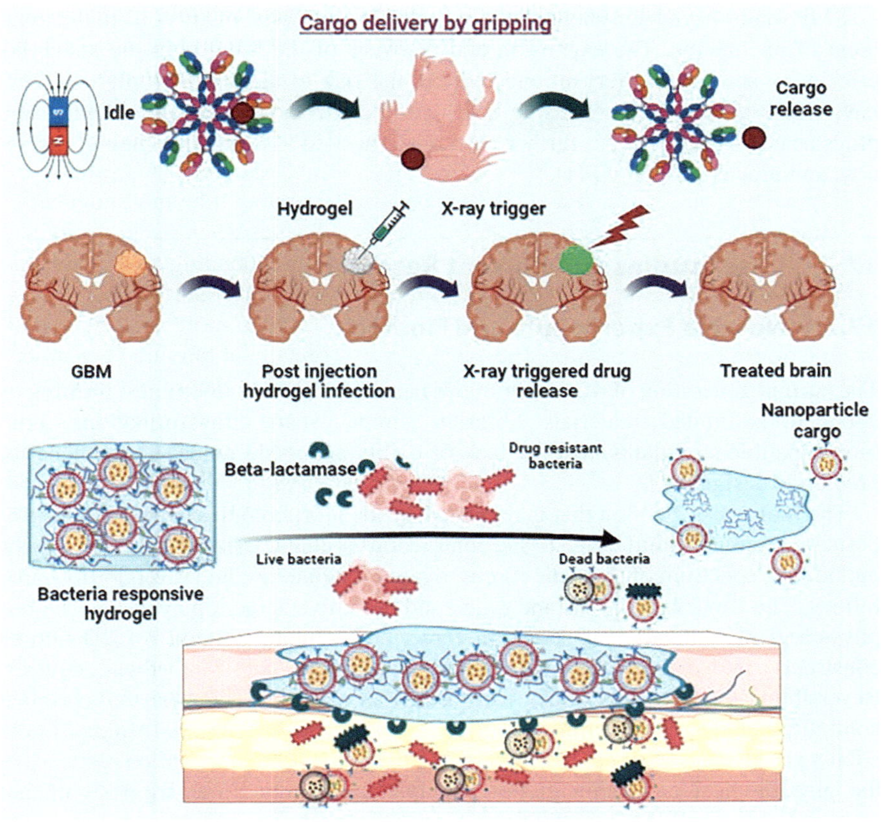

Fig. 17.2 4D bioprinting for drug delivery

17.6.3 Personalized Medicine

Soft materials are becoming more popular for applications that involve interacting with delicate tissues, thanks to their tissue-like mechanics and viscoelastic properties. This shift is driving advancements in soft-robotic technology across various fields, such as medical devices, wearable robots, prostheses, actuators, biohybrid devices, and tissue and organ simulators.

The potential of 4D printing is significant in creating self-contained soft-robotic systems that can respond to stimuli without needing an electrical or pneumatic source. Self-strengthening sutures based on biodegradable SMPs could react to physiological heat and effectively seal wounds at specific pressures, leading to improved wound healing and reduced scarring. SMP-based stents can be delivered by catheters in a transient, tiny state. They may then be triggered and restored at body temperature when they reach the target, giving critical support to the injured spacecraft.

SMP foams have been shown to be superior to traditional metal coils in the treatment of aneurysms. The expansion and recovery of the SMP after the aneurysm effectively seals the aneurysm and reduces the risk of dangerous ruptures. There have also been proposals for using SMP-based clot removal devices and occlusion plugs as contraceptives, but further research is needed to determine their effectiveness and biocompatibility [41].

17.7 Case Studies and Current Research

17.7.1 Notable Experiments and Findings

The current generation of 4D technologies has four major shortcomings, limiting its application: limited materials libraries, simple shape transformations, non-biocompatible stimulants, and the lack of highly adaptable modeling methods for predictive design [41].

The biological function that is regulated by the morphological transformation of tissues caused by stimuli (e.g., tissue contraction) is characterized by its complexity, including a spectrum of dynamic forces, temporal dynamics, and reversibility capabilities. The capacity to withstand quick and repetitive actuation cycles, as well as physiological standards for actuation force, are common criteria for 4D-printed constructs intended to replicate biological tissues or biomedical devices. Reversibility qualities are critical to ensuring that the material returns to its original configuration soon after stimulation is ceased, allowing for repeated stimulation to elicit a variety of responses. It's challenging to get the desired actuation response in the physiological environment. For example, hydrogels suffer from significant mechanical losses due to swelling [14].

The aim is to create composite designs with different properties and actuation methods in order to advance the development of synthetic tissues and biomedical devices.

Additionally, experimental data plays a crucial role in adjusting material models and refining simulation parameters, thereby enhancing the precision of virtual simulations. When 4D-printed structures alter their shape, the material properties respond to stimuli, which require integrating time-dependent characteristics into simulation models. Failing to accurately capture these dynamic changes can result in differences between simulated and experimental results, compromising the reliability of prediction models.

17.7.2 Comparative Analysis with 3D Printing

3D printing is a low-cost technique for product manufacturing, while 4D printing is an enhanced 3D printing technology capable of multifunctionality, self-repair, and self-assembly. 4D printing uses comparable technologies to 3D printing, adding a new dimension to the transformation process over time. It is a novel and innovative technology that is quickly being used in a wide range of technical sectors. The

Table 17.2 Comparative studies between 3D & 4D printing technology

Category	3D printing technology	4D printing technology
Printing method	Printing repeats a 2D structure	Printing is the extension of 3D printing
Printer type	3D printer	Multi- /smart-material 4D printer
Materials	Thermoplastics, food, polymers, paper, ceramics, nanomaterial metals, and biomaterials	Multi-material, self-assembled, smart material, self-actuating, shape memory polymers, self-sensing material, advanced, and magnetostrictive material.
Design concept	The 3D digital object with deformation feature-related equipment apparatus, material extrusion, and selective laser sintering	Selective laser, binder, and modified nozzle
Flexibility of product	No	Yes
State of product	Static structure	Smart, dynamic structure
Cost of equipment	Low	High
Outlook of market	Medium	Medium-high
Applications	Engineering and design, robotics, consumer items, military, education, medical, defense, and aerospace, fashion, industrial goods, and more.	Aerospace, construction, furniture, biomedical devices, medicine, soft robotics, transportation, aviation, and more

discussion covers the essential distinctions between 3D and 4D printing, as well as the necessary printing procedures. 4D printing integrates mathematical, stimuli, and interactive elements utilizing intelligent materials, which differs significantly from 3D printing. It is crucial to assess and contrast the technologies of 3D and 4D printing, along with their distinct features and market potential [17].

The information provided in Table 17.2 delves into the technologies of 3D and 4D printing, encompassing printing techniques, materials, design principles, equipment costs, associated machinery, market patterns, and uses. It also illustrates the evolution of 4D printing from 3D printing. The expansion of 3D printing has been considerable in recent years, potentially leading to an increased demand for 4D printing in the coming decade. The advancement of 4D printing and intelligent materials is poised to have a substantial influence on various industrial sectors [17].

17.8 Future Directions

The progression of 3D printing into 4D printing is an inventive method for producing smart medical implants and gadgets that adapt to the patient's growth through the use of smart materials. Patient data is scanned utilizing CT, MRI, and other scanning technologies and printed layer by layer with 4D printing technology. The

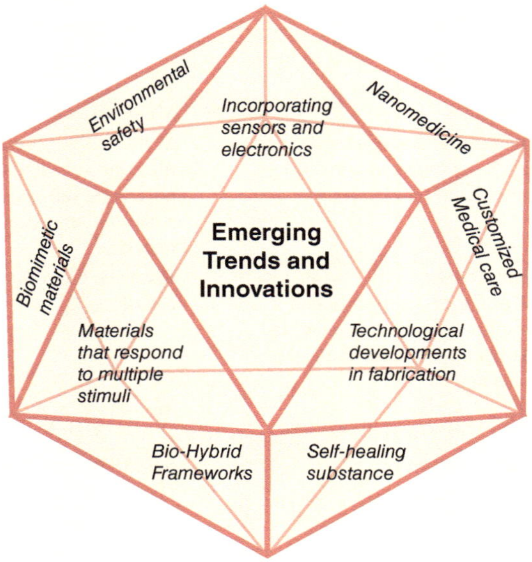

Fig. 17.3 Emerging trends and innovations of 4D bioprinting

form of the implant might alter throughout time or in response to the body's growth. It is quite good at producing organs and stents that can alter their shape over time to suit the needs [28].

The field of biomedical engineering has enormous potential for growth as 4D printing technology develops. This section outlines the field's potential future prospects for 4D printing while providing cutting-edge answers to urgent clinical problems [6].

17.8.1 Emerging Trends and Innovations

Creating smart materials through 4D printing allows them to gradually alter their characteristics or form in response to outside stimuli. Future developments in 4D printing in biomedical engineering are anticipated to be shaped by a number of new trends and research topics as this field of study advances. These are represented in Fig. 17.3.

17.8.1.1 Incorporating Sensors and Electronics

In the realm of 4D printing, a significant focus lies on integrating sensors and electronics directly into printed structures. This incorporation enables continuous monitoring of device performance, collection of vital patient health data, and the facilitation of responsive actions. For instance, implants created through 4D printing can incorporate sensors that monitor healing progress, detect potential complications, and deliver real-time feedback to healthcare providers, thereby enhancing the customization and efficacy of treatment plans.

17.8.1.2 Biohybrid Frameworks

It is possible to create biohybrid systems that have the required properties of both biological tissues and artificial materials by fusing living cells with 4D-printed components. In order to create living, 4D-printed structures that can respond to their surroundings and develop, researchers are looking into the possibilities of doing so. This might lead to new applications in tissue engineering and regenerative medicine. This method offers useful substitutes created from a patient's own cells, which may lessen the need for organ transplantation [4].

17.8.1.3 Self-Healing Substance

Biomedical engineering has advanced with the development of self-healing materials for 4D printing. The durability and dependability of 4D-printed devices are increased by these materials' capacity to self-heal damage [2]. This invention has great promise for prostheses and implants, since self-healing features may lessen the need for replacements and require less intrusive procedures.

17.8.1.4 Customized Medical Care

By making it possible to create devices that are tailored to each patient, 4D printing is transforming customized medicine. With the use of this technology, patients can have prostheses and implants that are exactly made to match their anatomy, as well as medicines that are accurately targeted and maximize dosage. The broad application of 4D printing in customized medicine holds forth the prospect of better patient outcomes and more potent therapies [65].

17.8.1.5 Environmental Safety

In biomedical engineering, the emphasis is moving toward eco-friendly and biodegradable materials for 4D printing because of increased concerns about waste management and environmental effects. Researchers are looking at biodegradable synthetic polymers as well as materials that are obtained naturally, such as chitosan and cellulose. These developments have the potential to improve sustainable healthcare practices and reduce the environmental impact of biomedical devices [27].

17.8.1.6 Materials That Respond to Multiple Stimuli

Multi-stimulus responsive materials are being investigated by researchers for use in biomedical 4D printing. These materials can adjust to different stimuli, such as light, pH, temperature, or magnetic fields, which makes it possible to create functional and adaptable 4D-printed devices. To improve treatment efficacy and customization, drug delivery systems composed of these materials, which might customize the release and targeting of medicines based on certain biological parameters [46].

17.8.1.7 Biomimetic Materials

Biomedical engineering is developing biomimetic materials for 4D printing that are modeled after natural systems. These materials provide benefits in biocompatibility, functionality, and adaptability by mimicking the characteristics and functions of biological tissues. Tissue engineering, regenerative medicine, and the development of implants and prostheses that closely mimic natural tissues are among the applications. Through the use of biomimetic materials in 4D-printed structures, scientists want to develop gadgets that blend in with the body naturally and aid in healing and recovery [50].

17.8.1.8 Nanomedicine

The design, synthesis, and utilization of materials and technologies at the nanoscale are the main goals of nanomedicine. Targeted medication delivery systems and complex, responsive nanostructures will be possible thanks to the developments in 4D printing. Personalized medicine is made possible by these nanoscale structures, which can also increase treatment efficacy and decrease negative effects. By combining 4D printing and nanomedicine, novel approaches to illness detection, treatment, and prevention might be developed, transforming the medical field and enhancing patient outcomes [69].

17.8.1.9 Technological Developments in Fabrication

Innovation in 4D printing is mostly driven by improvements in fabrication processes. One such noteworthy advancement is multi-material and multi-process printing, which expands the uses of 4D printing in biomedical engineering and smart materials by combining several materials and processes to produce multifunctional structures with a variety of features [54]. Precision and functionality are enhanced by high-resolution printing, which makes complex structures at the micro- or nanoscale possible. This is important for tissue engineering and drug delivery systems. By combining processes like electrospinning and 3D printing, hybrid manufacturing techniques create structures with improved characteristics that are perfect for tissue engineering. Important for adaptive 4D printing, self-assembly and self-folding methods produce dynamic structures without external manipulation by using material features and ambient variables. Smart structures that react to stimuli may be created using 4D-printed structures thanks to embedded sensors and actuators that allow for real-time monitoring and control. Biofabrication advancements, like bioprinting, enable the integration of biomolecules and live cells, which is crucial for tissue engineering and regenerative medicine [57]. Efficient production of intricate 4D-printed structures is made possible by machine learning and AI-driven design, which forecast material behavior and streamline workflows [59]. The last factor that makes 4D printing more affordable and accessible for a wide range of biomedical applications is automation and scalability, which enhance high-throughput production and quality control.

17.8.2 Potential Challenges and Solutions

Since 4D printing is still in its infancy, there are still a lot of obstacles to be solved. Some of the potential challenges are discussed along with solutions:

- The limited supply of smart materials that are acceptable for printing, particularly those that are biocompatible and hence appropriate for biomedical applications, is one of the major challenges of 4D bioprinting [55].
- Even if the cost of additive manufacturing printers has decreased, a significant amount of research funding is still required for 4D printed structures [28]. Further limiting time and expense are the complex simulations required to understand how a material or structure responds to changes in a way that isn't directly proportional and varies over time.
- Large-scale clinical trials will be necessary before these devices are patient-ready, as the current research is small scale. Hence, 4D printing technology still has a long way to go before being used in therapeutic settings.
- Unclear regulatory frameworks are causing delays in the real-world development. Therefore, the clinical use of biomedical equipment manufactured with 4D printing technology is still a ways off [12].
- Accurate micro/nanoscale design characteristics are essential for biomedical devices, and their large-scale manufacture cannot be achieved unless these features are improved. Improvements are required to increase the structures' longevity and endurance since frequent actuation between configurations might weaken them [12].
- Limited resolution in 4D printing makes it difficult to produce small-scale vascular structures, which is a key difficulty in tissue engineering [38]. The solution for this is either combining 4D printing with other techniques (lithography or microfabrication) or improving design software to provide more accurate control and printing process simulation.
- The use of high temperatures in the biomaterial 4D printing has constraints, since it hinders cell printing and necessitates an additional stage for cell seeding [40]. To prevent harming the cells, biomaterials that can be printed at lower temperatures should be employed. Another solution may be the use of curing methods based on light or UV light, which do not require high temperatures to harden printed materials [30].
- One of the major obstacles with regard to design-based challenges is the absence of specialized software for 4D printing. As of right now, the majority of the software that is available, including design and slicing tools, was created with earlier fabrication techniques like 3D printing in mind. No robust software has yet been developed to satisfy the demands of 4D printing technology. For instance, the majority of slicing software now in use, such as Cura and Simplify3D, was created to operate with fused deposition modeling 3D printers and filament-based

materials, which do not satisfy the prerequisites for 4D bioprinting [55]. For future projects, it is advised to introduce and create strong software in order to achieve more significance and efficiency in 4D printing technology.

- Among the design-based constraints is the inability to regulate the biological components that are implanted in the human body in terms of when and how quickly they respond to stimuli. In light of this, future research can leverage artificial intelligence (AI) and internet of things (IoT) technologies to address these problems [15].
- The commercialization of 4D bioprinting has significant challenges related to scalability, price, manufacturing, and user-friendliness. It is important to take these concerns into account early in the development phase in order to facilitate the translation of 4D bioprinting [8, 9].
- Issues with validation and cryopreservation of printed tissues in large-scale manufacturing may also exist [8, 9].
- The ability to provide contactless stimulations to 4D-printed materials in vivo is currently limited, and many of the contactless stimuli on the market are incompatible with the cellular environment. Shape-changing features are frequently achieved with the application of thermal stimuli. Exact response prediction is hampered by the unpredictability of novel and unusual stimuli as well as the unpredictable behavior of printed materials after repeated exposure to a stimulus. Moreover, the optimal performance of printed material in vivo is challenged by the diverse and unexpected inputs found in biological systems [10].
- Another matter that needs the biomedical community's attention is the availability of suitable bio-ink materials. Applications for 4D bioprinting have been used in tissue grafting when it's necessary to create novel bioink materials with dynamic behavior, cellular adhesion, good multistimuli, sensitivity, and sufficient stiffness for in vitro testing. Novel bioprinters, mechanisms, and structural designs are also in need of 4D bioprinting technology. The landscape of the bioprinting business will change as a result of the low-cost bioprinters that certain companies have recently produced being widely available [11].
- Improvements in 4D bioprinting technology notwithstanding, vascular tissue grafts' biomechanical performance still needs to be improved. The biological activity and structural intricacy of in vivo vascularization still require replication. Another issue that has to be addressed by scientists is the integration of vascular tissues with living materials. In the future, biomedical engineers should take non-thrombogenic cardiovascular tissue engineering into account to regulate biological activity [11].

With the help of these fixes and other creative adjustments, 4D printing will become immaculate in the future.

17.9 Ethical and Regulatory Considerations

17.9.1 Ethical Implications

A wide range of ethical issues, including informed consent, equity, access, and respect for the rights of humans and animals, are taken into account while using 4D bioprinting. Educating patients on the nature, advantages, and dangers of 4D bioprinted medicines is crucial. In particular, during clinical trials, patients need to be made fully aware of the experimental nature of these treatments. Assuring that cutting-edge medical technology is accessible to all areas and socioeconomic groups while preventing the escalation of healthcare inequities depends on affordability and fair access. Reducing animal usage and upholding ethical standards like the 3Rs (replacement, reduction, and refinement) are important ways to address the ethical issues of animal experimentation [54].

To safeguard the rights and safety of participants, human trials must adhere to strict ethical requirements. For the purpose of comprehending possible difficulties, continued study and monitoring are necessary about the long-term ramifications, including the lifespan and integration of bioprinted tissues in the human body. When using this technology ethically, therapeutic advantages should take precedence over non-therapeutic additions. Furthermore, the way the public views and accepts 4D bioprinting may have a big impact on how technology develops and is used, which is why public outreach and education are crucial. The use of 4D bioprinting must be guided by cultural awareness to ensure respect for various customs and beliefs.

17.9.2 Regulatory Guidelines

To guarantee the security and effectiveness of the tools and structures being created, every new medical technology, including 4D printing, must pass stringent testing and receive regulatory agency certification before being made available. Medical items, including those made using 4D printing, are regulated by organizations like the European Medicines Agency (EMA) and the US Food and Drug Administration (FDA) in many nations. It can be difficult to navigate the complicated regulatory environment since 4D-printed biomedical device clearance processes sometimes entail several steps, such as preclinical research, clinical trials, and post-market surveillance [10].

Furthermore, considering the novelty of 4D printing technology, it's possible that some laws already in place need to be updated or new rules should be created in order to handle the particular characteristics of 4D-printed products, such as their flexibility and shape-changing abilities. For 4D-printed biomedical devices to be approved and developed a thorough grasp of the requirements and approval procedures, makers and researchers must collaborate closely with regulatory bodies. This entails making certain that the devices exhibit safety and efficacy in preclinical and clinical testing, that the materials utilized are biocompatible, and that the production methods adhere to quality standards.

17.10 Conclusion

The area of 4D bioprinting is at the forefront of tissue engineering and regenerative medicine because of its capacity to create dynamic and responsive biological constructions. The production of more functional and lifelike tissues that can adapt to their surroundings and resemble the complexity of genuine biological systems is made possible by the addition of time as a transformational dimension. The application of smart biomaterials, which can alter their characteristics in response to outside stimuli, is revolutionary and presents hitherto unheard-of opportunities for the advancement of precision and customized medicine. These developments hold the potential to enhance drug delivery methods, promote the development of functioning tissues and organs, and result in more tailored and efficient therapeutic treatments. But as we advance, it is imperative that we confront the moral and legal issues raised by these developments. Strong guidelines and ongoing monitoring are needed to ensure the 4D bioprinting technologies are used safely, effectively, and ethically.

With continued development, this technology is expected to significantly advance biomedical engineering, improving patient outcomes and revolutionizing medical procedures in the process. The success of these developments will be largely dependent on industrial collaborations, interdisciplinary cooperation, and public participation and education. With further study and development, 4D bioprinting has great potential for revolutionizing the design and development of medical equipment, medicines, and treatments—essentially ushering in a new age in healthcare.

References

1. Abbas G, Hanif M, Khan MA. pH responsive alginate polymeric rafts for controlled drug release by using box behnken response surface design. Designed Monomers and Polymers. 2017;20(1):1–9. https://doi.org/10.1080/15685551.2016.1231046.
2. Abdullah T, Okay O. 4D printing of body temperature-responsive hydrogels based on poly(acrylic acid) with shape-memory and self-healing abilities. ACS Applied Bio Materials. 2023;6(2):703–11. https://doi.org/10.1021/acsabm.2c00939.
3. Ahmar K, Mir Javid I, Saima A, Humaira B, Aneeza N, Bushra M, Mahak Deep K, Khan A. 4D printing: the dawn of "smart" drug delivery systems and biomedical applications. Jddtonline Info. 2021;11(S):131–7. https://doi.org/10.22270/jddt.v11i5-S.5068.
4. Ding A, Jeon O, Cleveland D, Gasvoda KL, Wells D, Sang Jin Lee EA. Jammed micro-flake hydrogel for four-dimensional living cell bioprinting—Ding—2022—advanced materials—Wiley Online Library.pdf. In: Advanced materials. Wiley; 2022. p. 1–14.

5. Ali MH, Abilgaziyev A, Adair D. 4D printing: a critical review of current developments, and future prospects. Int J Adv Manuf Technol. 2019;105(1–4):701–17. https://doi.org/10.1007/S00170-019-04258-0.
6. Amiri E, Sanjarnia P, Sadri B, Jafarkhani S, Khakbiz M. Recent advances and future directions of 3D to 6D printing in brain cancer treatment and neural tissue engineering. Biomed Mater (Bristol) 2023;18(5):052005. https://doi.org/10.1088/1748-605X/ace9a4.
7. Amukarimi S, Rezvani Z, Eghtesadi N, Mozafari M. Corrigendum to "smart biomaterials: from 3D printing to 4D bioprinting". Methods. 2022;205(2022):191–9. https://doi.org/10.1016/j.ymeth.2022.10.004. [(S1046202322001608), (10.1016/j.ymeth.2022.07.006)]. Methods, 208(September), 27
8. Antezana PE, Municoy S, Ostapchuk G, Catalano PN, Hardy JG, Evelson PA, Orive G, Desimone MF. 4D printing: the development of responsive materials using 3D-printing technology. Pharmaceutics. 2023a;15(12) https://doi.org/10.3390/pharmaceutics15122743.
9. Antezana, P., Municoy, S., Ostapchuk, G., & Catalano, P. (2023b). 4D printing: the development of responsive materials using 3D-printing technology. https://ri.conicet.gov.ar/handle/11336/227739.
10. Appuhamillage GA, Ambagaspitiya SS, Dassanayake RS, Wijenayake A. 3D and 4D printing of biomedical materials: current trends, challenges, and future outlook. Explor Med. 2024;5(1):17–47. https://doi.org/10.37349/emed.2024.00203.
11. Arif ZU, Khalid MY, Zolfagharian A, Bodaghi M. 4D bioprinting of smart polymers for biomedical applications: recent progress, challenges, and future perspectives. React Funct Polym. 2022;179(August):105374. https://doi.org/10.1016/j.reactfunctpolym.2022.105374.
12. Bajpai A, Baigent A, Raghav S, Brádaigh C, Koutsos V, Radacsi N. 4D printing: materials, technologies, and future applications in the biomedical field. Sustainability (Switzerland). 2020;12(24):1–32. https://doi.org/10.3390/su122410628.
13. Battogtokh G, Y., K. T. Active-targeted pH-responsive albumin–photosensitizer conjugate nanoparticles as theranostic agents. J Mater Chem B. 2015;48:1–6.
14. Champeau M, Heinze DA, Viana TN, de Souza ER, Chinellato AC, Titotto S. 4D printing of hydrogels: a review. Adv Funct Mater. 2020;30(31) https://doi.org/10.1002/ADFM.201910606.
15. Chen J, Virrueta C, Zhang S, Mao C, Wang J. 4D printing: the spotlight for 3D printed smart materials. Mater Today. 2024;June:1–9. https://doi.org/10.1016/j.mattod.2024.06.004.
16. Cheng T, Thielen M, Poppinga S, Tahouni Y, Wood D, Steinberg T, Menges A, Speck T. Bio-inspired motion mechanisms: computational design and material programming of self-adjusting 4D-printed wearable systems. Adv Sci. 2021;8(13):1–12. https://doi.org/10.1002/advs.202100411.
17. Choi J, Kwon OC, Jo W, Lee HJ, Moon MW. 4D printing technology: a review. 3D Printing and Additive Manufacturing. 2015;2(4):159–67. https://doi.org/10.1089/3DP.2015.0039.
18. Choong YYC, Maleksaeedi S, Eng H, Yu S, Wei J, Su PC. High speed 4D printing of shape memory polymers with nanosilica. Appl Mater Today. 2020;18(March):1–8. https://doi.org/10.1016/j.apmt.2019.100515.
19. Cooperstein MA, Canavan HE. Assessment of cytotoxicity of (N-isopropyl acrylamide) and poly(N-isopropyl acrylamide)-coated surfaces. Biointerphases. 2013;8(1):1–12. https://doi.org/10.1186/1559-4106-8-19.
20. Espalin D, Ramirez JA, Medina F, Wicker R. Multi-material, multi-technology FDM: exploring build process variations. Rapid Prototyp J. 2014;20(3):236–44. https://doi.org/10.1108/RPJ-12-2012-0112/FULL/HTML.
21. Faber L, Yau A, Chen Y. Translational biomaterials of four-dimensional bioprinting for tissue regeneration. Biofabrication. 2024;16(1):12001. https://doi.org/10.1088/1758-5090/acfdd0.
22. Gugulothu SB, Chatterjee K. Visible light-based 4D-bioprinted tissue scaffold. ACS Macro Lett. 2023;12(4):494–502. https://doi.org/10.1021/acsmacrolett.3c00036.
23. Guo N, Tian J, Wang L, Sun K, Mi L, Ming H, Zhe Z, Sun F. Discussion on the possibility of multi-layer intelligent technologies to achieve the best recover of musculoskeletal injuries: smart materials, variable structures, and intelligent therapeutic planning. Front Bioeng Biotechnol. 2022;10(September):1–20. https://doi.org/10.3389/fbioe.2022.1016598.

24. Gupta P, Vermani K, Garg S. Hydrogels: from controlled release to pH-responsive drug delivery. Drug Discov Today. 2002;7(10):569–79. https://doi.org/10.1016/S1359-6446(02)02255-9.
25. Hoarau-Véchot J, Rafii A, Touboul C, Pasquier J. Halfway between 2D and animal models: are 3D cultures the ideal tool to study cancer-microenvironment interactions? Int J Mol Sci. 2018;19(1) https://doi.org/10.3390/ijms19010181.
26. Jang J, Park HJ, Kim SW, Kim H, Park JY, Na SJ, Kim HJ, Park MN, Choi SH, Park SH, Kim SW, Kwon SM, Kim PJ, Cho DW. 3D printed complex tissue construct using stem cell-laden decellularized extracellular matrix bioinks for cardiac repair. Biomaterials. 2017;112(January):264–74. https://doi.org/10.1016/j.biomaterials.2016.10.026.
27. Jang S, Park S. 4D printed untethered milli-gripper fabricated using a biodegradable and biocompatible electro- and magneto-active hydrogel. Sensors Actuators B Chem. 2023;384(June):1–9. https://doi.org/10.1016/j.snb.2023.133654.
28. Javaid M, Haleem A. 4D printing applications in medical field: a brief review. Clin Epidemiol Global Health. 2019;7(3):317–21. https://doi.org/10.1016/j.cegh.2018.09.007.
29. Kabirian F, Mela P, Heying R. 4D printing applications in the development of smart cardiovascular implants. Front Bioeng Biotechnol. 2022;10(May):1–11. https://doi.org/10.3389/fbioe.2022.873453.
30. Kalogeropoulou M, Díaz-Payno PJ, Mirzaali MJ, van Osch GJVM, Fratila-Apachitei LE, Zadpoor AA. 4D printed shape-shifting biomaterials for tissue engineering and regenerative medicine applications. Biofabrication. 2024;16(2):022002. https://doi.org/10.1088/1758-5090/ad1e6f.
31. Khoo ZX, Teoh JEM, Liu Y, Chua CK, Yang S, An J, Leong KF, Yeong WY. 3D printing of smart materials: a review on recent progresses in 4D printing. Virtual Phys Prototyp. 2015;10(3):103–22. https://doi.org/10.1080/17452759.2015.1097054.
32. Kilian D, Ahlfeld T, Akkineni AR, Lode A, Gelinsky M. Three-dimensional bioprinting of volumetric tissues and organs. MRS Bull. 2017;42(8):585–92. https://doi.org/10.1557/mrs.2017.164.
33. Koetting MC, Peters JT, Steichen SD, Peppas NA. Stimulus-responsive hydrogels: theory, modern advances, and applications. Mater Sci Eng R: Report. 2015;93:1–49. https://doi.org/10.1016/j.mser.2015.04.001.
34. Kolesky DB, Truby RL, Gladman AS, Busbee TA, Homan KA, Lewis JA. 3D bioprinting of vascularized, heterogeneous cell-laden tissue constructs. Adv Mater. 2014;26(19):3124–30. https://doi.org/10.1002/adma.201305506.
35. Kumar S, Singh R, Singh AP, Wei Y. Three-dimensional printed thermoplastic polyurethane on fabric as wearable smart sensors. Proceedings of the Institution of Mechanical Engineers, Part L. J Mater: Design Appl. 2023;237(7):1678–92. https://doi.org/10.1177/14644207221149693.
36. Kumari G, Abhishek K, Singh S, Hussain A, Altamimi MA, Madhyastha H, Webster TJ, Dev A. A voyage from 3D to 4D printing in nanomedicine and healthcare: Part i. Nanomedicine. 2022;17(4):237–53. https://doi.org/10.2217/nnm-2021-0285.
37. Li YC, Zhang YS, Akpek A, Shin SR, Khademhosseini A. 4D bioprinting: the next-generation technology for biofabrication enabled by stimuli-responsive materials. Biofabrication. 2017;9(1):27910820. https://doi.org/10.1088/1758-5090/9/1/012001.
38. Lukin I, Musquiz S, Erezuma I, Al-Tel TH, Golafshan N, Dolatshahi-Pirouz A, Orive G. Can 4D bioprinting revolutionize drug development? Expert Opin Drug Discov. 2019;14(10):953–6. https://doi.org/10.1080/17460441.2019.1636781.
39. Lv C, Sun XC, Xia H, Yu YH, Wang G, Cao XW, Li SX, Wang YS, Chen QD, De Yu Y, Sun HB. Humidity-responsive actuation of programmable hydrogel microstructures based on 3D printing. Sensors Actuators B Chem. 2018;259(April):736–44. https://doi.org/10.1016/j.snb.2017.12.053.
40. Ma Y, Shih C, Bao Y. Advances in 4D printing of biodegradable photopolymers. April: Respons Mater; 2024. p. 1–20. https://doi.org/10.1002/rpm.20240008.
41. Mandal, A., B, K. C.-J. of M. C., & 2024, undefined. (n.d.). 4D printing for biomedical applications. Eprints Iisc Ac In. Retrieved July 15, 2024, from https://eprints.iisc.ac.in/84434/

42. Momeni F, Mehdi Hassani M, N, S., Liu X, Ni J. A review of 4D printing. Mater Des. 2017;122(May):42–79. https://doi.org/10.1016/j.matdes.2017.02.068.
43. Moroni L, Boland T, Burdick JA, De Maria C, Derby B, Forgacs G, Groll J, Li Q, Malda J, Mironov VA, Mota C, Nakamura M, Shu W, Takeuchi S, Woodfield TBF, Xu T, Yoo JJ, Vozzi G. Biofabrication: a guide to technology and terminology. Trends Biotechnol. 2018;36(4):384–402. https://doi.org/10.1016/j.tibtech.2017.10.015.
44. Morouço P. Four-dimensional bioprinting for regenerative medicine: mechanisms to induce shape variation and potential applications. EMJ Innovation, January 2019; 2019. p. 36–43. https://doi.org/10.33590/emjinnov/18-00070.
45. Morouço P, Azimi B, Milazzo M, Mokhtari F, Fernandes C, Reis D, Danti S. Four-dimensional (bio-)printing: a review on stimuli-responsive mechanisms and their biomedical suitability. Appl Sci (Switzerland). 2020;10(24):1–30. https://doi.org/10.3390/app10249143.
46. Narupai B, Smith PT, Nelson A. 4D printing of multi-stimuli responsive protein-based hydrogels for autonomous shape transformations. Adv Funct Mater. 2021;31(23) https://doi.org/10.1002/adfm.202011012.
47. Nishiguchi A, Zhang H, Schweizerhof S, Schulte MF, Mourran A, Möller M. 4D printing of a light-driven soft actuator with programmed printing density. ACS Appl Mater Interfaces. 2020;12(10):12176–85. https://doi.org/10.1021/acsami.0c02781.
48. Osouli-Bostanabad K, et al. Traction of 3D and 4D printing in the healthcare industry: from drug delivery and analysis to regenerative medicine. ACS Publications; n.d.. Retrieved July 19, 2024, from https://pubs.acs.org/doi/abs/10.1021/acsbiomaterials.2c00094
49. Osouli-Bostanabad K, Masalehdan T, Kapsa RMI, Quigley A, Lalatsa A, Bruggeman KF, Franks SJ, Williams RJ, Nisbet DR. Traction of 3D and 4D printing in the healthcare industry: from drug delivery and analysis to regenerative medicine. ACS Biomater Sci Eng. 2022;8(7):2764–97. https://doi.org/10.1021/ACSBIOMATERIALS.2C00094.
50. Pan HM, Goto A. Topology-dependent pH-responsive actuation and shape memory programming for biomimetic 4D printing. Macromol Rapid Commun. 2023;44(9):36880381. https://doi.org/10.1002/marc.202300074.
51. Patdiya J, Kandasubramanian B. Progress in 4D printing of stimuli responsive materials. Polymer-Plastics Technol Mater. 2021;60(17):1845–83. https://doi.org/10.1080/25740881.2021.1934016.
52. Pei E, Loh GH. Technological considerations for 4D printing: an overview. Prog Additive Manufac. 2018;3(1–2):95–107. https://doi.org/10.1007/S40964-018-0047-1.
53. Pingale P, Dawre S, Dhapte-Pawar V, Dhas N, Rajput A. Advances in 4D printing: from stimulation to simulation. Drug Deliv Transl Res. 2023;13(1):164–88. https://doi.org/10.1007/S13346-022-01200-Y.
54. Ramezani M, Mohd Ripin Z. 4D printing in biomedical engineering: advancements, challenges, and future directions. J Funct Biomater. 2023;14(7) https://doi.org/10.3390/jfb14070347.
55. Sahafnejad-Mohammadi I, Karamimoghadam M, Zolfagharian A, Akrami M, Bodaghi M. 4D printing technology in medical engineering: a narrative review. J Braz Soc Mech Sci Eng. 2022;44(6) https://doi.org/10.1007/s40430-022-03514-x.
56. Schuurman W, Levett PA, Pot MW, van Weeren PR, Dhert WJA, Hutmacher DW, Melchels FPW, Klein TJ, Malda J. Gelatin-methacrylamide hydrogels as potential biomaterials for fabrication of tissue-engineered cartilage constructs. Macromol Biosci. 2013;13(5):551–61. https://doi.org/10.1002/mabi.201200471.
57. Sonatkar J, Kandasubramanian B, Ismail SO. 4D printing: pragmatic progression in biofabrication. Eur Polym J. 2022;169(April):1–9. https://doi.org/10.1016/j.eurpolymj.2022.111128.
58. Subeshan B, Baddam Y, Asmatulu E. Current progress of 4D-printing technology. Prog Addit Manuf. 2021;6(3):495–516. https://doi.org/10.1007/S40964-021-00182-6.
59. Sun X, Yue L, Yu L, Forte CT, Armstrong CD, Zhou K, Demoly F, Zhao RR, Qi HJ. Machine learning-enabled forward prediction and inverse design of 4D-printed active plates. Nat Commun. 2024;15(1):1–15. https://doi.org/10.1038/s41467-024-49775-z.

60. Suriano R, Bernasconi R, Magagnin L, Levi M. 4D printing of smart stimuli-responsive polymers. J Electrochem Soc. 2019;166(9):B3274–81. https://doi.org/10.1149/2.0411909JES/META.
61. Uboldi M, Gelain A, Buratti G, Gazzaniga A, Melocchi A, Zema L. Development of 4D printed intravesical drug delivery systems: scale-up of film coating. J Drug Deliv Sci Technol, 2023;87:104875. https://doi.org/10.1016/j.jddst.2023.104875.
62. Wan Z, Zhang P, Liu Y, Lv L, Zhou Y. Four-dimensional bioprinting: current developments and applications in bone tissue engineering. Acta Biomater. 2020;101:26–42. https://doi.org/10.1016/j.actbio.2019.10.038.
63. Wang G, Xia H. Sensors and actuators B : chemical actuator and generator based on moisture-responsive PEDOT. PSS/PVDF composite film. 2018;255(February):1415–21.
64. Wang J, Sun L, Zou M, Gao W, Liu C, Shang L, Gu Z, Zhao Y. Bioinspired shape-memory graphene film with tunable wettability. Sci Adv. 2017;3(6):1–16. https://doi.org/10.1126/sciadv.1700004.
65. De Wild M, Dany S, John C, Schuler F. Smart 4D-printed implants and instruments. Curr Directions Biomed Eng. 2020;6(3):3–6. https://doi.org/10.1515/cdbme-2020-3053.
66. Zhang C, Cai D, Liao P, Su JW, Deng H, Vardhanabhuti B, Ulery BD, Chen SY, Lin J. 4D printing of shape-memory polymeric scaffolds for adaptive biomedical implantation. Acta Biomater. 2021;122(March):101–10. https://doi.org/10.1016/j.actbio.2020.12.042.
67. Zhang L, Liang H, Jacob J, Naumov P. Photogated humidity-driven motility. Nat Commun. 2015;6(May):1–12. https://doi.org/10.1038/ncomms8429.
68. Zhang Z, Demir KG, Gu GX. Developments in 4D-printing: a review on current smart materials, technologies, and applications. Int J Smart Nano Mater. 2019;10(3):205–24. https://doi.org/10.1080/19475411.2019.1591541.
69. Zhu W, Webster TJ, Zhang LG. 4D printing smart biosystems for nanomedicine. Nanomedicine. 2019;14(13):1643–5. https://doi.org/10.2217/nnm-2019-0134.
70. Zu S, Zhang Z, Liu Q, Wang Z, Song Z, Guo Y, Xin Y, Zhang S. 4D printing of core–shell hydrogel capsules for smart controlled drug release. Bio-Des Manuf. 2022;5(2):294–304. https://doi.org/10.1007/S42242-021-00175-Y.

GPSR Compliance

The European Union's (EU) General Product Safety Regulation (GPSR) is a set of rules that requires consumer products to be safe and our obligations to ensure this.

If you have any concerns about our products, you can contact us on ProductSafety@springernature.com

In case Publisher is established outside the EU, the EU authorized representative is:

Springer Nature Customer Service Center GmbH
Europaplatz 3
69115 Heidelberg, Germany

Batch number: 10703867

Printed by Printforce, the Netherlands